ISCHAEMIC COLITIS

JACQUES W.A.J. REEDERS, MD
  Chief, Gastro-intestinal Radiology Section, Academic Medical Centre,
  Hospital of the University of Amsterdam, Amsterdam, The Netherlands

GUIDO N.J. TYTGAT, MD
  Professor of Gastro-enterology, Chairman, Department of
  Gastro-enterology, Academic Medical Centre, Hospital of the
  University of Amsterdam, Amsterdam, The Netherlands

GERD ROSENBUSCH, MD
  Professor of Abdominal Radiology, St. Radboud Hospital, Catholic
  University of Nijmegen, Nijmegen, The Netherlands

SIBRAND GRATAMA, MD
  Chairman, Department of Pathology, Stichting 'Laboratorium
  Pathologische Anatomie Rotterdam-Noord', Rotterdam, The
  Netherlands

ISCHAEMIC COLITIS

JACQUES W.A.J. REEDERS, MD
GUIDO N.J. TYTGAT, MD
GERD ROSENBUSCH, MD
SIBRAND GRATAMA, MD

1984 **MARTINUS NIJHOFF PUBLISHERS**
a member of the KLUWER ACADEMIC PUBLISHERS GROUP
BOSTON / THE HAGUE / DORDRECHT / LANCASTER

Distributors

for the United States and Canada: Kluwer Academic Publishers, 190 Old Derby Street, Hingham, MA 02043, USA
for the UK and Ireland: Kluwer Academic Publishers, MTP Press Limited, Falcon House, Queen Square, Lancaster LA1 1RN, England
for all other countries: Kluwer Academic Publishers Group, Distribution Center, P.O. Box 322, 3300 AH Dordrecht, The Netherlands

Library of Congress Cataloging in Publication Data

```
Main entry under title:

Ischaemic colitis.

   Includes index.
   Bibliography: p.
   1. Ischemic colitis.  I. Reeders, Jacques W. A. J.
[DNLM: 1. Colon--Blood supply.  2. Ischemia.  3. Colitis.
WI 522 I77]
RC862.I82I85  1984      616.3'447       84-4193
ISBN-13: 978-94-009-6020-6     e-ISBN-13:978-94-009-6018-3
DOI: 10.1007/ 978-94-009-6018-3
```

Copyright

CONTENTS

VI

PART III:

FOREWORD

Ischemic colitis is becoming increasingly one of the most important conditions involving the colon. This is due to a combination of multiple factors: (1) increasing age of the world population due to improved public health conditions and advances in medicine; (2) diagnostic advances in recognizing the condition; and, (3) education of physicians who suspect the disease in elderly individuals with colonic symptoms. The disease is a great masquerader of other conditions and can be mistaken for ulcerative colitis, Crohn's disease or almost any other inflammatory disease of the large bowel. It can have shallow ulcers, deep ulcers, filiform polyps, and pseudomembrane. It can produce fistulae or toxic megacolon. The thumb-printing and other acute findings are not always seen and the site of involvement may be atypical.

It is therefore so important to have a book dealing with this condition extensively and in detail. This scholarly presentation based on large clinical experience significantly contributes to the knowledge of this important disease that will assume even more importance as other conditions involving the colon are successfully treated. As physicians, radiologists and even pathologists have difficulty in diagnosing this condition that appears under multiple guises the information contained here should be invaluable.

Alexander R. Margulis, M.D.
March 1984, San Francisco

PREFACE

First of all, I would like to congratulate the authors on their successful publication of this monograph with many diagnostic radiographs of new touch taken by the modern technique. This monograph is also of great significance because of comprehensively compiled publication in the country with long tradition of gastrointestinal radiology behind it.

The content of this monograph is so rich that we do not need to collect and read other articles on ischaemic colitis. If we keep it at hand and always expose ourselves to the fruitful content with special reference to historical review, we could know all about ischaemic colitis.

I have often heard that the authors have had vast experience with ischeamic colitis and have played a leading role in this field. When I was invited to the South African Medical Congress a few years ago, I had an opportunity to listen to the special lecture on ischaemic colitis by Professor Tytgat. I could learn a great deal from his lecture, and, in Bangkok, when I attended the 4th Asian-Oceanian Congress of Radiology last year, I was deeply impressed with the high-leveled presentation on ischaemic colitis by Dr. Reeders. Having read through this monograph, I have decided to keep it as my desk companion without hesitation.

The methodology of gastrointestinal radiology dates back to very many years ago but it is also vividly alive in the present. Even recently, radiological diagnosis of gastrointestinal disorders has been advanced gradually but steadily, and nowadays, it is indispensable for clinical gastroenterology. This monograph evidently shows a lot of positive proof of the indispensableness.

Gastrointestinal radiology, with continuous progress step by step in the past, was revolutionally advanced by the introduction of the modern double contrast technique. The value of the modern double contrast technique worth while mentioning is visualization of fine mucosal abnormalities as shown in this monograph, and the concept of interpretation of radiological manifestations was also revolutionally altered.

In spite of rapid advance in other diagnostic modalities such as endoscopy, ultrasonography or computed tomography, barium studies of the gastrointestinal tract still stay in the leading position in the diagnosis of gastrointestinal disorders by the support of the modern double contrast technique. At interpretation, abnormalities visualized by the double contrast technique can be analyzed by the concept common to all parts of the gastrointestinal tract, and therefore, a double contrast diagnosis can be always theoretically established.

Radiological manifestions shown in this monograph are visualized by the standard but high-leveled technique. Skill in faithfully visualizing the abnormalities is also emphasized by this monograph, and we should recognize the importance of cultivating our skill everyday.

The basic concept in analyzing the manifestations on the double contrast view can be summarized as follows: (1) ulcerative lesions can be classified into those at the point, line or area by their shape, (2) the number of ulcerative lesions (solitary, multiple or numerous) is also very important for a differential diagnosis and (3) the next factor to be analyzed is the distribution pattern of ulcerative lesions (diffuse, segmental, skip, scattered or isolated). By analyzing the above mentioned factors, the staging and clinical course of disorders can be possibly decided.

Ischaemic colitis is unequaled as scientific material for searching the theoretical diagnosis of gastrointestinal disorders, and it is not too much to say that ischemic colitis is the nucleus of the scientific work in gastrointestinal radiology, because of its multiformity of pathology. For instance, from radiological point of view, ulcerative lesions at the point, line or area, that are often difficult to theoretically analyze, are all radomly seen. Moreover, lesions at each stage or their transitional stage can be noted together. The course is usually rapid and changes of the lesions with the passage of time are also observed.

This monograph is brilliant enough to make us appreciating the value of radiology in the diagnosis of gastrointestinal disorders and the basic way of thinking in gastrointestinal radiology.

I should like to repeat to read this monograph keeping it as a desk companion.

H. Shirakabe, M.D.
March 1984, Tokyo

ACKNOWLEDGEMENTS

This retrospective clinical study was performed in the Department of Radiology, St. Radboud University Hospital, Nijmegen, The Netherlands.

I would like to thank Prof. Dr. Wm. Penn and Prof. Dr. H.O.M. Thijssen most sincerely for the freedom of approach which they have permitted me in the design and course of this study. I would like to thank many others of the medical and technical staff for their efficient and cordial cooperation.

The writing and production of a book involves many people in addition to the author. Several persons who have been especially vital to the success of this project and whom I wish to individually acknowledge and thank for their continuing encouragement are: Mrs. Ch. Suripatty-Mikx, my secretary for typing and organizing the manuscript; Mr. K. Jannink for his help in computerized analysis and Mr. H. Straatman for the statistical analysis.

I owe a special acknowledgement to the efforts and skillful help of artist Mr. J. Konings for the anatomical artwork and to Mr. W. Witte for the photographs. I am particularly indebted to my former colleague, Dr. J. Taams, surgeon at the St. Elisabeth Hospital, Willemstad, Curacao, Netherlands Antilles, who has provided me with the greatest inspiration for this study.

Much of the preliminary work leading up to the study described here, was carried out together with Dr. Th. van Leeuwen, Department of Pathology, Medical Centre, Alkmaar, The Netherlands, I am grateful for his criticism and advice during the period of our collaboration.

In thanking the above-mentioned, I am personally aware of doing an injustice to many others, who have contributed to this study in their own way. It is through their help that this work could be completed. I wish to thank them all.

I am greatly indebted to my publishers for their careful attention to this volume.

Jacques W.A.J. Reeders, MD

PHOTOGRAPHIC CREDITS

PHOTOGRAPHIC CREDITS

Figures 2-6; 2-7A; 2-7B; 2-8: Courtesy of Prof. Dr. R.J.A.M. van Dongen, Department of Vascular Surgery, Academic Medical Centre, Amsterdam, The Netherlands.

Figures 14-1A; 14-1B: Courtesy of L. te Strake, MD, Department of Radiology, Academic University Hospital Groningen (AZG), Groningen, The Netherlands.

Figure 24-1: Courtesy of Prof. Dr. S.G.M. Meuwissen, Department of Gastroenterology, Academic Hospital of the Free University, Amsterdam, The Netherlands.

Figures 24-3A; 24-3B; 24-4A; 24-4B: Courtesy of C.I. Bartram, MB, BS, MRCP, FRCR. Department of Radiology, St. Marks Hospital, London, England. (published in Gastrointest. Radiol., 4, 85–88., 1979.)

Figures 24-10A; 24-10B; 24-18: With permission of J. Odo Op den Orth, MD, Department of Radiology, St. Elisabeth's of Groote Gasthuis, Haarlem, The Netherlands.

Figures 24-13A; 24-13B; 24-21A; 24-21B; 24-22: Courtesy of B.W. Ike, MD, Department of Radiology, St. Elisabeth Hospital, Amersfoort, The Netherlands.

Figures 24-20; 24-23: Courtesy of M. Matsukawa, MD and Prof. Dr. H. Shirakabe, Department of Internal Medicine, Juntendo University, Tokyo, Japan.

Figures 25-1; 25-2; 25-3; 25-4; 25-5; 25-6; 25-7; 25-8: Courtesy of K. Huibregtse, MD, and J.W.F.M. Bartelsman MD, Department of Gastroenterology, Academic Medical Centre, Amsterdam, The Netherlands.

The light-micrographs Figures 26-5 to 26-45 were made with a C. Zeiss photomicroscop II, Ocular 8X; Histological staining: Haematoxylin-Axophloxin (HA); Elastica van Gieson (EG); Prussian Blue. Film: AGFA-Isopan professional; 25 ASA, type 135/36.

1. INTRODUCTION

'A supply of oxygenated blood appropriate to the tissue needs of the gut is essential to the maintenance of its vital functions. The splanchnic vascular system serves this purpose and much of our knowledge of ischaemic bowel disease has developed from studies of radiological and pathological abnormalities in this system' (Alschibaja and Morson, 1977). Boley et al. (1963) and later Marston et al., (1966) must be credited with the designation of ischaemic colitis as a new clinical entity to rank amongst other, already well-established, inflammatory disorders of the bowel.

A multiplicity of names may be found in the literature to describe colonic abnormalities which, in the light of present knowledge, almost certainly had an ischaemic origin.

The purpose of this monograph is:
- to summarize current information from the literature concerning the clinical manifestations, diagnostic (radiology, endoscopy, histopathology) and therapeutic procedures.
- to compare these data with the results of our own retrospective analysis of 199 patients with ischaemic colitis.
- to try to find an answer to the following questions:
  - Which is the most practical classification of ischaemic colitis to use?
  - Does any form of ischaemic colitis have a specific clinical presentation or may it be associated with the full spectrum of clinical symptoms and signs?
  - What is the contribution of radiological and/ or endoscopical examination in the diagnosis of ischaemic colitis, e.g. in the follow-up as a control of the therapy?
  - Why has angiography little to offer in the diagnosis of ischaemic colitis?
  - Is occlusion of one of the main mesenteric vessels such an important aetiopathogenic factor as frequently has been suggested in the literature?
  - Why is this disease regularly incorrectly diagnosed by clinicians, radiologists and pathologists as 'ulcerative colitis' or 'Crohn's disease of the colon' and the wrong therapy given in consequence?
  - In what features does the macro- and microscopical appearance of ischaemic colitis differ from other inflammatory ulcerative colonic diseases?
  - What is the usefulness of endoscopical biopsies in the diagnosis and follow-up respectively during conservative treatment?
  - What is the therapeutic method for the different forms of ischaemic colitis and is this dependent upon the depth of the ischaemic lesion?

The literature concerning ischaemic colitis collected from 1950–1982, has been reviewed. 1024 detailed patient reports were analysed. The articles used in this analysis are indicated in the references with a prefix O.

The analysis of our own patient material was based upon the study of 199 patients, (collected from 24 different hospitals in the Netherlands, during the period 1970–1980), in whom the diagnosis was made by radiological, endoscopical and/or histological examination. Most cases were collected from the archives of pathology (autopsy material and/or surgically removed diseased tissue and biopsies). Later the relevant clinical data were added and the patient cases analysed.

All patients diagnosed on clinical grounds alone were excluded from the study.

Information on the presenting clinical symptoms, the physical signs, the associated disease, the laboratory results and other diagnostic methods, as well as the applied method of treatment, was collected from the medical reports of each patient. The radiological data analysed in this study were collected from 75 (first) double- or single contrast barium enemas, from 33 angiographies and from 30 follow-up barium enemas, performed in different hospitals. Fifty-five barium enemas and all angiographies were reviewed by G. Rosenbusch, MD and J.W.A.J. Reeders, MD.

The radiological reports of a further 50 (first) barium enemas showed such a clear evidence of ischaemic colitis that these were also immediately included in our studies. The diagnoses in these 50 patients were later confirmed by histological examination. The endoscopy data were collected from (first) endoscopies of 39 patients and 26 follow-up endoscopies. The results were reviewed by G.N.J. Tytgat, MD.

The histological study comprised material from 82 resected colonic specimens, 108 autopsies and 32 biopsies. All the histological slides were reviewed by S. Gratama, MD and J.W.A.J. Reeders, MD.

The accumulated data from the clinical presentation, the diagnostic tests and the form of therapy employed were tabulated for all patients by using a purpose written computer program. Statistics for 2 way tables were made. If over 20% of the cells of the cross table had expected counts less than 5, the chi-square was assumed as being an invalid test. If less than 20% of the cells had expected counts less than 5, the chi-square test was used.

The limitation of our studies is that since more than half of the patient material is derived from autopsy studies, the numbers and percentages used in this analysis reflect a selected patient group and are not necessarily representative for the incidence and presentation of ischaemic colitis in the general population. We suggest nevertheless, that the correct interpretation of the results of clinically diagnostic tests and of the pathology of ischaemic bowel disease, requires systemic observation and a knowledge of the salient features of differential significance in each of the major enterocolitides. We hope that the results of our studies will help to illuminate these features.

Successful treatment of ischaemic colitis depends on 'early recognition, which requires a high index of suspicion for this common but frequently unrecognized entity' (Abel and Russell, 1983).

2. VASCULATURE OF THE COLON

Anatomically, the intestinal circulation is complex. The blood supply of the colon may be divided into 4 parts: the main arteries, the anastomosing arteries, the terminal arteries and the veins.

2.1 Main arteries

The colon is supplied with blood via 3 main arterial routes: the superior mesenteric artery (SMA), the inferior mesenteric artery (IMA) and the hypogastric arteries.

2.1.1 Superior mesenteric artery (SMA)

The SMA arises from the front of the aorta, usually at the vertebral level of the mid lumbar I-, or upper lumbar II vertebra. The SMA supplies the entire small bowel below the second part of the duodenum and, via its ileocolic and middle colic branches, the coecum, the ascending and proximal transverse colon.

After studying 156 abdominal preparations by arteriography, corrosion and dissection, Vandamme and van der Schueren (1976) found that the *ileocolic artery* was the most constant branch of the SMA, running to the right and supplying the ileocoecal region (Figures 2.1, 2.2).

The ileocolic artery has a complex pattern of ramification. It is a transitional vessel between the small and large intestine. The ileocolic artery usually ends in two coecal branches (86%).

Other branches are direct collaterals of the main stem (Vandamme and van der Schueren, 1976).

Superior and inferior colic branch. The inferior

4

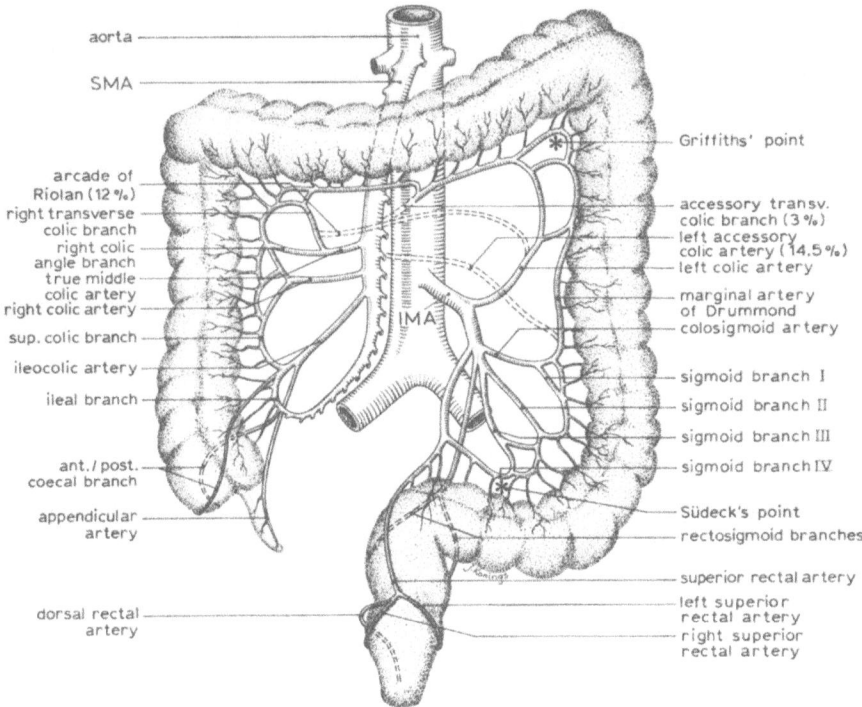

Fig. 2.1. Blood supply of the colon and rectum.

colic artery is a smaller and less constant (59%) branch.

The appendicular artery descends behind the ileum and along the free edge of the meso-appendix and is the sole arterial supply to the appendix.

The ileal branch anastomoses in the mesentery with other terminal branches of the SMA, to form an arcade from which straight branches serve the terminal part of the ileum.

The anterior and posterior coecal branches, which embrace the coecum.

The right colic artery is the second artery originating at the right side of the SMA. It courses to the right below the mesocolon and supplies the middle part of the ascending colon and the hepatic colic flexure (Fig. 2.1). The right colic artery is the most inconstant of the colic arteries (Sonneland et al., 1958; Vandamme and van der Schueren, 1976).

The middle colic artery is the first artery originating from the right side of the SMA (Fig. 2-1). It runs to the right between the layers of the meso-colon, then divides, its branches supplying the transverse colon and anastomosing with the right and left colic arteries. There is a degree of variability in the number of the middle colic arteries (Griffiths, 1956;

Sonneland et al., 1958; Michels et al., 1965; Vandamme and van der Schueren, 1976).

After a short common stem, the true middle colic artery divides up into a right colic angle branch and a right transverse colic branch.

The *right colic angle branch* runs towards the right colic flexure.

The *transverse colic artery* feeds the marginal arcade of Drummond at a point level with the middle of the transverse colon.

The right transverse colic artery is less frequently found (12% of cases) and is usually associated with another middle colic vessel (72% of cases) commonly the right colic angle artery.

An *accessory transverse colic artery* was found in 3% of patients studied by Vandamme and van der Schueren (1976); it supplies the distal part of the transverse colon (Fig. 2.1).

2.1.2 The inferior mesenteric artery (IMA)

Arising from the aorta at the level of the third lumbar vertebra, below the transverse segment of the duodenum, the IMA forms a 30 degree angle with the abdominal aorta and descends as a straight vessel beneath the peritoneum. It then runs to the

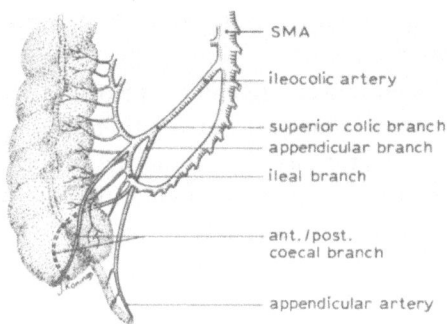

Fig. 2.2. Anatomic vascular network of the coecal region.

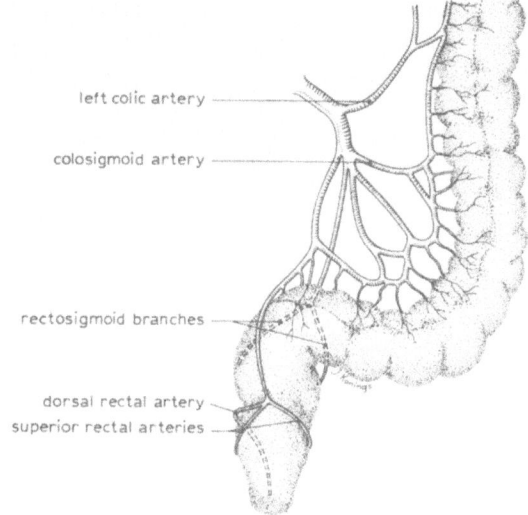

Fig. 2.3. Blood supply of the recto-sigmoid region.

left and supplies the distal part of the transverse colon and proximal part of the descending colon via the left colic branches: the distal part of the descending colon and the sigmoid are supplied via the sigmoidal branches, and the proximal rectum via the superior rectal (hemorrhoidal) artery.

The left colic artery is the first branch of the IMA. After a short descending course, the left colic artery turns upwards to the splenic flexure (Fig. 2.1). It reaches the splenic flexure in 86–89% of the cases, where, via the 'Arc of Riolan', it anastomoses with the middle colic artery, which arises from the SMA (Griffiths, 1956; Michels et al., 1965). Along its course the left colic artery usually gives off 3 branches, each of which anastomoses with the marginal artery of Drummond.

The ascending left colic artery bifurcates at the splenic flexure; its right branch joins the left branch of the middle colic artery and its left branch joins the marginal artery of Drummond. The left colic artery presents aberrant patterns (17% of cases) (Vandamme et al., 1982), and a variability in course (Steward and Rankin, 1933), or can be absent altogether (6–12%) (Griffiths, 1956; Vandamme et al., 1982).

When the left colic artery is small or has a high course, both the sigmoid colon and the lower part of the descending colon are irrigated by a large, constantly observed and clearly identifiable artery, the *colosigmoid artery,* originating separately from the IMA (48%), or common with the left colic artery (14%) or as an anastomosis of the latter (38%) (Fig. 2.3). Sigmoidal branches arise from the colosigmoid artery, the left colic artery, the IMA or the superior rectal arteries. The rectosigmoid section of the colon is provided by a *rectosig-*

moid artery, which arises separately from the IMA between the sigmoidal artery and the terminal bifurcation of the IMA (Fig. 2.3, 2.4). The rectosigmoid artery usually bifurcates (80%) into 2 descending branches, one for each side of the bowel. They arise on the dorsal side of the intestine but run progressively more laterally whilst their branches encircle the wall of the intestine.

The *rectum* is supplied by a variable number of small arterial branches originating from the right and left superior rectal (hemorrhoidal) artery, from the middle and inferior rectal arteries (from the hypogastric arteries) and by a variable number of branches of the middle sacral artery.

The *superior rectal artery,* the continuation of the IMA, divides near the upper end of the rectum into 2 branches, a right and a left superior rectal artery (Fig. 2.4), which can then further anastomose (in 8% of cases) (Vandamme et al., 1982).

Small vessels supply the bowel in the gap between the termination of the marginal artery in the lower portion of the sigmoid and the division of the superior rectal artery, at the rectum. These small vessels encircle the anterior aspect of the bowel and run more or less parallel with the longitudinal axis of the rectum on its lateral and anterior aspects. In contrast to the colic arteries, which form anastomosing arcades before penetrating the intestinal wall, the branches of the rectal arteries enter the intestinal wall directly, where they form a rich

6

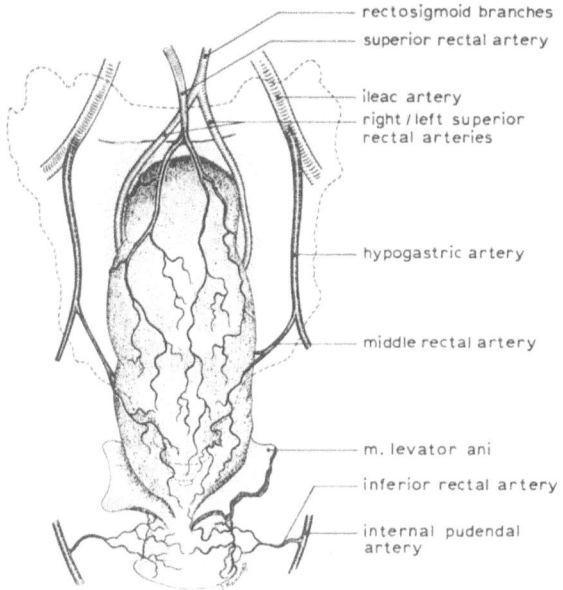

rectosigmoid branches
superior rectal artery
ileac artery
right / left superior
rectal arteries

hypogastric artery

middle rectal artery

m. levator ani
inferior rectal artery
internal pudendal
artery

Fig. 2.4. Blood supply of the rectum.

intramural anastomotic network (McGowan, 1955; Michels et al., 1965).

2.1.3 Hypogastric arteries

The middle rectal arteries are the first vessels to the large bowel to be derived from outside the splanchnic circulation (Fig. 2.4). Their origin is variable, coming either directly from the hypogastric artery, or from a common trunk containing the middle vesical, vaginal, prostatic or internal pudendal artery. The arteries course forward to the lateral aspect of the rectum along which they descend, sending into it small branches, some of which anastomose with the branches of the supe-

rior rectal and some with the vaginal, vesical or prostatic arteries.

The anal canal is supplied by the paired *inferior rectal arteries,* which are derived from the internal pudendal arteries, as major branches of the internal iliac arteries. Fine communications between the ramifications of all three rectal arteries extra- and intramurally, (Fig. 2.4) occur to a varying extent.

2.2 Anastomotic arteries between the SMA, IMA and hypogastric arteries

In the splanchnic circulation a number of anastomoses is present which function as a collateral blood supply when necessary. The main anastomotic arteries are: the 'Arc of Riolan' and 'the marginal artery of Drummond'.

2.2.1 The 'Arc of Riolan'
The 'Arc of Riolan' ('intermesenteric arcade', Vandamme et al., 1982) is a left colic arterial branch, which runs cephalad in the mesentery to anastomose more centrally with the middle colic artery near the splenic flexure (Diemel et al., 1964) (Fig. 2.1). The 'Arc of Riolan' is only clearly visible on arteriography when an occlusion is present at one of its limbs. Four types of the 'Arc of Riolan' have been described and are associated with different hemodynamics (Courbier et al., 1976) (Fig. 2.5):

Type 1:
The hypertrophic 'Arc of Riolan' associated with a small superior rectal artery, due to an occlusion near the orifice of the SMA or IMA. The blood

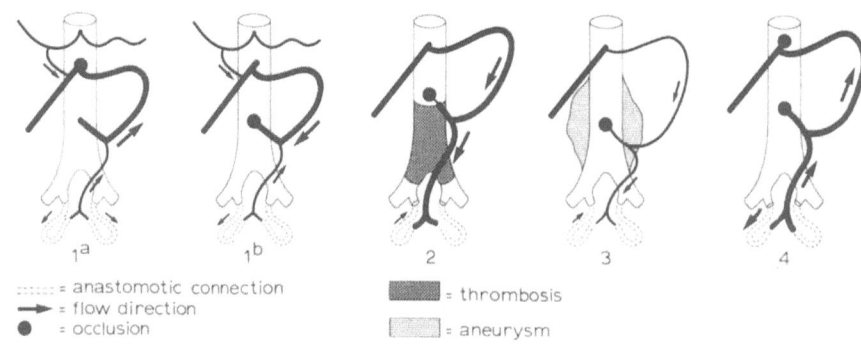

1ᵃ   1ᵇ   2   3   4

······· = anastomotic connection   ▓▓▓ = thrombosis
→ = flow direction
● = occlusion   ░░░ = aneurysm

Fig. 2.5. Four types of 'Arc of Riolan', and associated haemodynamics.

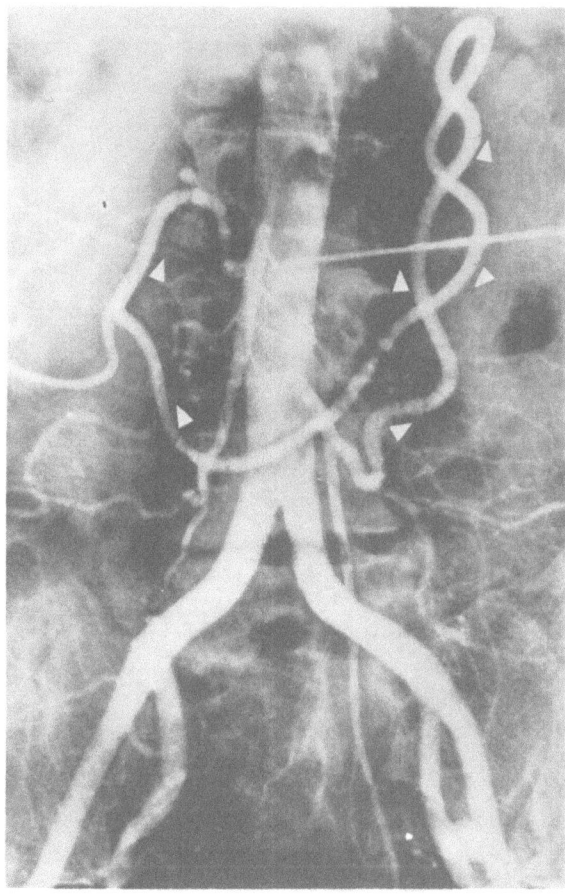

Fig. 2.6. Percutaneous aortography: Hypertrophic 'Arc of Riolan', due to an occlusion near the orifice of the SMA. The blood flow is ascendant. (from distally to proximally) (see arrowheads) (Type 1A).

flow is accordingly ascendant (Fig. 2.5, 1A) or descendant (Fig. 2.5, 1B). Frequently a hypertrophic pancreatico-duodenal arcade is also seen.

Type 2:
The hypertrophic 'Arc of Riolan' with a hypertrophic superior rectal artery is associated with two simultaneously occurring hemodynamic phenomena:
– occlusion at the orifice of the IMA and
– a pressure gradient between the SMA and hypogastric artery, due to thrombosis of the aorta beneath the level of renal arteries or obstruction of one of the iliac arteries. The blood flow is descendant (Fig. 2.5, 2). The 'Arc' functions as a collateral with the iliac artery.

Type 3:
An ill-developed 'Arc of Riolan' with an ill-developed superior rectal artery. This is associated with an isolated obstruction of the orifice of the IMA or an aortic aneurysm without an ileo-femoral obstruction. The left colon is dependent on the SMA. There is a descendant blood flow (Fig. 2.5, 3).

Type 4:
A hypertrophic 'Arc of Riolan' and a hypertrophic superior rectal artery with an ascendant blood flow. This type has been described by Kieny (1979) and is due to an obstruction at the orifice of both mesenteric arteries. The ascendant blood flow is supplied from the superior rectal arteries to revascularize the two mesenteric territories (Fig. 2.5, 4). In summary, it may be said, that when the SMA is occluded, blood can be supplied from the coeliac trunk by way of the pancreatico-duodenal arcade or from the IMA via the hypertrophic 'Arc of Riolan'. When the IMA is occluded, blood can be supplied by way of the hypogastric and middle rectal artery, which anastomoses with the sigmoid and via the 'Arc of Riolan'.

2.2.2 The 'marginal artery of Drummond'
The 'marginal artery of Drummond' also called 'the functional vessel of the colon' (Drummond, 1913; Griffiths, 1961) is an anastomotic paracolic artery which runs along the mesocolic surface of the colon, often from the coecum up to the sigmoid and connecting the 5 main arteries from the SMA and IMA (Fig. 2.1). The marginal artery gives off the vasa recta to the bowel.

A poorly developed connection in this marginal artery is most likely to be found between the ileocolic and right colic branches of the SMA or between the middle colic branch and the left colic artery near the splenic flexure (Sonneland et al., 1958). There is a congenital absence of such a marginal artery in about 5% of normal individuals (Griffiths' point).

Meyers (1976) defined the *Griffiths' critical point* as 'the site of

1 communication of the ascending left colic artery with the marginal artery of the descending colon at the splenic flexure; and
2 anastomotic bridging between the right and left

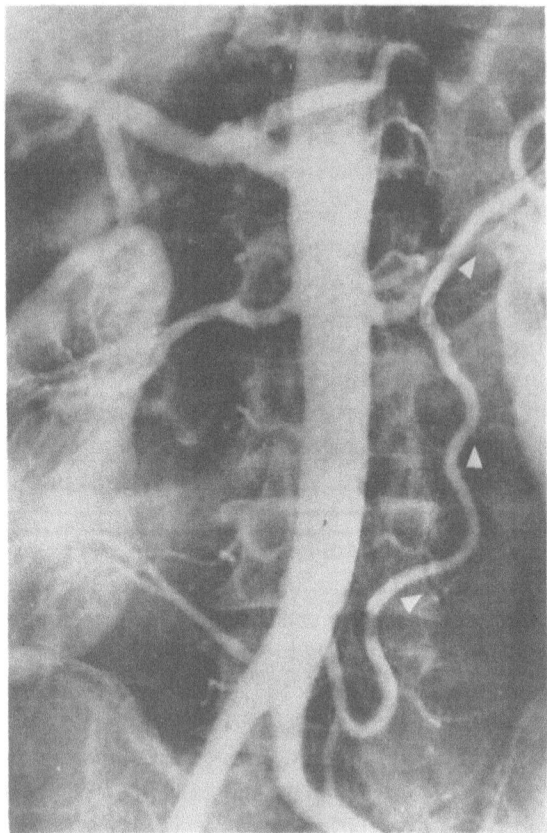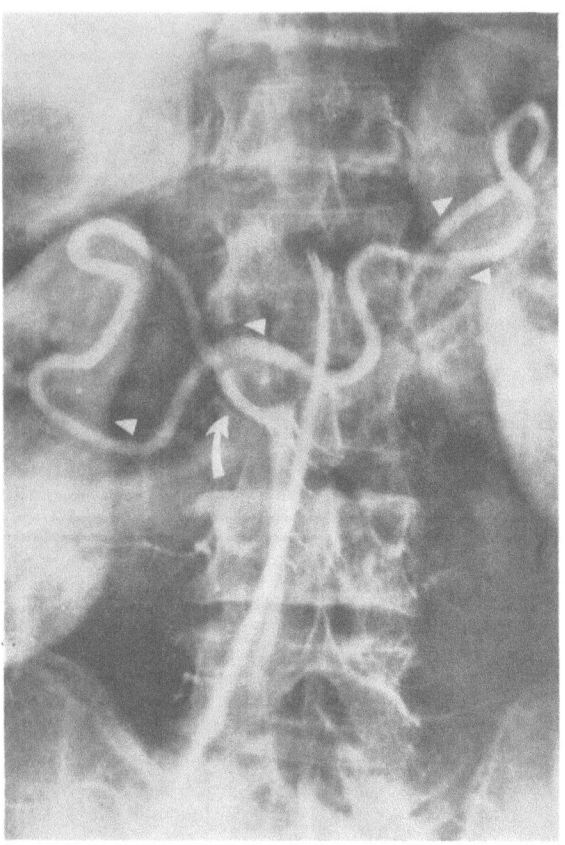

A   B

Fig. 2.7A, B. Aortography using Seldinger technique (A and B) Hypertrophic 'Arc of Riolan', due to an occlusion of the SMA. The blood flow is ascendant (from distally to proximally) (small arrowheads). Note that the SMA steals blood from this 'Arc' via the medial colic artery (large arrow) (Type 1A).

terminal branches of the ascending left colic artery'.

Analysis of selective arteriographic studies in 46 patients by Meyers (1976) showed that an anastomotic connection at Griffiths' point was present in only 22 (48%) of the cases, poor or tenuous in 4 (9%) of the cases and absent in 20 (43%) of the cases.

Within the mesentery of the sigmoid colon (pelvic mesocolon) several sigmoidal branches form by anastomosing arcades the distal extent of the marginal artery. The point of bifurcation between the lowest sigmoidal branch contributing to the marginal artery and the superior rectal artery has been called '*Südeck's critical point*' (Südeck, 1907): this is of theoretical rather than of practical interest (McGowan, 1955; Michels et al., 1965).

2.3 Terminal arteries

The branches of the terminal arteries (vasa recta) usually originate independently from the marginal artery and run directly to the colon, but occasionally 2 branches may have a common origin. Terminal arteries are most numerous in the coecum and ascending colon. The size of the terminal arteries in the transverse and descending colon is slightly smaller, and the density of vasculature is less than in the ascending portion. The terminal arteries of the colon may be either in the form of long or of short branches or as a combination of both long and short branches (Fig. 2.9).

2.3.1 Long branches
The *long* branches divide near the mesocolic taenia; one branch courses in the haustra on the ante-

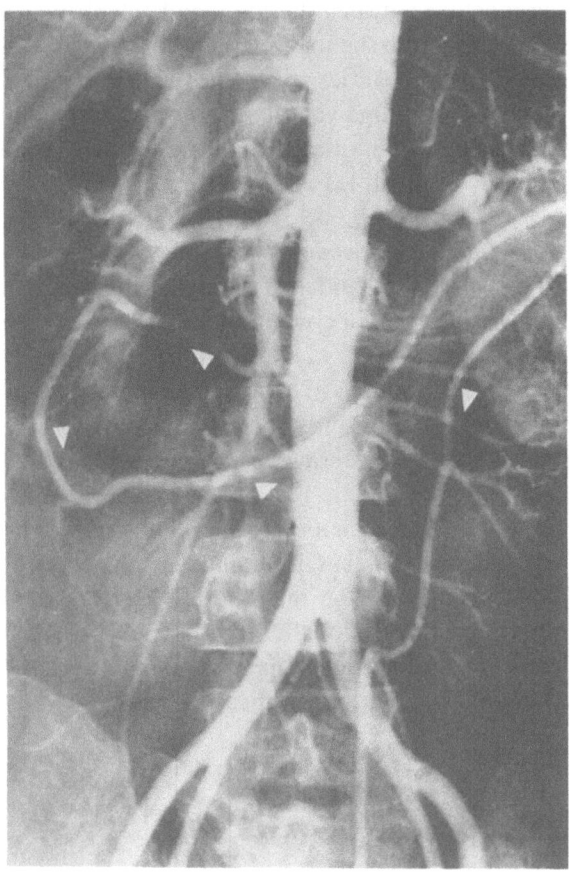

Fig. 2.8. Aortography using Seldinger technique. Hypertrophic 'Arc of Riolan', due to an occlusion near the orifice of the IMA. The blood flow is accordingly descendant. (Type 1B) (see arrowheads).

rior aspect, and the other on the posterior aspect of the wall of the colon. In this part of their course the arteries lie in the serosa and give off short branches to the (sub)mucosa, the circular muscle, the serosa, the peritoneum and to the epiploic appendages at the antimesenteric side of the colon. In the submucosa the long branches anastomose with the short branches.

2.3.2 Short branches

The *short* branches are smaller and four or five times as numerous as the long branches.

The first short branches pierce the mesocolic longitudinal band, giving offshoots to serosa and muscle en route and thence passing directly to the submucosa.

The other short branches lie in the serosa where they have a tortuous distribution and anastomose through the circular muscle to the submocusal plexus at various points. Vasa recta rarely anastomose and there is little longitudinal spread of their submucosal ramifications.

2.4 Veins

In general the veins of the colon follow directly the course of the corresponding arteries. There are always at least 2 veins for each peripheral artery. The marginal peripheral vein of the colon follows

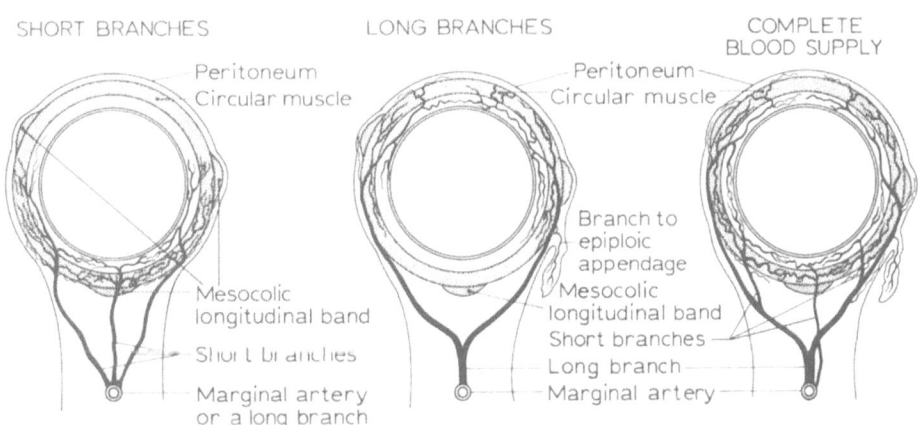

Fig. 2.9. Terminal arteries of the colon.

closely the marginal peripheral arteries, usually lying posterior and slightly medial to the artery.

2.4.1 Superior mesenteric vein (SMV)

The three colic tributaries of the *superior mesenteric vein* (SMV) return blood from the right, or proximal half of the colon. The SMV, coursing to the right of its artery, ascends in front of the inferior vena cava and receives branches from the small intestine. At the level of the second lumbar vertebra and behind the head and neck of the pancreas, the SMV joins the splenic vein to form the portal vein.

2.4.2 Inferior mesenteric vein (IMV)

The *inferior mesenteric vein* (IMV), beginning as the superior rectal (hemorrhoidal) vein and then receiving flow from the left colic vein, ascends at the left of the artery and usually empties in the splenic vein. An alternative course carries the IMV medially across the root of the SMA to join directly the juncture between the SMV and splenic veins. The veins of the sigmoid region follow the general course of the arteries in all the smaller ramifications until the large veins are formed. These unite near the base of the mesosigmoid, and join with the left colic vein and IMV.

2.4.3 Internal/external rectal venous plexus

The lower rectum and anal canal are supplied by a rich venous network which is comprised of the *internal rectal plexus* in the submucosa at the level of the rectal columns of Morgagni and of the *external rectal plexus* in the subcutaneous tissue at the anal verge. The internal rectal plexus is drained chiefly by the middle rectal vein, which is much more important than its corresponding artery. The external rectal plexus is drained by the inferior rectal vein. Both the middle and inferior rectal veins are branches of the hypogastric veins, and lead into the inferior vena cava. There are free communications between these plexuses.

3. PATHOPHYSIOLOGY OF ISCHAEMIC COLITIS

Pathological changes of the colonic wall similar in their histology and radiological image to those changes observed in ischaemic colitis in man have been produced experimentally in animals, particularly in the presence of prolonged impaired arterial perfusion of the intestine (Boley et al., 1963; De Villiers, 1966; Ranninger and Scheiner, 1967; Marston et al., 1969; Möller and Stjernvall, 1971; Whitehead, 1972; Marcuson et al., 1972; Parks, 1974; Horie et al., 1976; Matthews and Parks, 1976; Robinson et al., 1981; Griffen and Hagihara, 1982).

In spite of its clinical importance, colonic ischaemia has been the subject of far fewer experimental studies than the corresponding lesion of the small intestine (Robinson et al., 1981).

There is a close parallel between clinical and experimental observations in colonic ischaemia (Boley et al., 1963, 1965; Marston et al., 1969; Rausis et al., 1973; Parks, 1974). Reduction of the colonic arterial blood pressure after vessel occlusion, small vessel disease, 'low flow' state and increased intralumenal pressure secondary to obstruction (Fig. 3.1) will lead to (sub)mucosal blood flow reduction, (sub)mucosal hypoxia, capillary wall damage, interstitial oedema and haemorrhage and finally to necrosis. The severity of the ischaemic involvement is dependent upon the severity, duration and the extent of the blood flow impairment. As a result there is a great heterogeneity in response of the colonic wall to hypoxia.

Functional and morphological examination of the ischaemic colon have led to the conclusion that the colonic mucosa is less sensitive to ischaemia than is the small intestinal mucosa (De Villiers, 1966; Marston et al., 1969; Robinson et al., 1972; Rausis and Robinson, 1973). Studies of mucosal structure and function during recovery showed that damaged colonic mucosa, regenerates more slowly than small intestinal mucosa.

than small intestinal mucosa.

Robinson et al., (1981) showed that after colonic ischaemia of one hour only superficial lesions developed (necrosis of the epithelium and of the lamina propria of the mucosa) accompanied by a slight reduction in functional capacity. Almost complete recovery was observed one day later (Robinson et al., 1975).

After colonic ischaemia of $1^1/_2$ hours in rats, Rijke and Gart (1979) were able to demonstrate the development of accelerated proliferation of cells during the recovery phase. Recovery was complete 24 to 48 hours after ischaemia. Robinson et al., (1981) showed that after ischaemia of 2 hours in the dog colon, 7 days were necessary for complete functional recovery. They compared the response of ileum and colon after the same degree of ischaemia and suggested that the colon recovered more slowly. The damage caused by these short periods of total ischaemia were readily reversible within a short time.

After a colonic ischaemia of 3 hours there was a variable response of the colonic mucosa (Robinson et al., 1972, 1981). In some cases, structural and functional recovery occurred within 2 to 4 weeks whereas in other cases a stenosis of the colonic wall developed (Rausis et al., 1973; Robinson et al., 1981) after 4 weeks. In yet other cases, there was no regeneration of the mucosa and muscularis mucosae and in some cases colonic gangrene developed with perforation of the colonic wall.

It is questionable how far intrinsic vessel damage after releasing the clamps is a contributing factor to the severity of such experimentally imposed ischaemic colonic damage.

During the ischaemic episode there is vasodilatation with capillary necrosis.

Secondary plasma loss and haemorrhage in the mucosa/submucosa and colon lumen can lead to

12

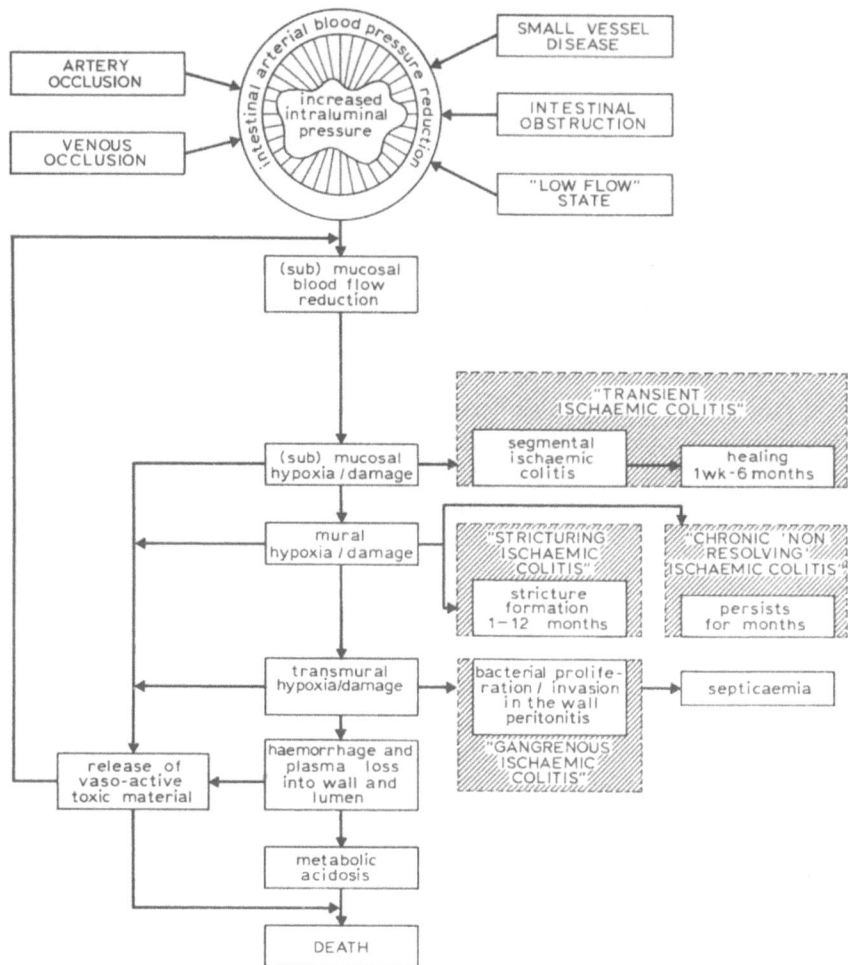

Fig. 3.1. Pathophysiology of ischaemic colitis.

metabolic acidosis, submucosal oedema, lumen narrowing, ileus, hypovolaemia and eventually to shock or death.

The intramural circulation may further deteriorate due to gas production in the ischaemic colonic segment. Bacterial proliferation or invasion in the colonic wall, release of endotoxins and vaso-active toxic material may lead to bacterial septicaemia and endotoxic shock and will have a negative influence on the intramural blood flow (Bounous, 1974), thus causing extension of the lesion in depth as well in length. This accounts for the fact that an initially mild hypovolaemia can lead to severe ischaemic colonic destruction.

If the hypoxia or damage is limited to the mucosa a segmental usually 'transient' or 'evanescent' ischaemic colitis will develop.

A sufficient collateral blood supply allows complete restoration of the mucosa without any adverse sequelae. When there is also damage to parts of the muscularis propria, and the collateral blood supply is just sufficient to prevent transmural gangrene, but is inadequate to allow healing of mucosa, the 'stricturing form' or 'chronic non resolving form' of ischaemic colitis will develop (see 5.2).

In case of prolonged severe ischaemia with insufficient collateral circulation, the muscularis propria becomes involved. A transmural gangrene develops which can lead to perforation and peritonitis ('gangrenous ischaemic colitis'). The colonic tissue has needs other than oxygen – such as proteins, carbohydrates, lipids, water, electrolytes etc. The capacity of cells to obtain these nutrients and to extract oxygen from the blood is intimately associated with their membrane structure and internal metabolism (Alschibaja and Morson, 1977). Ischaemia profoundly affects these structures and their functions. 'The pathogenesis of ischaemic colitis can be defined at the level of molecular biology and pathology as the balance between increased tissue needs as caused by diminished blood flow, anoxic injury and infection, and the capacity of the body to deliver the substances necessary to compensate for all serious deficiencies in cell structure and function.

Conditions which create the imbalance in the vital economy of colonic tissues and cells, may be primarily within the wall of the bowel itself (intrinsic causes), or in the major and intermediate vessels of the splanchnic circulation or in disorders of the general cardiovascular and related systems (extrinsic process). These conditions may act alone or together and they may be simultaneous or discontinuous' (Alschibaja and Morson, 1977).

The progress of the ischaemic process and the different aetiopathogenic factors, which can play an important role are summarized in Fig. 3.1.

PART I:

LITERATURE REVIEW (1950–1982)

4. AETIOLOGY OF ISCHAEMIC COLITIS

4.1 *Occlusive aetiopathogenic factors*
  4.1.1 Arterial occlusion
    4.1.1.1 Iatrogenic occlusion
      Ligation of IMA in aortic reconstruction/abdominal aortic aneurysm surgery
      Abdomino-perineal excision of rectum
      Abdomino-aortic angiography
      Transcathether embolotherapy
    4.1.1.2 Non iatrogenic occlusion
      Obliterative atherosclerosis/thrombosis
      Embolism
      Dissecting aneurysm of aorta
      Compression of mesenteric arteries
      Thrombangitis obliterans
      Fibromuscular hyperplasia
      Takayasu's disease
  4.1.2 Venous occlusion
    Portal thrombosis
    Oral contraceptives
    Hypercoagulable states
    Pancreatitis
    Pylethrombosis

4.2 *Non occlusive aetiopathogenic factors*
  4.2.1 'Low flow state':
    Congestive heart failure, myocardial infarction, valvular disease, myocarditis
    Arrhythmia
    Functional vasospasm
    Drugs causing vasoconstriction:
      Ergotamine
      Digitalis
      Antihypertensives
      Other drugs
    Postoperative haemorrhagic shock
    Posttraumatic cause
    Septic shock
    Dehydration (diuretics)
  4.2.2 Small vessel disease
    Vasculitis
      Systemic lupus erythematosus
      Rheumatoid arthritis
      Polyarteritis nodosa
      Dermatomyositis, Wegener's granulomatosis
    Irradiation vasculopathy/vasculitis
    Malignant atrophic papulosis
    Amyloidosis
    Proliferative hyperplasia of intima
    Organ transplantation
    Haemolytic uraemic syndrome
    Dissiminated intravascular coagulation
  4.2.3 Increased intralumenal pressure secondary to colonic obstruction
    Carcinoma
    Diverticulitis
    Faecal impaction

A deficient blood flow to the colon may arise from the following iatrogenic- or non iatrogenic-, occlusive- or non occlusive groups of aetiopathogenic factors.

Occlusive aetiopathogenic factors:
Arterial occlusion;
Venous occlusion.

Non occlusive aetiopathogenic factors:
'Low flow state'
Small vessel disease
Increased intralumenal pressure secondary to obstruction.

One or more combinations of these 5 mechanisms

Table 4.1. Aetiopathogenic factors for ischaemic colitis.

ARTERIAL OCCLUSION

non-iatrogenic
- obliterative atherosclerosis
- thrombosis
- embolism
- compression of mesenteric arteries:
  tumour (carcinoid, carcinoma, lymphoma)
  median arcuate ligament
  dissecting aortic aneurysm
  haematoma
  other conditions
- fibromuscular hyperplasia
- Takayasu's disease

iatrogenic
- ligation of IMA in aortic reconstruction or abdominal aortic aneurysm surgery
- abdomino-perineal excision of the rectum
- abdominal angiography
- transcatheter embolotherapy

INCREASED INTRALUMENAL PRESSURE SECONDARY TO COLONIC OBSTRUCTION

- stricturing colon carcinoma
- stricturing diverticular disease
- faecal impaction
- intussusception
- adhesions
- colostomy strictures
- volvulus

(central diagram: ring labelled "intestinal arterial blood pressure reduction" surrounding core labelled "increased intraluminal pressure")

VENOUS OCCLUSION

- venous thrombosis
  portal thrombosis
    livercirrhosis
    hepatocellular carcinoma
  pylethrombosis:
    appendicitis
    diverticulitis
    necrotizing pancreatitis
  oral contraceptives
- hypercoagulable states:
  thrombocytosis
  polycythaemia vera rubra
  macroglobulinaemia
  antithrombin iii deficiency
  migratory thrombophlebitis
  neoplasm
  stickle cell anaemia
- mechanical compression of mesenteric veins
  see arterial occlusion

SMALL VESSEL DISEASE

- proliferative intima hyperplasia (diabetes, hypertension)
- vasculitis
  systemic lupus erythematosus
  rheumatoid arthritis
  polyarteritis nodosa
  dermatomyositis
  anaphylactoid purpura (Henoch-Schönlein)
- malignant atrophic papulosis (Degos' disease)
- amyloidosis
- irradiation-vasculopathy
- organ transplantation
- cholesterol emboli
- dissiminated intravascular coagulation
  haemolytic uraemic syndrome

LOW FLOW STATE

- cardiogenic causes
  - congestive heart failure
  - myocardial infarction
  - valvular disease
  - myocarditis
  - cardiac arrhytmia
- haemorrhage
- septic shock
- dehydration
- other causes:
  functional vasopasm with hypotension
  drugs:
    ergotamine
    cardioglycosides (digitalis)
    antihypertensives
    diuretics
    efedrine
    others

can often be found. The different aetiopathogenic factors with subdivisions are summarized in table 4.1.

4.1 Occlusive aetiopathogenic factors

4.1.1 Arterial occlusion

4.1.1.1 Iatrogenic occlusion. Abdominal aortic prosthesis for aneurysm or *aorta reconstruction*: ligation of the IMA in absence of a well developed collateral circulation is usually the main cause of the development of ischaemia of the descending colon or sigmoid.

Moore (1954) and Cannon (1955) were the first to describe ischaemic colonic lesions after aortic aneurysm surgery: many groups have since made similar observations (Table 4.2).

The literature on ischaemia of the colon following ligation of the IMA during resection of abdominal aortic aneurysm or aortic reconstruction was reviewed in 1974 by Johnson and Nabseth who found an overall incidence of 99 cases (1.6%) in 6,100 patients at risk. Papadopoulos et al., (1974) found in a group of 282 patients that had undergone surgery of the abdominal aorta 3 patients (1.1%) with colonic ischaemia. Ernst et al., (1976) reported an incidence of 1–2%. There is a marked variation in the reports of the frequency of occurrence of frank necrosis, ranging from 0.25% to nearly 10% (Smith and Szilagyi, 1960; Miller and Knox, 1966; Kilpatrick et al., 1968), but this variation may be partly related to differences in operative technique and the following concomitant factors:

- atheromatous lesions of the coeliac, superior mesenteric and hypogastric arteries;
- abnormalities of the marginal artery of Drummond preventing sufficient flow from the SMA;
- improper ligation of the IMA, preventing adequate blood flow from the SMA to the IMA;
- ligation of one or both hypogastric arteries, particularly when there is an aneurysm of the iliac artery bifurcations, without re-establishment of arterial continuity (Shaw and Green, 1953; Wald, 1964; Rob and Snyder, 1966; Papadopoulos et al., 1974).

In the vast majority of the population a rich collateral circulation will enable acute occlusion of the IMA to be well tolerated with very few associated problems (Mavor et al., 1962).

Thomas and Wellwood (1973), described one patient who developed ischaemic colitis following *abdomino-perineal excision of the rectum* for carcinoma.

Later, Wittenberg et al., (1975) described 4 cases of ischaemic colitis occurring at intervals from 3 months to 7 years after abdomino-perineal resection.

Earlier ligation of the IMA will reduce the blood flow through the marginal artery of Drummond rendering the remaining colon more vulnerable to ischaemic damage; thus patients who pass bright red blood through a colostomy following abdomino-perineal excision of the rectum for carcinoma, may have ischaemic colitis rather than a recurrence of the neoplasm.

Joyeux et al., (1950) and Courty and Carli (1950) were the first to report *abdomino-aortic angiography* as a cause of ischaemic damage of the colon. Using Ténébryl as a contrast agent, they described necrosis of the sigmoid after aortic angiography: more cases have subsequently been reported (Fineberg et al., 1958; Mc. Dowell and Thompson, 1959; Padhi, 1960; Knox and West, 1961; Guilfoil, 1963; Puylaert, 1965; Killen et al., 1967; Anderson, 1969). It is not clear whether the contrast medium, the trauma of catheterization or the high injection pressure is the causative factor.

Experimental work suggests that the gut is very tolerant to concentrated angiographic media and the presently used agents are less toxic than those previously used. In postmortem studies multiple cholesterol emboli may be found microscopically after angiography as a result of trauma or of high pressure injection (Gratama, 1982).

Acute colonic mucosal necrosis developed in 3 of 23 patients following *transcatheter embolotherapy* for colonic haemorrhage (Shenoy, 1981; Rosenkrantz et al., 1982). Injury of the intima during catheterization was suggested as being one of the main causes.

Postembolization arteriography in each of these ischaemic colons demonstrated large segments of devascularisation. The authors concluded that the presence or absence of persistent small vessel per-

Table 4.2. Distribution of ischaemic disease of the colon and rectum following aortic bifurcation-prosthesis for abdominal aortic aneurysm. Review of the literature: 1954–1983.

Author	Year	Number of patients	Surgical procedure	Result	
				Death	Recovery
Sigmoid/colon					
Bernstein and Bernstein;	1963	1	Colostomy	1	–
Birnbaum et al.;	1964	1	resection/colostomy	–	1
Bicks et al.;	1968	19	16× none	9	7
			3× hemicolectomy	1	2
Papadopoulos et al.;	1971	1	reimplantation IMA	–	1
Ottinger et al.;	1972	13	not known	11	2
Papadopoulos et al.;	1973	2	2× resection	1	1
Papadopoulos et al.;	1974	1	resection/colostomy	–	1
Rötzcher et al.;	1976	1	resection (Hartmann)	1	–
Rückert and Buckmann;	1982	1	resection	–	1
Kim et al.;	1983	18	18× resection	10	8
		58		34	24
Descending colon					
Barnes;	1958	1	none	1	–
McKain and Schumacker;	1958	1	none	1	–
Bernatz;	1960	2	none	2	–
Smith and Szilagyi;	1960	1	none	1	–
Young et al.;	1962	1	none	1	–
Birnbaum et al.;	1964	1	none	–	1
Papadopolous et al.;	1974	2	1× resection	1	–
			1× reimplantation IMA	–	1
Ernst et al.;	1976	27	27× resection	–	27
Launer et al.;	1978	1	resection	1	–
Hagihara et al.;	1979	12	12× resection	7	5
Rückert and Buckmann;	1982	1	none	1	–
		50		16	34
Rectum					
Moore;	1954	1	none	–	1
Movius;	1955	2	none	–	2 (stricture)
Smith and Szilagyi;	1960	1	Colostomy	–	1 (stricture)
Young et al.;	1962	1	none	1	–
Rötzcher et al.;	1976	1	none	–	1 (stricture)
Quesada et al.;	1980	1	none	1	–
		7		2	5
Rectosigmoid					
Smith/Szilagyi;	1960	6	5× none	1	4 (1 stricture)
			1× resection and colostomy	–	1
Perdue and Lowry;	1962	3	2× none	1	1
			1× resection	1	–
Bernstein and Bernstein;	1963	1	none	–	1
Birnbaum et al.;	1964	2	1× none	–	1
			1× Colostomy	–	1
Rötzcher et al.;	1976	1	resection	1	–
Launer et al.;	1978	1	resection	1	–
Quesada et al.;	1980	2	1× none	1	–
			1× resection	1	–
Rückert and Buckmann;	1982	4	3× resection	3	–
			1× colostomy	–	1 (stricture)
		20		10	10

Table 4.2. Continued.

Author	Year	Number of patients	Surgical procedure	Result	
				Death	Recovery
Sigmoid					
Cannon;	1955	1	none	1	–
McKain and Schumacker;	1958	1	resection	–	1
Bernatz;	1960	1	resection	1	–
Smith and Szilagyi;	1960	2	1× none	–	1
			1× exteriorization	1	–
McVaugh;	1961	1	none	1	–
Young et al.;	1962	2	1× none	1	–
			1× resection	–	1
Perdue and Lowry;	1962	1	resection	1	–
Bernstein and Bernstein;	1963	1	none	1	–
Goodman;	1965	1	resection	–	1
Rückert and Buckman;	1982	1	resection	1	–
		12		8	4

fusion after embolisation has important prognostic implications regarding the likelihood of infarction.

4.1.1.2 Non iatrogenic occlusion. Non iatrogenic occlusion may lead to a diminished flow in the mesenteric arteries for many reasons:

Obliterative atherosclerosis and *thrombosis* (Russell, 1950; Engelhardt and Jacobson, 1956; Marshak et al., 1965; Varga and Currie, 1965; Kilpatrick et al., 1968; Karmody et al., 1976; Langeron and Thery, 1976) can cause gradual obstruction of the SMA, IMA and hypogastric arteries and eventually lead to colonic ischaemia. Lambana et al., (1973) and later Saegesser et al., (1979) described stenosing colonic lesions of an ischaemic nature secondary to atheromatous plaques in the IMA; the SMA was normal. In a study of 88 patients with colonic ischaemia, examined as a consecutive unselected postmortem series, Reiner et al., (1963) found that 77% had evidence of atherosclerosis of the mesenteric vessels. Stenosis or occlusion involved the SMA in 39, the IMA in 30, branches of the IMA in 16, and the middle colic artery in 14 patients. Severe mesenteric involvement was almost exclusively associated with severe aortic atheroma.

They found a high incidence of diabetes mellitus in cases with severe atherosclerosis and a close correlation between mesenteric arteriopathy, aortic atheroma, coronary disease and peripheral arterial disease.

Three cases of ischaemic colitis with terminal uraemia in patients with an end-stage kidney disease have been reported by Aubia et al., (1981). They suggested that the accelerated arterial disease (premature-and accelerated atherosclerosis) presented by terminal uraemic patients and the coincidental factors of constipation and intestinal motility disturbances might be responsible for this complication. Acute occlusion of the mesenteric arterial system due to *embolism* (Wang and Reeves, 1960; Farman, 1966; Karmody et al., 1976) and *dissecting aneurysm of the aorta* (Young et al., 1963; Bernstein and Bernstein, 1963; Wald, 1964) are rare causes of ischaemic colitis. This is firstly because the IMA is an unusual site for an embolism and secondly because there is usually a sufficient collateral blood supply in most patients via the 'Arc of Riolan', the pancreatico-duodenal- and ileomesenteric arcades. Therefore ischaemic lesions due to an acute occlusion of the IMA by an embolus may be mild, asymptomatic and heal without significant residual damage. Only a few cases of IMA emboli have been reported in the literature (Brown and Dey, 1932; Ferguson, 1932; Carvajal, 1967).

The SMA is more commonly a trap for emboli compared to the IMA, owing to its greater diameter and less steep angle of origin (Demos et al., 1962; Dickson, 1968). The origin of the middle colic artery is the most usual site for an embolus. Emboli of the ileocoecal branch of the SMA, causing reversible coecal infarction have been documented angiographically (Dunbar et al., 1966).

Mesocolon haematoma due to peripheral arterial injury (Corbett, 1957; Mays and Noer, 1966; Renton, 1967; Huber, 1972; Poupon and Bonnefond, 1973; Rickert et al., 1974; Humphreys and Graham, 1977) and expanding tumours (carcinoid, carcinoma, lymphoma and dissecting aneurysm) (Young et al., 1963; Wald, 1964; Anthony, 1970) have been mentioned as a cause of ischaemic colitis due to *compression of the large mesenteric arteries and veins*. An additional but rare cause which can lead to ischaemic colitis is *thrombangitis obliterans* (Buerger's disease) (Ferguson, 1932; Rijsbosch, 1958; McCort, 1960; Herrington and Grossman, 1968; Guay et al., 1976).

Fibromuscular hyperplasia represents a general arterial dysplasia of unknown aetiology rather than a process limited to the renal arteries.

Also the coeliac artery and mesenteric arteries may be involved (Najafi, 1966; Claiborn, 1970).

Irregular thickening of the vessels by proliferation of smooth muscle and fibrous tissue of the media and intima may lead to colonic ischaemia. If the inflammatory aortic wall lesions in case of *Takayasu's* disease extends into the ostia or main branches of the abdominal aorta with secondary marked narrowing of the mesenteric vessels, colonic ischaemia may occur (Lupi Herrera et al., 1977).

4.1.2 Venous occlusion

Ischaemic colitis due to mesenteric venous thrombosis is rare (Demuth et al., 1959; Demos et al., 1962; Irwin, 1965; Dickson, 1968). Often no cause of mesenteric venous occlusion can be found.

However, mesenteric venous thrombosis can be seen in combination with *portal thrombosis* and livercirrhosis (Demuth et al., 1959; Demos et al., 1962; Irwin, 1965; Varga and Currie, 1965; Grendell and Ockner, 1982). Occlusion of the mesenteric veins can precipitate colonic ischaemia through obstruction of outflow. The capillary flow is consequently arrested and arterial obstruction eventually follows. Obstruction of the Inferior Mesenteric Vein (IMV) is of less clinical importance than obstruction of the Superior Mesenteric

Vein (SMV). The IMV has an extensive collateral circulation and venous blood may be shunted directly into the systemic circulation (Trotter, 1913).

Reed and Coon (1963) suggested that there might be a correlation between mesenteric vein thrombosis and *oral contraceptives*.

They described a patient with extensive gangrene of the colon after use of oral contraceptives. Since then this association has regularly been mentioned in the literature (Brennan et al., 1968; Ward and Stevenson, 1968; Kilpatrick et al., 1968; Hurwitz et al., 1970; Civetta and Kolodny, 1970; Cotton and Thomas, 1971; Miller, 1971; McClennan, 1976; Martin et al., 1977; Nesbit and deWeese, 1977; Ghahremani et al., 1977; Lescher and Bombeck, 1977; Barcewicz and Welch, 1980).

The question of why estrogens may have a thrombogenic effect has not been answered. Although reduced antithrombin in III activity has been reported in patients on oral contraceptives (Wessler et al., 1976) other studies have failed to substantiate this finding (Carvalho et al., 1977).

Although the precipitating factor in mesenteric venous thrombosis is uncertain, there seems to be a positive correlation between the dose of estrogen and the incidence of venous occlusion.

Oral contraceptives containing 100 μg or more of estrogens are known to be associated with a greater risk of deep vein thrombosis (Inman et al., 1970; Rose, 1972). Ischaemic colitis may be more common than is realized with the increasing usage of conjugated estrogen preparations in menopausal women and of stilboestrol in elderly men treated for prostatic cancer.

Hypercoagulable states which predispose to thrombosis can cause both venous and arterial occlusion. Polycythaemia rubra vera has been associated with ischaemic colonic ulceration (Fitts et al., 1960; Ostermiller et al., 1969). Essential thrombocytosis, sickle cell anaemia, macroglobulinaemia and antithrombin III deficiency are also mentioned as causes of venous thrombosis, leading to colonic ischaemia (Grendell and Ockner, 1982; Gage and Gagnier, 1983).

Pancreatitis as a possible cause of mesenteric venous thrombosis has been mentioned in the literature in association with colonic ischaemia by several authors (Lindahl et al., 1972; Raven, 1973; Agrawal et al., 1974; Katz et al., 1974; Hunt and Mildenhall, 1975; Thompson et al., 1977; Dallemand et al., 1977).

The association of ischaemic strictures of the colon with pancreatitis is rare and only a few cases have been found in literature (Katz et al., 1974; Hunt and Mildenhall, 1975; Fagniez et al., 1976).

Venous occlusion by compression of mesenteric veins or/and a period of circulatory disturbance associated with an acute attack of pancreatitis may precipitate ischaemic colitis.

Pylethrombosis can be associated with abdominal inflammatory conditions as diverticulitis, appendicitis, necrotizing pancreatitis etc.

4.2 Non- occlusive aetiopathogenic factors

4.2.1 'Low flow state'
In 'low flow state' a diminution in the circulating blood volume causes shunting of blood to more vital organs (brain) and spasm of the splanchnic vessels. A high incidence of cardiac failure as a cause of small and large bowel ischaemia has been reported in the literature. Haemorrhage, sepsis and dehydration are other causes of the low flow state.

Congestive heart failure, myocardial infarction, valvular disease, myocarditis – all diseases which result in low left ventricular cardiac output are frequent and important predisposing causes of colonic ischaemia (Hamilton et al., 1955; Ende, 1958; Hoffman et al., 1960; Gazes et al., 1961; Polansky et al., 1964; Musa, 1965; Morin, 1967). During low cardiac output blood will be shunted away from the bowel to more vital centers and this will lead to a reduction of blood flow to the mucosa, submucosa and muscle layer of the colonic wall. A concomitant mesenteric vasoconstriction may develop which will ultimately result in irreversible necrosis of the colon.

The importance of *cardiac arrhythmia* in reducing cardiac output and precipitating small bowel damage has been underlined by Britt and Cheek (1969) who were able to demonstrate experimentally an abrupt fall in mesenteric flow following induced atrial fibrillation. Later Frenkel (1969) demonstrated the relationship of cardiac arrhythmia and colonic ischaemia secondary to a drop in mesenteric blood flow. Renton (1972) found low flow states secondary to arrhythmias in more than 50% of the patients in his series of studies.

Functional vasospasm of small or large mesenteric vessels in combination with hypotension can lead to ischaemia of the colon wall.

Vasospasm can also potentiate ischaemic damage of the colon wall in cases of thrombo-embolic states. This has been frequently shown by the discrepancy between the localisation of vessel occlusion and the extent of colonic ischaemia (van Dongen et al., 1982). From results of animal experiments, Parks (1972), concluded that hypotension and hypovolaemia, which lead to splanchnic vasoconstriction, can result in mucosal colonic necrosis, especially if there are some predisposing factors.

Drugs causing vasoconstriction
Predisposing factors such as administration of ergotamine, digitalis and antihypertensive medication will potentiate the hypotensive effects in cardiac patients.

Prolonged *ergotamine medication* can give rise to colonic ischaemia, due to the chronic vasoconstrictive effect (Stillman et al., 1977; van Blankenstein and Gratama, 1979; Huibregtse et al., 1980).

Cardiac glycosides, such as *digitalis* have a selective vasoconstrictive action on the splanchnic circulation and can cause a significant increase in peripheral vascular resistance (Todd and Pearson, 1963; Polansky et al., 1964; Ferrer et al., 1965; Fogarty and Fletcher, 1965; Muggia, 1967; Renton, 1972; Shanbour and Jacobson, 1972; Pawlik and Jacobson, 1974).

The pathogenic mechanism is still a subject of controversy. Digitalis has been shown to further decrease mesenteric blood flow in experimental haemorrhagic and endotoxin shock (Gazes et al., 1961; Bhagwat and Hawk, 1966; Ulano et al., 1971).

Ischaemic involvement of the colon has been reported in 9–15% of postmortem studies of hypertensive patients using *antihypertensive* medication (Moritz and Oldt, 1937; Brown and Szakas, 1959; Granata et al., 1961; O'Connell, 1976).

Prolonged vasoconstriction in the bowel wall following efedrine injection has been postulated as the cause of an ischaemic stricture in an asthmatic patient (Deloyers, 1970).

Non-occlusive ischaemic colitis has been described in a patient after an i.v. injection of Diconal® (dipipanone HCl and cyclicine HCl) (Turnbull and Isaacson, 1977), or Distalgesic® (dextropropoxyphene and paracetamol) (Briggs et al., 1977). The hypotensive 'low flow' state secondary to drug abuse can be potentiated by alcohol (Turnbull and Isaacson, 1977).

In addition to a low flow state and vasoconstriction there are also other aetiopathogenic splanchnic factors such as increased levels of catecholamines in the blood (Braunwald and Chidsey, 1965). Brown et al., (1959) and Brown and Borowsky (1960) were the first to correlate the increased output of catecholamines by phaeochromocytomas with serious gastrointestinal complications. (Roach, 1959; Rosati and Augur, 1971).

Reversible ischaemic colitis has been described in a patient, who received intravenous vasopressin for oesophageal variceal haemorrhage. Vasopressin reduces the splanchnic blood flow and decreases portal pressure (Lambert et al., 1982).

Ischaemic colitis in the *postoperative* phase can be caused by *haemorrhagic shock* (Demuth et al., 1959; Laufman et al., 1964; Sakai et al., 1980). Ischaemic colitis has been described frequently following abdominal and orthopaedic surgery (Penner and Bernheim, 1939; Penner and Druckermann, 1948; Foster and Dadey, 1956; Horton et al., 1968; Whitehead, 1971; Renton, 1972; Mazingarbe, 1973; Rosen and Cooter, 1973; LeGall et al., 1973; Prandi, 1975; Balz and Minton, 1975; Aldrete, 1977).

Ischaemia of the colon has also been observed in the postoperative phase of cardiac and thoracic vascular surgery or after correction of coarctation of the aorta (Horton et al., 1968; Renton, 1972; Pradhan and Ikins, 1975; Aldrete, 1977).

Hill et al., (1971) reported 3 cases of colonic

ischaemia following aortic valve replacement and suggested that the sudden decrease in the pulse pressure and the rise of diastolic pressure caused instability and vasospasm in the mesenteric vessels.

Ischaemic colitis can also be caused by *septic shock,* secondary to urosepsis or diverticulitis in elderly patients (Demuth et al., 1959; Laufman et al., 1964). *Posttraumatic ischaemic colitis* has been reported secondary to shock and septicaemia (Mays and Noer, 1966; Humphreys and Graham, 1977; Rickert et al., 1974; Guly and Stewart, 1982).

Dehydration especially in older patients with a generalized atherosclerotic disease, may lead to ischaemic colitis.

Abuse of *diuretics* which in 3 patients had led to a massive extracellular volume deficit and haemoconcentration leading to colonic ischaemia was reported by Sharefkin and Silen (1974). A prolonged medication of diuretics in older patients may therefore be dangerous.

4.2.2 Small vessel disease

Small vessel disease is, in combination with a diminished circulatory blood volume and an already compromised splanchnic circulation, an important aetiopathogenic factor for non-occlusive ischaemic colitis. Vasculitis secondary to systemic lupus erythematosus, rheumatoid arthritis or polyarteritis nodosa can lead to focal ischaemia of the colon.

Systemic lupus erythematosus may also affect small blood vessels. Vasculitis has been implicated in small bowel ischaemia, but similar changes may occur in the colon (Pollak et al., 1958; Finkbiner and Decker, 1963; Phillips and Howland, 1968; Matolo and Albo, 1971; Zizic et al., 1975; Tsuchiya et al., 1975; Kleinman et al., 1976; Yoshioka, 1982; Kirks, 1982).

Kistin et al., (1978) reported a 26-year-old woman with systemic lupus erythemasosus, who developed massive rectal bleeding which failed to respond to medical treatment. Pathological examination of the subtotal colectomy specimen showed a normal small intestine and a gangrenous large intestine with ischaemic ulcerations and the extensive fibrinoid vasculitis typical of systemic lupus erythematosus.

In a report of 33 patients with ischaemic enterocolitis by McGovern and Goulston (1965) four patients with *rheumatoid arthritis* were described: in three of these, the entire small and large intestine showed thrombi and submucosal haemorrhages.

A correlation between rheumatoid arthritis and colonic and/or small intestinal ischaemia has also been described by other authors (Finkbiner and Decker, 1963; Hingorani and Graham, 1963; Ottinger and Austen, 1967; Mogadam, 1972).

In 20–50% of cases of *polyarteritis nodosa* inflammatory lesions of the intestinal arcades, proximal vessels and intramural arteries are found (Arkin, 1930; Jernstrom and Stasney, 1952; McKeown and Ganguli, 1956; Bane and Austin, 1963; Finkbiner and Decker, 1963; Couris, 1964; Bircher et al., 1966; Bienenstock et al., 1967; Wood et al., 1979; Huber, 1981). Proctoscopical ischaemic changes in a patient with polyarteritis nodosa have been described by Felsen (1941).

Inflammatory lesions of intramural colonic vessels and mucosal ulcerations of the colon wall have also been described in association with other diseases such as *dermatomyositis* (Boyland and Sokoloff, 1960; Finkbiner and Decker, 1963; Levesque et al., 1981), *Henoch-Schönlein's Syndrome* (Handel and Schwartz, 1957) and *Wegener's granulomatosis* (Girst and Muller, 1953; Maas et al., 1971). These inflammatory vascular lesions are triggered by immunological mechanisms.

Enterocolitis secondary to *irradiaton vasculopathy* may become manifest either shortly after, or alternatively many years after radiotherapy treatment (Qan, 1968). In 75–90% of cases with irradiation vasculopathy, the large bowel is involved, most commonly after irradiation for gynaecologic cancer (Anderson et al., 1955).

A rare cause of ischaemic colitis is *malignant atrophic papulosis* (Degos' disease) (Degos, 1954; Naylor et al., 1960; Nomland and Layton, 1960; Sidi et al., 1960; Strole et al., 1967; Roenigk and Farmer, 1968; Rodriguez, 1977). The development of skin lesions is followed by multiple ischaemic ulcers of the colon.

Ischaemic colonic necrosis and ulceration, due to a narrowing of mesenteric vessels secondary to *amyloidosis* are occasionally encountered (Symmers, 1956; Brody et al., 1964; Gilat and Spiro, 1968; Perarnau et al., 1982). Brom et al., (1969) presented a case of ischaemic colitis secondary to amyloid involvement of the peripheral mesenteric vessels.

Proliferative hyperplasia of the intima in the distal mesenteric arteries has been cited as a cause of ischaemic colitis: it most frequently occurs in association with diabetes and/or hypertension, often in combination with a low flow state (Felsen, 1941; Aboumrad et al., 1963; Castagnoli, 1965; Ambruoso and Feraro, 1967; Williams et al., 1969; Detry et al., 1979).

Arosemena and Edwards (1967) described 13 patients with proliferative intima hyperplasia: in 2 cases there was intestinal arterial occlusion.

Colonic ischaemia has been reported as a complication of *organ transplantation* (Penn et al., 1970; Powis et al., 1972; Perloff et al., 1976).

Most usually affected were patients who experienced a difficult post-transplantation course and who received high doses of immunosuppressive agents for repeated episodes of rejection.

Whether the intestinal lesions are a result of tissue sensitization following the transplantation or whether the immunosuppresive therapy lowers mucosal resistance to bacterial invasion, is not clear.

Histological studies suggest that small colonic arteries may become occluded by endarteritis and fibrosis.

Four cases of ischaemic colitis associated with *haemolytic uraemic syndrome* have been presented (Bar-Ziv et al., 1974; Peterson et al., 1976; Sawaf, 1978; Kirks, 1982). The pathologic process of ischaemia is due to occlusion of the intestinal microvasculature by fibrin deposits.

Recent evidence suggests that *dissiminated intra-*

26

vascular coagulation may play a part in the pathogenesis of non-occlusive ischaemia.

In a study of 20 cases of ischaemic enterocolitis Whitehead (1971) found microthrombosis in the capillary/venous circulation of the necrotizing mucosa/submucosa, and also in many other organs, such as the lungs and the kidneys. Margaretten and McKay (1971) have postulated that ischaemic necrosis may be a manifestation of disseminated intravascular coagulation because of the presence of capillary and venous thrombi in the bowel of patients with this condition. These findings could not be confirmed by Brandt et al., (1976), who performed a retrospective study of the significance of fibrin-thrombi in the vessels of the bowel wall. They noted that fibrin-thrombi were a characteristic feature of ischaemic necrosis. Mechanisms triggering intravascular coagulation are complex and numerous. Small quantities of endotoxin absorbed from the mucosa are presumably harmless but diminished mucosal resistance as a result of splanchnic hypoxia may lead to absorption of larger amounts, which could initiate intravascular coagulation (Whitehead, 1972).

Multiple traumata, severe burns, abdominal septic conditions (appendicitis, pelvic inflammatory disease, diverticulitis etc.) and anaphylaxis may be recognized as predisposing factors for ischaemic colitis due to dissiminated intravascular coagulation.

The Schwartzman reaction (a manifestation of sensitivity to gram negative endotoxins) is another potent cause of dissiminated intravascular coagulation. A generalized Schwartzman phenomenon could well be an important factor in the causation of intestinal ischaemia.

4.2.3 Increased intralumenal pressure secondary to colonic obstruction

The occurrence of ischaemic colitis, proximal to a colonic stenosis caused by *carcinoma of the colon*, *diverticulitis* or *faecal impaction* has been documented intermittently since the early 1960's.

Table 4.3 shows a review of the literature between 1950 and 1982 on the association between ischaemic colitis and colonic carcinoma.

(The articles used for this study are marked with an □ in the references). The incidence of this association is between 1 and 4.7% in the case material of most authors (Nix et al., 1952; Glotzer and Phil, 1966; Rutledge, 1969; Stellamor et al., 1977). For some authors the occurrence of this association is less than 1% (Hurwitz and Khafif, 1960; Ganchrow et al., 1971; Saegesser and Sandblom, 1975; Lewin et al., 1979).

On the other hand Schwartz and Boley (1972)

Table 4.3. A review of the literature between 1950–1982 on the association between ischaemic colitis and colonic carcinoma.

Reports in literature (see references marked with □)	Number of cases	Sex-ratio	Mean age	Localization of colon carcinoma in %	Localization of ischaemic colitis in %	Presence of normal segment between carcinoma and ischaemic colitis	Barium enema	Pathological diagnosis
1950–1982	36 (not detailed reports: 46)	45% F 55% M	70 62			31%	20%	74%

reported that 9 of their 90 patients (10%) with ischaemic disease of the colon had an associated stenosing neoplasm. Hurwitz and Khafif (1960) reported thirteen patients with 'acute necrotizing colitis' proximal to a carcinoma of the colon which had caused incomplete large bowel obstruction. Several other authors (Kremen, 1945; Killingback and Williams, 1961; Herrmann et al., 1965; Goulston and McGovern, 1965; Ambruoso and Feraru, 1967; Bryk, 1968; Dencker et al., 1969), described cases in which long segments of gangrenous colon were found proximal to carcinoma involving the rectosigmoid region.

Various terms, such as 'necrotic colitis', 'pseudomembranous colitis', 'colitis and antecedent carcinoma' or 'ulcerative colitis' were used in describing the condition. Ganchrow et al., (1971) presented a case of obstructive carcinoma of the colon in which stenosing ischaemic lesions were found.

Distension and increased intralumenal pressure (Glotzer and Phil, 1966; Boley et al., 1969; Dencker et al., 1969; Schwartz and Boley, 1972; Saegesser, 1972; Saegesser and Sandblom, 1975) are considered to be the most important causative factors in such circumstances.

Almost all experiments designed to study the consequences of increased intra-enteric pressure have been carried out in the small intestine. Van Zwalenburg (1907) found capillary stasis occurring at an intralumenal pressure of 30 mmHg; at 60 mmHg the venous circulation was arrested and at 130 mmHg all circulation ceased.

These experiments were repeated by Gatch and Gulbertson (1935) working with dogs and by Oppenheimer and Mann (1943) using rats; all circulation ceased at 80 mmHg.

Noer and Derr (1949) found experimentally that in rats a rise of intra-enteric pressure to 70 mmHg or higher prevents the filling of the blood vessels of the distended intestine even when all the mesenteric vessels remain intact. Later, Noer et al., (1951) obtained the same results with rabbits. In their experiments an intralumenal pressure of 50 mmHg was high enough to produce irreversible changes in the circulation of the intestinal wall. Rapid distension of the bowel interfered first with the blood flow in the small veins; only after marked increase of the intralumenal pressure did the small

arteries become affected. Angiographic studies in the dog by Dencker et al., (1969) showed that the layers close to the serosa retain their flow longer. Competence of the ileocoecal valve – which allows intestinal contents to enter the coecum, but prevents the reverse flow of faecal contents into the ileum – is obligatory for distension of the colon proximal to an obstruction (Kremen, 1945).

When early decompression of the obstructed bowel does not occur, a slow increase of the intralumenal pressure in this 'closed loop' can lead to massive distension, interruption of the circulation, causing gangrene of a colonic segment and eventually to perforation.

The blood flow through the mucosa, the muscular layer and the serosa react differently to elevation of the intralumenal intestinal pressure. The inner layers (mucosa) are the first to show reduced flow as a result of compression. The serosal circulation does not cease even at extremely high intraenteric pressure. The severity of the ischaemic changes depends upon:

- the degree of bowel distension and of intralumenal pressure (P);
- the duration of the distension;
- the tension in the colonic wall of each segment (F);
- the diameter of the bowel lumen (D) (La Place law: $F = D \times P \times \pi$);
- the vascular condition of the patient (Boley et al., 1969; Saegesser, 1972; Stillwell, 1973);
- the virulence of bacterial overgrowth.

In addition to mechanical factors, bacterial proliferation in stagnant faecal material should also be considered as an important factor in the aetiology of colonic ischaemia (Julien, 1965; Glotzer and Phil, 1966; Roy and Jobard, 1966; Tonitza and Ionescu, 1966; Senturia et al., 1967; Boley et al., 1978).

By 1960, Hurwitz and Khafif had already proposed that partial tumorous obstruction can lead to stagnation of colonic contents, possibly with subsequent bacterial proliferation, which ultimately results in colonic inflammation and ulceration. Whatever the extent of tissue damage caused by hypoxia, the diminution in tissue viability inevitably results in diminished resistance to invasion by intestinal microorganisms (Addleman, 1963; Saegesser et al., 1972). However, Glotzer et al., (1963) believe that faecal stasis is not important. When prestenotic colonic ulcers were produced in 50% of dogs after high-grade distal stenosis with a surgical tape, the stool flora changed neither quantitatively, nor qualitatively. Other investigators have found bacteria to be very scarce in areas of ulceration.

In addition to causing an elevation of intraluminal pressure and bacterial invasion, obstruction of the colon can also affect colonic motility and lead to alteration of the defaecation pattern with hypermotility, repetitive straining and increased muscle spasms with subsequent direct deleterious effect on mural circulation (Glotzer and Phil, 1966; Saegesser et al., 1972, 1974, 1975; Boley et al., 1978). There are also reports of colonic ulceration and inflammatory changes proximal to benign obstructive lesions such as adhesions (Bryk, 1968; Dietz, 1969).

Hirschsprung's disease (Swenson, 1959; Bill and Chapman, 1962; Hope et al., 1965; Berry, 1969), incarcerated inguinal hernia (Carlin and Manashil, 1973), diverticulosis (Lenz, 1962; Thijn, 1973), obstruction or narrowing at the site of colostomy (Thayer and Spiro, 1962; Thomas and Wellwood, 1973), sigmoid volvulus (Hermanek and Mühe, 1971), intussusception (Demuth et al., 1959; Avnet and Elkin, 1961; Varga and Currie, 1965; Meyers and Ghahremani, 1977; Maroy et al., 1982), ileus and congenital megacolon (Boley et al., 1969; Carasquilla and Arbula, 1970).

De Boer and van Unnink (1968) and later Clark et al., (1972) and Hay (1978) described colon-gangrene due to faecal impaction after prolonged use of phenothiazine derivatives (chlorpromazine).

5. CLASSIFICATION OF ISCHAEMIC COLITIS

5.1 Introduction

In 1962 Marston reviewed the then existing literature on ischaemia of the colon (Marston, 1962); in 1966 they reported on 16 patients with similar clinical, radiological and pathological findings associated with vascular disease of the distal colon and designated this entity 'ischaemic colitis'. (Marston et al., 1966.) Other nomenclature such as 'postoperative colitis', (Penner et al., 1939), 'haemorrhagic enterocolitis' (Wilson and Qalheim, 1954), 'necrotizing colitis' (Killingback and Williams, 1961), 'reversible vascular occlusion of the colon' (Boley et al., 1963), 'pseudomembranous enterocolitis' (Goulston and McGovern, 1965), 'ischaemic enterocolitis' (McGovern and Goulston, 1965), 'Cl. Welchii colitis' (Tate and Thompson, 1965) have been used when describing ischaemic lesions of the colon and should be regarded as synonyms for ischaemic colitis.

Marston et al., (1966) were the first to classify the clinical syndrome in accordance with the degree of ischaemic damage of the colon in the 'gangrenous form', the 'transient form' and 'the stricturing form'.

Since then several different or modified classifications have been introduced by different authors, based upon clinical or pathological or endoscopical findings.

5.2 Clinical classification

Brown (1968) and later van Dongen et al., (1982) modified Marston's classification and considered two principle forms of ischaemic colitis, based upon clinical findings:

5.2.1 a 'non gangrenous' form, subdivided into a 'transient' and a 'stricturing' form and

5.2.2 a 'gangrenous' form subdivided into a partially gangrenous form (mucosal slough) and a transmural gangrenous form.

5.2.1 Non gangrenous ischaemic colitis

Marston et al., (1966) defined the *transient form* as a form which involves morphological changes of the mucosa with oedema, submucosal haemorrhage and diffuse superficial ulcerations. A sufficient collateral circulation allows complete regeneration and complete structural and functional recovery, within 1-2 weeks.

In some cases, however, mucosal ischaemia of a segment may represent only a temporary stage with subsequent evolution into more severe ischaemia with deeper involvement of the bowel wall.

If the muscle layer is involved and the collateral bloodsupply is sufficient to prevent progression to transmural ischaemia, but insufficient to allow regeneration to proceed, the *chronic 'non resolving' form* with or without stenosis (*'stricturing form'*) can develop within 4 weeks-3 months. Tubular stenosis occurs in areas where ulceration and subsequent fibrotic scarring involve the entire circumference of the colon.

When the damage affects only part of the circumference multiple sacculations (pseudodiverticula) with a rigid, flaccid bowel wall at the mesenteric side will ensue. The stricturing form may lead to obstruction of the colon.

5.2.2 Gangrenous ischaemic colitis

Van Dongen et al., (1982) suggested that in some cases the ischaemic necrosis is limited to the inner layers without involvement of the muscularis and serosa. Consequently a chronic ulcerative process can persist after sloughing of necrotic layers (*partially necrotizing form* or mucosal slough).

If a severe episode presents (for example, in the event of acute mesenteric artery occlusion after ligation of a large mesenteric vessel in the course of aortic reconstruction, or as a result of acute thrombosis or embolism and the collateral circulation is insufficient), necrosis can extend across all wall layers (*transmural necrotizing form*). The severe gangrenous form of ischaemic colitis, which is also referred to as 'necrotizing colitis' usually occurs in patients over 60 years. These patients frequently have a history of cardiovascular disease; precipitating features include congestive cardiac failure, cardiac arrhythmia, myocardial infarction, aneurysm, pulmonary embolism, aortic or mitral valve replacement for rheumatic heart disease, hypoten-

sion, shock and digitalis intoxication (chapter 4).

Within these forms defined above, many variations and combinations are possible, depending upon the severity and duration of the ischaemia.

Under certain favourable conditions of the collateral circulation it is possible that a severe low flow state will only lead to a condition of reversible ischaemia. Conversely, it is also possible that under unfavourable conditions a mild low flow state will be followed by transmural necrosis (Marcuson, 1972; van Dongen et al., 1982).

A correct judgement can thus be made only when the degree of damage of the ischaemic lesion has been assessed by radiology, endoscopy, or at operation (van Dongen et al., 1982). Sometimes, one must wait for several months until the nature of the lesion can be established and a correct classification made.

Miller et al., (1971) described a syndrome of 'evanescent colitis of the young adult', similar to ischaemic colitis. The syndrome affects young patients, usually in their 20's (Friedland and Filly, 1974; Dewbury, 1976; Heron et al., 1981).

Because of its similar pathology, *'evanescent colitis'* is regarded as a part of the spectrum of diseases typified by transient ischaemic colitis.

5.2.3 Literature review

In the existing literature the clinical classification after Marston et al., 1966 has been frequently used. A review of the collected literature (the articles used in this study are indicated in the references with a prefix ○) between 1950 and 1982 reveals that of the cited 1,024 patients with ischaemic colitis, in 744 cases the form had been mentioned. There were 355 cases of gangrenous ischaemic colitis, and 389 cases of non gangrenous ichaemic colitis, i.e. 283 cases of transient ischaemic colitis and 106 cases of stricturing ischaemic colitis.

5.3 Histological classification

5.3.1 Swerdlow's classification

Swerdlow et al., (1981) proposed a histological classification of colon ischaemia which was based solely on the depth of necrosis in the colon wall, independent of cause or distribution.

This classification emphasizes the effects of ischaemic injury of the bowel.

The authors classified ischaemic colitis as mucosal ischaemia, mural ischaemia and transmural ischaemia. An ischaemic lesion is classified as mucosal if the necrotic process extends no deeper than the muscularis mucosae; as mural if necrosis extends into the submucosa or into, but not through the muscularis propria, and as transmural if it extends through the muscularis propria with or without serosal involvement.

5.3.2 Morson's classification
Morson (1971), however, based his classification on the histopathological changes, observed at progressive phases of ischaemic colitis, i.e. in the early ischaemic phase, in the reparative phase (subacute or chronic) and in the stricturing phase.

5.4. Endoscopical classification

5.4.1 Classification according to severity (Favier et al., 1976)

Favier et al., (1976) classified the ischaemic lesions observed at endoscopy in 3 stages according to their *severity:* stage I is characterized by non confluent petechiae, separated by normal mucosa; stage II is characterized by extensive haemorrhagic plaques with small central ulcerations and larger haemorrhages in an oedematous mucosa; stage III is characterized by ulceration with polypoid lesions and necrosis.

5.4.2 Classification according to duration (Scowcroft et al., 1981)
Scowcroft et al., (1981) proposed an endoscopical classification of ischaemic colitis according to the *duration* of the ischaemic process, i.e. an acute, subacute and chronic stage.

The heterogeneity of the different and modified classifications may cause confusion. The practical usefulness of these different classifications will be discussed in chapter 28.

6. VARIATIONS IN THE INCIDENCE OF ISCHAEMIC COLITIS WITH AGE AND SEX OF THE PATIENTS STUDIED IN THE LITERATURE

In reports of 1,024 patients (the articles used in this study are indicated in the references by the prefix ○) collected from the literature the age was mentioned in 676 cases. The average age was 60 years.

In 721 patients the sex was mentioned. The sex distribution between men and women was in the ratio 1.5:1 (428 men and 293 women). Recently Andersen and Eklöf (1981) reported 2 children of 4 and 9 years old with clinical and radiological manifestation highly suggestive of ischaemic colitis.

Twenty-nine cases (14 men and 15 women) of ischaemic colitis in patients below 36 years of age have been reported to date (Millar, 1965; Miller, 1971; Clark et al., 1972; Dharia, 1973; Friedland and Filly, 1974; Rickert, 1974; Guay, 1976; Sawaf et al., 1978; Barcewicz and Welch, 1980; Archibald et al., 1980; Duffy, 1981; Gage and Gagnier, 1983).

7. ASSOCIATED DISEASES

Associated diseases
The more frequent occurrence of ischaemic colitis in older patients may be correlated with the increased incidence of atherosclerotic vasculopathy, progressive peripheral arterial insufficiency, tortuosity of the intramural blood vessels of the colon and diminishing cardiac function (Aboumrad et al., 1963; Ambruoso and Feraru, 1967; Détry et al., 1979).

According to Marcuson (1972) it is nearly always possible to find a single predisposing factor in patients below 50 years of age. In patients above 50 years of age in Marcuson's study, such factors were discernable in about half of the patients, but since several such symptoms were often present, it was difficult to identify a single causal agent.

Atheroma, cardiac disease, diabetes, hypertension, hypotensive episodes and arrhythmia were found, often in combination, in 98 (80%) of the 122 patients above 50 years of age.

8. CLINICAL PRESENTATION

8.1 *Introduction*

8.2 *Clinical symptoms*
    8.2.1 'Non gangrenous form'
        'Transient (mucosal) form'
        'Stricturing (mural) form'
    8.2.2 'Gangrenous form'
        'Gangrenous (transmural) form'

8.1 Introduction

The following clinical signs were found to be suggestive of ischaemic colitis:

– acute onset of intermittent abdominal colicky pain, mostly localized in the left hypochondrium and periumbilical region, accompanied by tenesmus;
– passage of dark or bright red rectal blood within 24 hours after onset;
– diarrhoea;
– nausea, vomiting.

Neither the severity of pain, nor the frequency of diarrhoea, nor the character of the rectal bleeding are dependent upon the clinical stage or type of ischaemic colitis. Severe abdominal pain might be found in a 'transient (mucosal) form' of ischaemia for example, while a case of the 'gangrenous (transmural) form' may present with a complete lack of clinical symptoms.

Swerdlow et al., (1981) examined the usefulness of their histological classification by correlating the major clinical features of 25 patients with acute colonic ischaemia with the histological findings in the surgical specimens. The series contained 6 men and 19 women with an average age of 70 years. The cases were easily categorized as mucosal ischaemia in 4 cases, mural ischaemia in 4, and transmural ischaemia in 17 cases. They concluded that there is no correlation between depth of ischaemic damage and severity of clinical symptoms.

Therefore, it seems that any form of ischaemic colitis can be associated with the full spectrum of clinical symptoms and signs, or on the contrary may go completely unnoticed.

8.2 Clinical symptoms

Table 8.1 represents the frequency of occurrence of various clinical symptoms in 712 patients with ischaemic colitis reported in the literature. (The articles used in this study are indicated in the references with a prefix ○).

Abdominal colicky pain, diarrhoea and rectal bleeding were the most frequent signs of ischaemic colitis.

Table 8.1. Clinical symptoms in 712 patients with ischaemic colitis reported in the literature.

abdominal pain	72%
diarrhoea	63%
rectal blood	61%
nausea/vomiting	18%
tenesmus	2%

8.2.1 *'Non gangrenous form'*
The transient (mucosal) form is more commonly reported in the literature than the stricturing (mural) form.

'Transient (mucosal) form'
All the symptoms characteristic of ischaemic colitis

(as described above) may be found, e.g. lower abdominal pain, often of a colicky nature, tenesmus, diarrhoea and the passage of blood or mucus. The severity of the abdominal pain is quite variable, although it is usually mild (in some cases, discomfort is so slight as to pass unnoticed by the patient).

The rectal bleeding is quite characteristic; it differs from the massive bright bleeding which occasionnally complicates diverticular disease and from haemorrhoidal bleeding, which is usually small in volume, bright red and unmixed with the stool.

In ischaemic colitis the bleeding is moderate in amount, dark or bright red mixed with stools and may contain blood clots. In the acute phase of the disease where there is severe intramural bleeding, the mucosa of the ischaemic colon segment will separate from the inner layer and a mucosal cast can be passed with the stool (mucosal slough).

Nausea and vomiting may be present. Physical signs examination will usually elicit some abdominal tenderness and muscle guarding in the lower abdomen, particularly in the left iliac fossa and in epigastrio. Peristalsis may be normal. Rectal examination frequently discloses blood on the finger stall.

There can be mild fever and a rise in pulse rate. After 2 days all symptoms may disappear and after 1–2 weeks, when the submucosal haemorrhage and oedema are resorbed, the patient can be fully recovered.

'Stricturing (mural) form'
Colicky abdominal pain, paradoxical diarrhoea and rectal bleeding can occur. Hyperperistalsis or ileus signs may be found. Progressive stricture formation can lead to incomplete or complete bowel obstruction. The most critical time for stricture formation is about 6 weeks after the onset of ischaemia.

8.2.2 *'Gangrenous form'*

'Gangrenous (transmural) form'
In this form patients present with a short history, usually of less than 18 hours duration. Abdominal pain is mostly acute, severe and colicky: it may be localized in the left iliac fossa or may be generalized.

However, there may also be a complete lack of pain. Diarrhoea may be present with or without rectal bleeding. The most important signs usually are shock and generalized peritonitis.

There is tenderness and muscle guarding. On examination the temperature may be subnormal and there may be tachycardia. There is usually no time for detailed laboratory investigation at this stage, as immediate resuscitation and laparotomy are necessary.

9. ANATOMICAL DISTRIBUTION OF ISCHAEMIC COLITIS

9.1 *Predisposition*

9.2 *Left colonic ischaemia*

9.3 *Right colonic ischaemia*

9.4 *Rectal ischaemia*

9.5 *Correlation aetiology – distribution*

9.6 *Extent of ischaemic damage*

9.7 *Focal, segmental, massive involvement*

9.1 Predisposition

The splenic flexure, descending colon and the sigmoid show a predisposition for ischaemia. The transverse, ascending colon and the rectum are less frequently involved (Table 9.1).

9.2 Left colonic ischaemia

The marginal artery of Drummond as the direct connection between the middle colic artery and the left colic artery serves as the major connection between SMA and IMA. At the splenic flexure (Griffiths' point, page 7) this vessel was present in 48%, poorly developed or tenuous in 9% and absent in 43% of patients with ischaemic colitis (Meyers, 1976).

The blood flow at the splenic angle can therefore be precarious.

A flow reduction in the middle- or left colic artery, due to atherosclerosis, thrombosis or compression may then lead to ischaemia of a colonic

Table 9.1. Distribution of ischaemic lesions in the larger groups of patients described in the literature between 1962 and 1981, and in our series.

Author(s)	Year	Ascending colon	Transverse colon	Splenic flexure	Descending colon	Sigmoid	Rectum	Total number of patients
Young et al.	1962	5.8%	5.8%	5.8%	40.4%	30.8%	11.4%	40
McGovern and Goulston	1965	18.2%	22.7%	9.1%	27.3%	11.4%	11.3%	31
Marston et al	1966	4.2%	4.2%	54.2%	33.2%	4.2%	–	16
Egger and Kellock	1970	–	30.8%	30.8%	30-8%	7.6%	–	16
Whitehead	1971	20.7%	18.4%	16.1%	18.4%	18.4%	8%	20
Thomas	1972	5.7%	17.1%	35.7%	24.4%	17.1%	–	32
Boley and Schwartz	1971	6.8%	12.1%	22.7%	30.2%	24.3%	3.8%	87
Marcuson	1972	6.0%	14.7%	28.0%	25.9%	21.1%	4.3%	122
Brown	1972	–	17.2%	34.5%	41.4%	6.9%	–	17
Wittenberg et al.	1975	6.3%	3.2%	9.5%	33.3%	31.7%	16%	41
O'Connell et al.	1976	11.4%	6.8%	45.5%	22.7%	13.6%	–	26
Cogbill et al.	1977	13.9%	11.1%	11.1%	25.0%	27.8%	11.1%	15
Hagihara et al.	1977	5.9%	5.9%	29.4%	23.5%	32.4%	2.9%	18
Huber	1981	7.2%	27.0%	19.8%	24.3%	20.7%	1.0%	109
Our own series	1983	14.9%	19.3%	14.8%	25.1%	22.3%	3.6%	199

38

segment near the splenic flexure. This is the reason that ischaemic colitis occurs with the highest frequency on the left side of the colon and particularly around the splenic flexure. In a review of 1,024 patients* collected from the literature in 23% the splenic angle, in 27% the descending colon and in 23% the sigmoid colon were involved in ischaemic colitis (see Fig. 9.1).

9.3 Right colonic ischaemia

The transverse colon and the ascending colon are less frequently involved than the left side, due to the rich collateral network at the right side of the colon.

In 1,024 patients mentioned in the literature, the ascending colon was involved in 8% and the transverse colon in 15% of the cases (Fig. 9.1).

Right sided ischaemic colitis can be found in case of distal colonic obstruction, in cases where there is an embolus in the main branch of the SMA, and in young adults.

* The articles used in this study are indicated in the references with a prefix O.

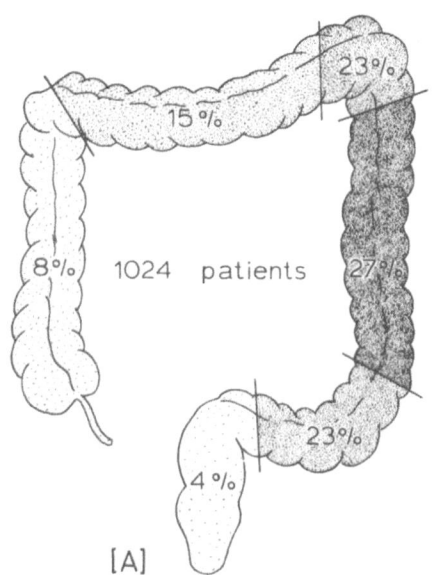

[A]

Fig. 9.1. Anatomical distribution of ischaemic colitis in 1024 patients as described in the literature (1950–1982).

9.4 Rectal ischaemia

While most authors initially considered rectal ischaemia rare or non-existent (Marston et al., 1966; Egger and Kellock, 1970; Thomas, 1972; Brown, 1972; O'Connell, 1976) some groups suggested that rectal involvement represented 4–16% of the cases (Roberts, 1965; Farman, 1966; Kilpatrick et al., 1968; Boley and Schwartz, 1971; Parks et al., 1972; Wittenberg et al., 1975; Heller et al., 1977; de Witte et al., 1977; Rasmussen and Thordsen, 1982).

Although Farman et al., (1968) found that rectal ischaemic disease was always accompanied by involvement of the sigmoid colon, isolated proctitis caused by ischaemia has been described by several authors (Shearburn et al., 1955; Carter et al., 1959; Littman et al., 1963; Kilpatrick et al., 1968; Montesori and Liepa, 1970; Dawson and Schaeffer, 1971; Orr and Jones., 1982; Rasmussen and Thordsen., 1982). In 4% of the 1,024 cases reviewed in the literature, rectal ischaemia was present. The lower incidence of rectal ischaemia compared to ischaemia in other parts of the colon can be explained by the particular vascularisation of the rectum. Branches of the superior rectal artery originating from the IMA, anastomose directly with the middle rectal and inferior rectal arterial branches, which originate from the hypogastric arteries (Fig. 2.4).

Because of the elaborate provision for collateral circulation when required there would need to be major obstruction of sacral artery branches before rectal ischaemia would develop.

9.5 Correlation aetiology – distribution

In many cases a correlation between aetiopathogenic factors and localisation can be found.

– Cardiogenic or hypovolaemic shock may be additional factors in patients with severe arteriosclerosis in precipitating colonic ischaemia around the splenic flexure because of their effect in lowering the forward pressure and thus further decreasing the already marginal flow to this point.
– In patients with aneurysmal aortic lesions ligation of the IMA, in the absence of a well de-

veloped collateral circulation, most frequently leads to ischaemia of the sigmoid (63%) (Papadopoulos et al., 1974).

- Demos et al., (1962) showed that the IMA was stenosed at its origin in 65% of postmortem cases. This high incidence can be correlated with the presence of severe atherosclerosis of the aorta at the distal end with secondary narrowing or occlusion of the ostium of the IMA. This might be a predisposing condition for ischaemic involvement of the sigmoid.
- The higher frequency of right sided colonic ischaemia in cases of distal colonic obstruction and embolus of the SMA has already been discussed in chapter 9.3.

9.6 Extent of ischaemic damage

The extent of colon damage produced by ischaemia depends upon:

- the cause of circulatory impairment;
- the localisation of vessel obstruction (main arteries or branches);
- the rapidity of onset of ischaemia;
- the duration of the ischaemic period;
- the capacity of the collateral mesenteric circulation and the general vascular condition of the patient;
- the metabolic requirements of the affected bowel;
- the quantity and virulence of intestinal bacterial flora;
- the degree and duration of distension due to intramural pressure proximal to an obstruction.

(Boley et al., 1969; Boley and Schwartz, 1971; Stillwell, 1973; Hagihara et al., 1977; Marston, 1977; van Dongen et al., 1982).

9.7 Focal, segmental, massive involvement

In cases of *vasculitis* or the presence of cholesterol-microemboli (multi) focal ischaemic lesions can be found throughout the colon.

Atheromatous lesions often lead to (short) segmental colonic ischaemia. In this slowly progressive atheromatous disease, a rich collateral network is frequently seen to have developed.

Since there is little opportunity for the development of an alternative blood supply when an *embolus* obstructs one or both of the main mesenteric arteries, the resulting colonic ischaemia is massive. When there is a generalised circulatory *'low flow state'*, segments of the left side of the colon are more usually affected by ischaemia; the right side being protected by blood flow via the Arc of Riolan. Should the inadequacy of blood flow to the mesenteric main system persist in the long paracolic artery of Drummond, massive ischaemia of the colon may develop.

10. LABORATORY INVESTIGATIONS

10.1 *Blood examination*
    10.1.1 Leucocyte (WBC) count
    10.1.2 Erythrocyte Sedimentation Rate
        (ESR)
10.1.3 Serum enzyme studies
10.1.4 Haemoglobin/Haematocrit/
       Urea/Potassium

10.2 *Stool examination*
    10.2.1 Stool cultures
    10.2.2 Guajac test

Laboratory investigations offer little help in making the diagnosis. Most findings are non specific.

10.1 Blood examination

10.1.1 Leucocyte (WBC) count
A high total lcucocyte count of up to 30×10^9/L with a high percentage of polymorphs is commonly found in acute colonic ischaemia.

Similar counts may occur in other inflammatory bowel diseases.

10.1.2 Erythrocyte Sedimentation Rate (ESR)
The ESR is usually high, up to 100 mm/hr.

10.1.3 Serumenzyme studies
Changes in transaminase, amylase and lactic dehydrogenase levels may occur. The results of the experimental work of Marcuson et al., (1969) suggested that elevations of the serum alkaline phosphatase level occur in the first few days after acute colonic ischaemia. In Marston's (1977) experience, however, it was usually normal.

10.1.4 Haemoglobin/Haematocrit/Urea/Potassium
There is usually progressive haemoconcentration with a rise in haematocrit and increase in blood viscosity, accompanied by metabolic acidosis with elevated blood urea and potassium.

10.2 Stool examination

10.2.1 Stool cultures
These do not usually contribute useful information to the diagnosis.

10.2.2 Guajac test
In the acute and also the chronic phase of colonic ischaemia this is usually positive.

11. RADIOLOGICAL ASPECTS OF ISCHAEMIC COLITIS

11.1 Plain film of the abdomen

Sometimes no changes are visible in the initial phase of ischaemic colitis on the plain film of the abdomen. Usually however, after 8 hours to 1 week (Marston et al., 1966; Marshak and Lindner, 1968; Marston, 1977), submucosal oedema and submucosal haemorrhage can change the configuration of the normally haustrated colon wall (Fig. 24-1). Gas within the lumen may accentuate the outline of submucosal oedema which is observed as 'nodular filling defects' (Marston et al., 1966), 'thumbprints' (Boley et al., 1963) or 'pseudotumors' (Schwartz et al., 1964). As oedema increases, the lumen narrows and the haustral pattern may disappear.

A splenic flexure, descending colon or sigmoid without haustral folds and with obvious irregular filling defects and marked contraction are suggestive of ischaemic colitis.

Segmental dilatation and gas in the colonic wall due to infection with gas-forming organisms during an acute stage of ischaemic colitis are indicative of the gangrenous form (Hannan et al., 1964; Marshak et al., 1965).

'Curvilinear streaks of gas in the bowel wall' (Tomchik et al., 1970), gas in the portal vein (Samuel and Sinclair, 1968), linear pneumatosis intestinalis (Gore et al., 1979), or fluid levels (Lister and Jungmann, 1956; Miller et al., 1970) are suggestive of transmural intestinal ischaemia. When perforation occurs, free air is present intraabdominally (Standard, 1952; Marrash et al., 1962; Marston et al., 1966; Marshak and Lindner, 1968; Marston, 1977).

11.2 Barium enema (single/double contrast)

11.2.1 Review of the literature
A review of the collected literature* on 1,024 patients between 1950 and 1982 reveals that of the 402 barium enemas performed and described in detail, 368 (92%) showed one or more positive signs for ischaemic colitis.

In 34 cases (8%) ischaemic colitis could not be diagnosed on the barium enema. It should be noted that in most case reports the time interval between the onset of symptoms and the time of performing the barium enema was not mentioned.

In 77 cases (19%) a repeat enema was perform-

---

* The articles used in this study are indicated in the references with a prefix ○.

ed. In 45 cases pathological lesions had disappeared between 1 week and 3 months after therapy. In 24 cases in which the barium enema was repeated 3 months or later after the first barium examination, strictures and/or sacculations were found.

In 8 cases described the ischaemic changes in the colonic segment involved did not change and the lesion persisted.

11.2.2 Indications/contra-indications

When there is radiological evidence of gas in the bowel wall or when peritonitis is clinically suspected, barium studies are contra-indicated.

In this situation, especially when a perforation is suspected, a water soluble contrast agent or air can be used (Tytgat, 1982).

Only in patients with the non gangrenous form of ischaemic colitis should a barium enema be performed.

11.2.3 Scheduling of a barium enema

The barium enema should be performed in the early stage of the disease, preferably within 5 days after onset of symptoms (Ross, 1972; Gore et al., 1979). When diagnostic doubt exists even after the barium enema, a repeat barium enema is recommended by Brown (1972) to demonstrate the evolutional changes which can distinguish ischaemic lesions from other ones. A follow-up barium enema can be performed after 1 to 3 months to exclude a stricturing lesion or tubular narrowing.

11.2.4 Problems

Irritability and intensive spastic contraction in some patients may render it difficult to fill the affected colonic segment. Because such patients cannot be cleansed normally, blood clots and retained stool may result in extensive artefacts. Frequently there is a good catharsis due to bloody diarrhoea.

11.2.5 Radiological signs

Barium enema usually shows up changes of the splenic flexure, descending colon and sigmoid (Schwartz et al., 1964; Marston et al., 1966; Marston, 1971) with sharp demarcation from the normal colon. Depending on the form of ischaemic colitis and time at which the barium enema was performed, the following signs may be observed:

Thumbprinting. 'Thumbprinting' is a polypoid change, giving a scalloped margin to the bowel wall with translucent oval or rounded filling defects extending into the lumen in the filled phase of the barium enema, and presenting as soft tissue masses in the air-barium double contrast studies' (Marston et al., 1966) (Fig. 24.2 and 24.3). These marginal indentations resemble digital impressions. Thumbprinting, a term introduced by Boley et al., (1963), is due to submucosal haemorrhage and submucosal oedema (Marshak and Lindner, 1968; Sherbon, 1970; Thomas, 1972; Wittenberg et al., 1975; Benacerraf et al., 1976; Gore et al., 1979; Schmutz et al., 1980). Different synonyms have been used for the term thumbprinting such as 'pseudopolyposis' (Thomas, 1972), 'scalloping' (Thomas, 1972), or 'pseudotumors' (Schwartz, 1964).

The thumbprints usually have a diameter of 10–30 mm at the base (Schmutz et al., 1980) and may be asymmetrically located on the anterior and posterior bowel wall. They may be temporary and disappear after 48–72 hours by resorption of submucosal blood and oedema, or they may persist for weeks (Gore et al., 1979). They are usually accompanied by spasm of the involved segment (Marston, 1977). Thumbprinting in an incompletely filled colon in single contrast studies becomes diagnostic only when it remains in an optimally filled colon (Schwartz et al., 1964).

The degree of thumbprinting in double contrast studies can vary with the amount of intralumenal pressure after air insufflation (Bartram, 1979) (Figs. 24.3 and 24.4).

Transverse ridging. Deep transversal contractions ('transverse ridging') are sometimes visible, running perpendicular to the colonic axis; the width of the ridges varies but seldom exceeds 1 cm (Fig. 24.14).

These contractions result from spasms of the colon musculature (Schwartz et al., 1963). They may occur alone or in combination with thumbprinting (Boley et al., 1963; Schwartz et al., 1963). Disappearance of the central portion of a 'transverse ridge' may result from the use of highly concentrated barium sulphate suspension. As 'ridging' is distributed symmetrically over the wall of the colon, this phenomenon is easily distinguished from thumbprinting, which usually has an asymmetrical distribution.

Loss of haustration. Due to submucosal haemorrhage and oedema in the acute stage of ischaemic colitis and fibrosis in a later stage, the normal haustrations can disappear in the involved segment of the colon (Sherbon, 1970).

Ulceration. The colon can show a 'spiculation' or 'ragged saw tooth irregularity of the (sub)mucosa' (Marston et al., 1966; Marshak and Lindner, 1968; Thomas, 1972), 1–3 weeks after the initial symptoms of ischaemic colitis as a result of diffuse superficial ulcerations (Figs. 24.11 and 24.12). The ulcerations may vary in number and form and may be distributed either symmetrically or asymmetrically over the colonic circumference: the ulcerated bowel frequently has a spiculated appearance. The ulcerations may be superficial or deep, with a diameter between 1–4 mm and characteristically are surrounded by submucosal oedema. In the acute phase the ulcerations are solitary: at later stages, they may be solitary, confluent or longitudinal (Schmutz et al., 1980) (chapter 12.5). These radiological findings are in accord with the endoscopical observations (chapter 12).

Intramural barium. Distribution of barium within the damaged mucosa of the ischaemic colon segment was first described in 1976 by Greves et al. Where the mucosa is damaged heavily, it becomes elevated, allowing the barium to infiltrate and thereby to dissect the submucosa; this presents as linear collections of intramural barium on the barium enema (Chino et al., 1974; Lazarovitch et al., 1980) (Figs. 24.7 and 24.8). There can be a prolonged persistence of intramural barium sulphate on the barium enema lasting up to 1 week after the barium enema (Greves et al., 1976).

Tubular narrowing and/or stricturing. Tubular narrowing and stricturing are the final stages of ischaemic colitis and are due to progressive fibrosis and (sub)mucosal reorganisation. It takes place 3 weeks to 12 months after the onset of colonic ischaemia (Marston et al., 1966; Marshak and Lindner, 1968; Williams, 1971; Gore et al., 1979) (Figs. 24.15,

16, 17). The submucosa of the ischaemic segment of the colon, usually 8–10 cm in length, is replaced by inflammatory cells and contracting fibrous tissue (Boley et al., 1963; Marston et al., 1966); narrowing of the bowel lumen ensues. The contour of the bowel can be smooth ('tubular narrowing') or irregular ('stricturing'). Finally a narrowing with proximal dilatation is seen. The merging of the narrowed section of the colon into the normal adjacent colon can be sharply demarcated (Fig. 24.6) or tapering and gradual ('funneling', Thomas, 1968) (Fig. 24.5). The stricture is usually shorter than the initially involved segment suggesting that there is more widespread ischaemic damage in the acute stage.

Sacculation. 'Sacculation' consists of shallow, wide mouthed, outpouchings or pseudodiverticula of the colonic wall' on the antimesenteric side (Marston et al., 1966; Marshak and Lindner, 1968; Greves et al., 1976) (Fig. 24.9). It develops when one margin of the colon is affected by structural damage more than the other, so that the antimesenteric margin becomes pleated. It occurs in a later stage of ischaemia, mostly after 1–3 months, and is commonly associated with tubular narrowing or stricturing (Fig. 24.15). In the investigation of Marston et al., (1966) thumbprinting and sacculation were the most consistently observed pathological features associated with ischaemic colitis and were therefore considered to be characteristic for ischaemic colitis.

In table 11.1 the frequency of radiological signs associated with ischaemic colitis as described by several authors is listed.

'Thumbprinting' has been most frequently found (67%), followed by 'spasm' in 56% of the cases. Ulceration has been found in 42%, tubular narrowing and/or stricture formation in 20% and loss of haustration in 19% of the cases.

Sacculation, one of the most constant radiographic signs in the series of Marston et al., (1966), – but frequently not mentioned in other series described in the literature – showed an overall frequency of 11%. Transverse ridging was found in 32% in the series of Wittenberg et al., (1975).

Table 11.1. The frequency of occurrence of the different radiological signs associated with ischaemic colitis as described by several authors and as found in our series.

Author(s)	Year	Number of patients	Number of patients with barium enema	Thumb-printing	Ulcer-ation	Tubular narrowing and/or strictu-ring	Saccu-lation	Loss of haus-tration	Trans-verse ridging	Spasm
Sherbon	1970	7	6	3	4	4	2	3	1	5
Brown	1972	17	17	17	–	5	3	–	–	17
Wittenberg et al.	1975	41	39	31	18	–	–	7	13	34
Benacerraf et al.	1976	8	8	4	3	4	1	2	–	–
O'Connell et al.	1976	26	16	5	11	2	–	–	–	6
Barcewicz and Welch	1980	10	8	7	1	–	–	–	–	1
Eisenberg et al.	1979	8	5	3	4	1	–	–	–	–
Bartram	1979	3	3	–	–	–	–	–	–	3
Cormier and Desouttier	1980	23	23	12	7	3	5	–	–	–
Schmutz et al.	1980	22	22	16	14	10	5	16	–	16
Total number in the literature		165	147 (89%)	98 (67%)	62 (42%)	29 (20%)	16 (11%)	28 (19%)	14 (10%)	82 (56%)
Total number in our own series		199	58 (29%)	33 (57%)	28 (48%)	10 (17%)	14 (24%)	30 (52%)	11 (19%)	13 (22%)

11.3 Angiography

11.3.1 Review of the literature

Review of the literature (indicated by the prefix ○ in the reference list) on patients with ischaemic colitis on whom an angiography had been performed, reveals that of the 1,024 cases covered, in only 96 cases were there indications of occlusion; stenosis of the main mesenteric vessels (with or without collaterals) occurred in 43 cases (45%) and in 53 cases (55%) the mesenteric vessels were patent.

11.3.2 Advantages

– Biplane abdominal angiography permits assessment of the orifices of the coeliac trunk, SMA and IMA and the visualization of the internal iliac arteries.
– Selective studies of the IMA and SMA may give more details of
 1 the peripheral vascularization, especially at Griffiths' point;
 2 the flow pattern in the marginal artery of Drummond; or

 3 the presence of a hypertrophic 'Arc de Riolan' (Meyers, 1976; Courbier et al., 1976).
– Preoperative aortography in patients with abdominal aneurysm, can give information about the condition of the main mesenteric vessels. If the IMA is the main or only vessel supplying the bowel and if there is stenosis or occlusion of the coeliac trunk or SMA, preoperative information allows the surgeon to anticipate the need for reimplantation of the IMA or revascularization of the SMA or coeliac artery.

11.3.3 Radiological findings

Atheromatous lesions, stenosis or occlusion at the orificium of one or both main mesenteric vessels may be found. Occlusion of the IMA can cause a low flow state in the sigmoid artery and left colic arterial system and lead to ischaemia of the left side of the colon. Stenosis or occlusion of branches of the SMA can lead to ischaemia of the right side of the colon. Occlusion of the coeliac trunk or compression of the main vessel by the medial arcuate ligament can reduce blood flow to a colonic segment (van Dongen et al., 1982), for instance by the blood flow in the SMA being appropriated by the pancreatic duodenal artery, resulting in hypoperfusion in the SMA. Stagnation of contrast agent in the small vessels of the colon wall and non opacification of the intramural vessels in the capillary phase in an early stage of the disease, are reported to be highly suggestive of gangrenous ischaemic colitis (Herlinger, 1972; van Dongen et al., 1982).

11.3.4 Disadvantages

Most authors (Engelhardt and Jacobson, 1956; Marston et al., 1962; Schwartz et al., 1963; De Dombal et al., 1969; Williams et al., 1969; Reuter et al., 1970; Sherbon, 1970; Boysen, 1971; Egger et al., 1971; Westcott, 1972; Lambana et al., 1973; Voegeli, 1974; Wittenberg et al., 1975; Williams et al., 1975), report that angiography is disappointing from a diagnostic point of view.

– It is often difficult to correlate clinical symptoms with the vessel occlusion shown by arteriography. The angiographic finding of a stenosis or occlusion of one of the colic arteries is not conclusive for the aetiology or presence of ischaemic colitis. A rich collateral network can prevent ischaemia of a colonic segment despite occlusion of one or more main colic vessels.

– Flow obstruction which can cause ischaemic colitis can occur in peripheral vessels too small to be identified by angiography, thus, a negative arteriography does not exclude ischaemic colitis.

– The diagnostic value of angiography is also dubious because of the dangers inherent in angiography for seriously sick patients (Marston et al., 1966; Williams and Wittenberg, 1975; Marston, 1977).

– Arteriography in the early stage of ischaemia usually does not show arterial or venous occlusion, but rather a paradoxical hypervascularity of the bowel wall (Fig. 24.19) (Williams et al., 1967, 1969; Reuter et al., 1970; Boysen, 1971; van Dongen et al., 1982). These findings may be explained by the rapid and intense inflammatory response in colon ischaemia. They are, however, *non specific* and can also be seen in other inflammatory disorders of the colon (Williams et al., 1969; Reuter et al., 1970).

– Bookstein et al., (1978) reported that angiography can show reduced blood flow to the colon, when colonic ischaemia is developing, but is not a sensitive method in the diagnosis of non occlusive ischaemia when the ischaemia is already established.

12. ENDOSCOPY IN DIAGNOSIS OF ISCHAEMIC COLITIS

12.1 Introduction

Barium enema examination and clinical presentation are the twin pillars of diagnosis in the detection of colonic ischaemia. Colonoscopy is the third diagnostic tool in the evaluation of patients with this condition. Owing to the risk of perforation of necrotic bowel, the use of colonoscopy in the diagnosis of ischaemic colitis is relatively uncommon. Carter et al., (1959) and Littman et al., (1963) were the first to describe the sigmoidoscopic observations of reversible vascular occlusion of the colon.

Colin et al., (1974) described the endoscopical appearance in 2 cases of transient ischaemic colitis. Since then several reports have been made of colonoscopy in ischaemic bowel disease (Favier et al., 1976; Favriel et al., 1977; Farinon et al., 1977, 1978; Hunt, 1978/79; Hunt and Buchanan, 1979; Archibald et al., 1980; Waye and Hunt, 1982; Tytgat and Reeders, 1982; Kühner et al., 1983). Ernst et al., (1976) in a retrospective study of 50 patients who had undergone abdominal aortic reconstruction operations (23 patients with occlusive disease and 27 patients with aortic aneurysmal disease) concluded that colonoscopy is valuable for early recognition of ischaemic damage at a stage when clinical manifestations of ischaemic damage are not evident.

12.2 Clinical value of endoscopical examination

The value of endoscopy in the evaluation of patients with suspected ischaemic colitis is:

1 to establish the diagnosis of colonic ischaemia in cases of rectal bleeding (Shinya et al., 1982);
2 to differentiate ischaemic colitis from other forms of inflammatory bowel disease such as ulcerative colitis and Crohn's colitis;
3 to exclude the presence of carcinoma and other obstructing lesions which can occur in patients with colonic ischaemia;
4 to obtain material for histological study;
5 to define the extent of mucosal ischaemia in a bowel which has a normal external appearance at surgery;
6 to diagnose and confirm the stages of evolution in chronic'non resolving'ischaemic colitis.

12.3 Contra-indications and risks

When the clinical presentation and the radiological examination are characteristic for ischaemic colitis, colonoscopy is rarely indicated. The procedure is contraindicated because of the danger of perforation, when there is clinical evidence of peritoneal inflammation, arising from transmural gangrenous colonic ischaemia.

12.4 Endoscopical classification

Favier et al., (1976) classified the ischaemic colonic

lesions seen at endoscopy into 3 stages according to their *severity* (chapter 5.4.1).

Scowcroft et al., (1981) proposed an endoscopical classification of ischaemic colitis according to *duration* (chapter 5.4.2).

Because different stages of ischaemic colitis may coexist simultaneously in immediately adjacent areas of a single segment of the colon, it is difficult to find any practical application for such classifications.

12.5 Endoscopical appearances

Observations made using a fibre-optic colonoscope in the first 24 hours of ischaemic colitis, include patchy areas of markedly oedematous hyperaemic, reddened mucosa and areas of pallor. The hyperaemic areas are friable, while the areas of pallor show minimal bleeding.

Superficial 1–4 mm ulcerations and small irregular pinpoint petechiae with a diameter of a few mm or larger may be observed; sometimes confluent bluish submucosal haemorrhages can develop.

Ulcerations are responsible for the spiculated appearance of the bowel wall on the barium enema.

When oedema and haemorrhage are prominent, large dark coloured bulbous protrusions may be seen, equivalent to the 'thumbprinting' seen on the barium enema.

Schmutz et al., (1980) concluded in their endoscopical series of 22 patients that 'thumbprinting' appeared in the first 2 weeks in 11 of the 16 cases. It persisted until the 4th week in 3 cases. In 1 case thumbprints persisted into the 6th week. In the initial stages of illness, the nodular protrusions may gradually disappear as a result of regression of oedematous swelling and spastic contraction. Depending on the state of vascular insult the ulceration may heal within 3–7 days.

Large echymoses with small central ulcerations may develop. The ulceration may elongate into well defined longitudinal or irregular shaggy serpiginous ulcerations covered with a greyish-white necrotic membrane surrounded by oedematous haemorrhagic mucosa. These ulcers are of varying surface area (1–2 cm width and 1–4 cm length) and depth and are quite irregularly distributed around the circumference of the bowel. These ulcerations can give the bowel wall a 'sawtooth irregularity' appearance on the barium enema.

Initially the ulcerations are surrounded by oedematous and haemorrhagic mucosa. In the en-

Table 12.1. Endoscopical findings in the different stages of ischaemic colitis (modified after Scowcroft et al., 1981).

	Endoscopical findings
Acute stage	– Patchy areas of oedema ('bulbous protrusions') – Hyperaemic friable mucosa – Bluish submucosal haemorrhage – Erythema – Non confluent pinpoint petechiae, separated by oedematous mucosa – Superficial fine ulcerations (2–4 mm)
	⇩
Subacute stage	– Oedema – Haemorrhage – Longitudinal and shaggy serpiginous ulcerations (1–2 cm wide, 3–4 cm long) – Sharp demarcation of abnormal mucosa – Necrotic slough
	⇩
Chronic stage	– Normal mucosa – Patchy areas of residual fine granularity – Stricture formation – Sacculation formation – Linear scars and fine intersecting lines – Residual scar formation

doscopical series of Schmutz et al., (1980) ulcerations were shown in 8 of the 10 cases in the first month. They persisted in 4 cases until the second month. In the mucosal form of ischaemic colitis the ulcers gradually show a tendency to reepithelialisation and finally to complete healing. The reepithelialisation starts from non-infarcted areas. Epithelial regeneration is an early and essential index of ultimate recovery. Complete mucosal healing may take place between 2 weeks–3 months, with an average of 4 weeks; if healing does not proceed, a chronic 'non resolving' stage of (mural) ischaemic colitis can develop.

When ulceration extends into the submucosa with destruction of the muscularis mucosae, then the areas between the ulcerations show cribriform pseudopolypoid elevations. After the ulcerative process has subsided, residual fine granularity or strictures can remain.

Stricturing or tubular narrowing may develop 3 weeks to 12 months after the first episode of ischaemia. Sacculation and pseudodiverticular formation mostly occur on the antimesenteric site from the third month onwards and are more easily visualized by barium enema than with endoscopy.

12.6 Identification of strictures by colonoscopy

A major problem that may not be solved by barium enema examination is the precise identification of strictures in patients with stricturing ischaemic colitis (Waye and Hunt, 1982).

Stricture formation – as a result of fibrosis, muscular hypertrophy and spasm – can be due to ulcerative colitis, granulomatous colitis, carcinoma or diverticulitis as well as ischaemic colitis.

The colonoscope can be passed up to and often through the stricture to determine its precise nature. Many strictures demonstrated on barium enema may be successfully negotiated with a small calibre endoscope.

A carcinomatous stricture (Fig. 24.21) should be suspected if, at endoscopy, the stricture is rigid, has an abrupt 'shelf like' edge or cannot be passed with the colonoscope (Waye and Hunt, 1982). The colonic wall in patients with stricturing ischaemic colitis may be thin with friable mucosa, which does not permit the longitudinal stretching which is tolerated by normal bowel. The endoscopist should therefore exert only minimal pressure when attempting to pass the scope through strictures in patients with ischaemic colitis, lest the bowel wall be traumatized and perforation result (Waye and Hunt, 1982).

13. HISTOPATHOLOGY OF ISCHAEMIC COLITIS

13.1 Introduction

When the colon is deprived of blood, histological changes follow which vary in accordance with the rapidity of onset and severity and duration of the ischaemic process.

The severity of ischaemia is dependent upon the cause, the level of arterial occlusion, the state of the collateral circulation and the virulence of the bacterial flora. The location and extent of ischaemic lesions of the colon is a reflection of the anatomy of the blood supply in the occlusive form, the decrease of circulating volume, and the state of the microvasculature (small vessel disease and spasm) in the non-occlusive form of ischaemic colitis, and of the level of intralumenal pressure elevation in obstructive ischaemic colitis.

The varying severity of ischaemia produces changes which range from microscopical lesions in the mucosa, to full thickness infarction or gangrene of the entire colonic wall. The lesions may vary according to depth and length of ischaemia. Distribution of the lesions (focal, segmental or massive) is dependent upon the cause of the ischaemic process (chapter 4). Focal ischaemic lesions are an early expression of colonic ischaemia, but are rare as established lesions and occur mostly as a sequence of occlusion of small vessels within the colonic wall or mesocolon, e.g. secondary to vasculitis, induced by the immune complex mechanism described by Whitehead in 1971, cholesterol emboli or thrombosis.

More frequently found are segmental ischaemic lesions of the colon which may be induced by occlusion of arterial branches of a larger calibre. They may occur as the result of embolism, thrombosis in combination with atherosclerosis, trauma or large vessel arteritis, they may also occur secondary to colonic obstruction and without demonstrable vascular occlusion in association with hypotensive periods or distal colonic obstruction. Massive ischaemic lesions are usually caused by occlusion of the SMA and/or IMA at or near their origin, but such lesions may also be of the non-occlusive type. Lesions having varying depth may occur within one colonic segment.

13.2 Histopathological classification after Morson and Whitehead

Morson (1971) divided the response to ischaemia of the colon into 3 phases:

- an acute phase which may comprise a transient ischaemia followed by total resolution or lesions extending across the full thickness of the colon wall causing massive necrosis;
- a reparative (subacute or chronic) phase, characterized by granulation tissue formation and reepithelialisation;
- residual pathology with persistent ulceration, fibrosis, ischaemic stricture and chronic complications.

13.2.1 Acute ischaemic phase
Macroscopical appearance. The macroscopical appearance of the ischaemic colonic wall varies with the depth of the ischaemic lesions. Severe ischaemic involvement secondary to e.g. main mesenteric artery occlusion will lead to a grey dilated colon with a friable wall which is usually thinner than normal. If the ischaemia persists, the wall becomes black, due to transmural necrosis and blood extravasation. Transmural necrosis, caused by a low flow state or venous thrombosis is visualized as a congested bowel wall which is purple and is thickened by blood extravasation, oedema and fibrin deposition. In an advanced stage the bowel wall will appear completely black. Early mucosal lesions are regularly found at autopsy as a consequence of preterminal circulatory collapse; they may manifest themselves as patchy red or purple slightly swollen or granular areas in the mucosal lining.

More serious early lesions of the non-transmural type comprise congestion and haemorrhage often with focal massive oedema of the submucosa which can give rise to haemorrhagic blebs; these correspond with the 'thumbprinting', seen on radiographs, in which the mucosa interspersed between the lesion retains a normal appearance. In a more advanced stage, larger areas are involved and the mucosa has the appearance of purplish cobblestones.

The depth of the necrosis will determine whether the serosa becomes involved. However, it should be noted that the extent of the ischaemic process may not be apparent from the deceptively normal looking serosa.

Microscopical appearance. In the early phase, the superficial capillaries dilate widely. The surface epithelium and parts of crypts become necrotic. There is haemorrhage and oedema in the lamina propria. The deeper intact capillaries adopt a ballooning appearance, due to sludging of red cells and subsequent stasis (Whitehead, 1972).

As a reaction to necrosis and due to the invasion of bacteria from the faecal bowel contents, a polymorphonuclear demarcation zone develops in the borderland between the necrotic inner zone and the hyperaemic viable bowel wall.

The necrotic mucosa assumes a 'ghostlike' appearance due to lysis of cells and loss of nuclei, while outlines of pre-existent structures such as crypts and vessels may still be faintly visible.

Fibrin thrombi may be present within mucosal capillaries and submucosal veins.

The ischaemic lesion may be limited to the mucosa, but with increasing severity and duration of ischaemia, progression to deeper layers and extension to adjacent bowel segments occurs.

In this case an ischaemic or haemorrhagic necrosis may occur, penetrating into the muscularis propria or into the serosa, initially without and later with a demarcating granulocytic infiltration. Bacterial invasion of the bowel wall – organisms of the mixed faecal type, but, in some cases, predominantly by e.coli, faecal streptococci, staphylococci or clostridia – may result in an extensive phlegmonous inflammatory reaction in the surviving bowel wall (McKinnell and Kearney, 1967; Bounous et al., 1969). Gas may be produced by the bacterial flora intramurally.

13.2.2 Reparative phase
Macroscopical appearance. The macroscopical appearance in this stage varies with the severity and depth of the ischaemia and with the stage of healing (Whitehead, 1972). Irregularly shaped areas of greenish grey mucosal necrosis develop when the ischaemia persists. Sloughing of the necrotic layers is followed by a stage of ulceration; longitudinal and serpiginous ulcers with a yellow or greyish base may involve large areas. Acute mucosal lesions not

involving the muscularis mucosae will heal without leaving scars.

Microscopical appearance. Healing occurs after the necrotic tissue of the colonic (sub)mucosa has sloughed away and the remnants are being removed by phagocytosis (Whitehead, 1971). Reepithelialisation takes place from the still viable parts of remaining crypts and from the surface epithelium at the margin of the ulcerated area. The lamina propria is reconstituted by a proliferation of capillaries and fibroblasts.

If the muscularis mucosae of the bowel wall, which has no power to regenerate, is preserved, acute colonic ischaemia is a self-limiting condition.

A sloughed superficial layer of mucosa may thus be reconstituted within a week. In more seriously damaged areas, complete healing does not occur and a mucosa in which glandular deformities or pseudopolyps are present may result. In deeper ulcerations the ulcer base consists of inflammatory granulation tissue, which is rich in capillaries and contains plasmacells, lymphocytes and histiocytes in large numbers. These infiltrates gradually de-

crease in density; macrophages containing haemosiderin from lysed erythrocytes may remain visible for quite some time and fibroblasts proliferate. Reepithelialisation starts from the ulcer margins, eventually producing a flat layer of undifferentiated epithelial cells, which seals off the granulating area from the lumenal contents.

If the muscularis propria is involved in the ischaemic process, muscle damage may be observed microscopically in the inner circular layer, varying from vacuolisation of cells and pycnosis of nuclei (Morson, 1971) to complete destruction of fibres.

This may be followed by patchy replacement of circular muscle fibres by granulation tissue ('splaying') and later by fibrosis.

13.2.3 Residual pathology with persistent ulceration, ischaemic stricture and chronic complications

Permanent morphological changes will result when the ischaemic damage involves a bowel segment short enough to be compatible with survival and when the lesion does not extend through the entire bowel wall, but penetrates deeper than the muscularis mucosae.

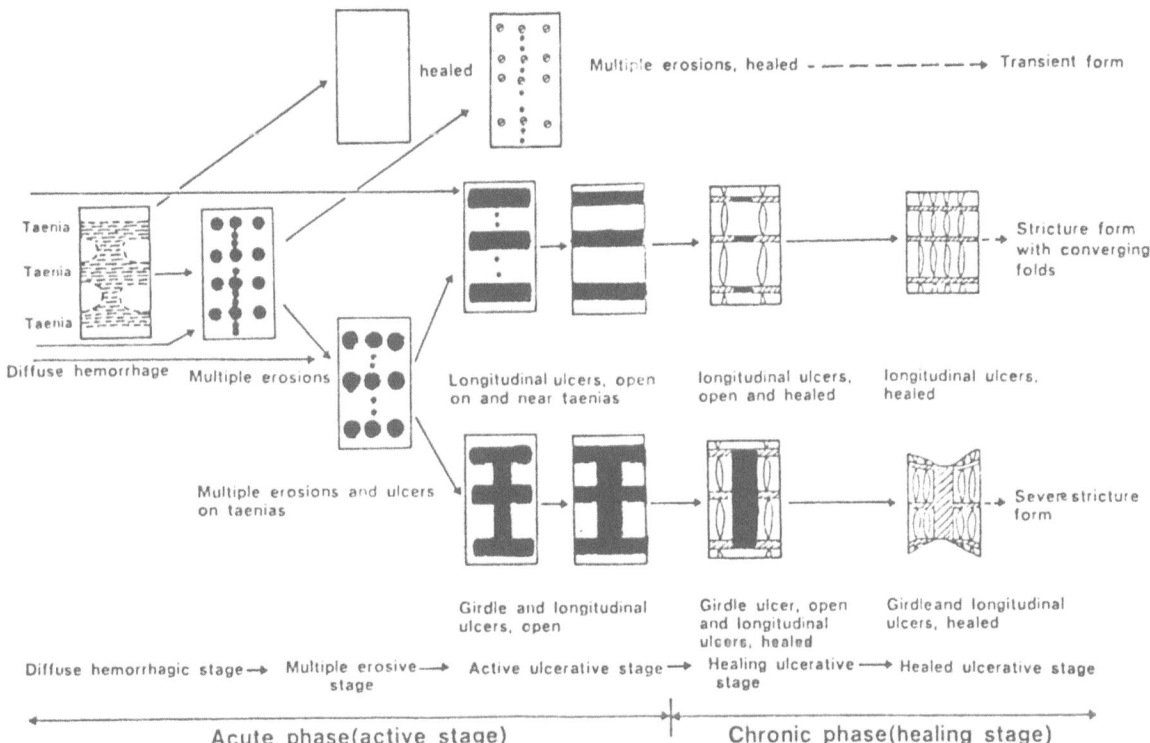

Fig. 13.1. Macroscopical changes of ischaemic colitis by lapse of time (Watanabe and Horimukai, 1982).

Such lesions encompass persistent ulcerations, sacculations, fibrosis and strictures.

The bowel wall ultimately becomes thickened with a narrowed lumen and, if, the ischaemic process is severe, a short or long smoothly contoured tubular or fusiform stricture of the colon with a granular ulcerating surface, tapering off gradually at both ends may develop. Sometimes a sacculation can be seen due to irregular fibrosis involving only part of the circumference of the bowel wall.

Watanabe and Horimukai (1982) have summarized the macroscopical changes of ischaemic colitis by lapse of time as shown in Fig. 13.1.

13.3 Ischaemic colitis secondary to distal colonic obstruction

13.3.1 Macroscopical appearance
Two different and separate forms may occur: the subacute, subchronic ulcerating form and the acute necrotic transmural form.

Subacute, subchronic ulcerating form. In these cases the colitis occurs proximal to the obstruction and is usually separated from it by a short segment of relatively normal mucosa. Eleven of 36 patients whose cases are reported in the literature (31%) with ischaemic colitis proximal to colon carcinoma had a normal segment of mucosa between the carcinoma and the beginning of the ischaemic involvement. Linear longitudinal ulcers can be seen covered with fibrino-purulent material. There is often congested intervening mucosa which is lifted up by oedema and haemorrhage (Morson, 1971).

Acute necrotic transmural form. Sometimes purple to yellow-greenish focal necrosis may occur in a severely dilated segment with a smooth mucosal lining and diminished folds.

13.3.2 Microscopical appearance
The two macroscopically identified stages of ischaemic colitis as described above have a correlated microscopically distinct histology.

Subacute, subchronic ulcerating form. The appearance is similar to the pattern described in 13.2.2.

Acute necrotic transmural form. The precise histological picture depends upon the severity of the ischaemic process. Acute focal transmural necrotizing ischaemia – particularly in the coecum and ascending colon – sometimes following a phlegmonous inflammation, may occur.

13.4 Peripheral mesenteric arterial disease

Disease of small peripheral mesenteric arteries may play an important role in exacerbating the deleterious effects of large vessel disease and of poor circulation. Most cases cited in the literature do not mention the presence of stenosing lesions in small mesenteric vessels. This suggests that small mesenteric vessels are rarely histologically examined at autopsy, or in resection material, even in patients with known ischaemic vascular disease.

Only a few studies have identified obstructive lesions of the distal mesenteric arteries as being important in the pathogenesis of colonic ischaemia. The occurrence of such stenosing or obstructive lesions has been frequently associated with diabetes and hypertension (Détry et al., 1979; McGregor et al., 1980). Intimal proliferation, medial hypertrophy and periarterial fibrosis have been described as potentiating ischaemic colonic damage (Aboumrad et al., 1963; Arosemena and Edwards, 1967; Williams et al., 1969; Pierce and Brokenbrough, 1970; Hansen et al., 1976; Raghunata et al., 1983). Intimal changes may lead to increased resistance to blood flow and to a proportionate decrease in the local blood supply and eventually to ischaemia. Diabetes, hypertension and age have been directly related to the degree of this type of small vessel involvement (Aboumrad et al., 1963; Pierce and Brokenbrough, 1970).

Other vascular processes which lead to narrowing of the lumen of the vessel may also play an important role. In addition to atherosclerosis, arteritis (lupus erythematosus, rheumatoid arthritis, polyarteritis nodosa), and vasculopathy secondary to collagenic disorders (scleroderma), amyloidosis, radiation etc. belong to the group of small vessel diseases.

13.5 Biopsies

13.5.1 Value

The usefulness of biopsies in the diagnosis of ischaemic colitis is limited, because of the superficial nature of the specimens and lack of specificity of the microscopical findings in the chronic ulcerating phase (Whitehead, 1973; Hunt and Buchanan, 1979).

13.5.2 Microscopical appearance

In biopsy tissues the appearance of the early necrotic lesion in ischaemic colitis may be characteristic.

Mild lesions will show an oedema, haemorrhage and necrosis of the superficial- and crypt epithelium.

More severe lesions will show ischaemic necrosis of the full thickness of the mucosa with extension into the deeper layers.

The histology of both types of lesions has been described earlier (13.2.1–13.2.3). In the chronic phase the ischaemic necrotic changes are not characteristic and are difficult to differentiate from other chronic ulcerating inflammatory bowel diseases.

14. OTHER DIAGNOSTIC PROCEDURES

14.1 *Ultrasound*

14.2 *Doppler ultrasound flow measurements*

14.3 *Computed tomography*

14.4 *Radionuclide imaging*

14.1 Ultrasound

Abdominal ultrasound has recently been employed in the diagnosis of colonic ischaemia. The oedematous colonic wall is thickened and shows low level echoes. The lumen is narrowed. The results of this method are however non specific and allow no differentiation of changes caused by ischaemic colitis from these caused by inflammatory bowel diseases or carcinoma (te Strake, 1983; Ike, 1983).

14.2 Doppler ultrasound flow measurements

It is difficult or impossible to discern the border between the involved and uninvolved colon in ischaemic colitis. However, techniques, whereby the blood in the colonic vessels may be measured intraoperatively are currently being reported in the literature, and may become important in helping to resolve this problem. Hobson et al., (1976) used Doppler ultrasound flow measurement to evaluate collateral mesenteric blood flow of the colon before and after temporary occlusion or division of the IMA during aortic surgery in man. Cooperman et al., (1979[1]) used Doppler ultrasound intra-oper-

atively in 117 patients undergoing small or large intestinal anastomosis, colostomy or enterostomy to determine the adequacy of blood supply at the margins of resection.

In 92% of the cases Doppler signals and clinical observation agreed (Cooperman et al., 1979[2]).

14.3 Computed tomography

Computed tomography (CT) performed on two patients with abdominal pain showed an irregular, segmental thickening of the submucosa of the colon that proved to be due to ischaemic colitis (Jones et al., 1982). In one case CT showed narrowing of the lumen of the right colon by a polypoid mass which was clearly the CT analog of thumbprinting. Jones et al., (1982) concluded that CT can be useful in the diagnosis and management of ischaemic colitis.

14.4 Radionuclide imaging

Experimental work, demonstrating the prominent acute inflammatory infiltrate in intestinal ischaemia prompted the study of a non-invasive method using radionuclides (^{99m}Tc pyrophosphate or ^{111}Indium labelled autologous leucocytes).

This work demonstrated the rapid (within 30 minutes) localisation of ischaemic bowel via the increase (sixfold) in radioactivity in ischaemic tissue compared to the normal intestine.

The technique has been only used experimentally in animals so far (Bardfeld et al., 1977; Barth et al., 1978, 1979; Dutcher et al., 1981).

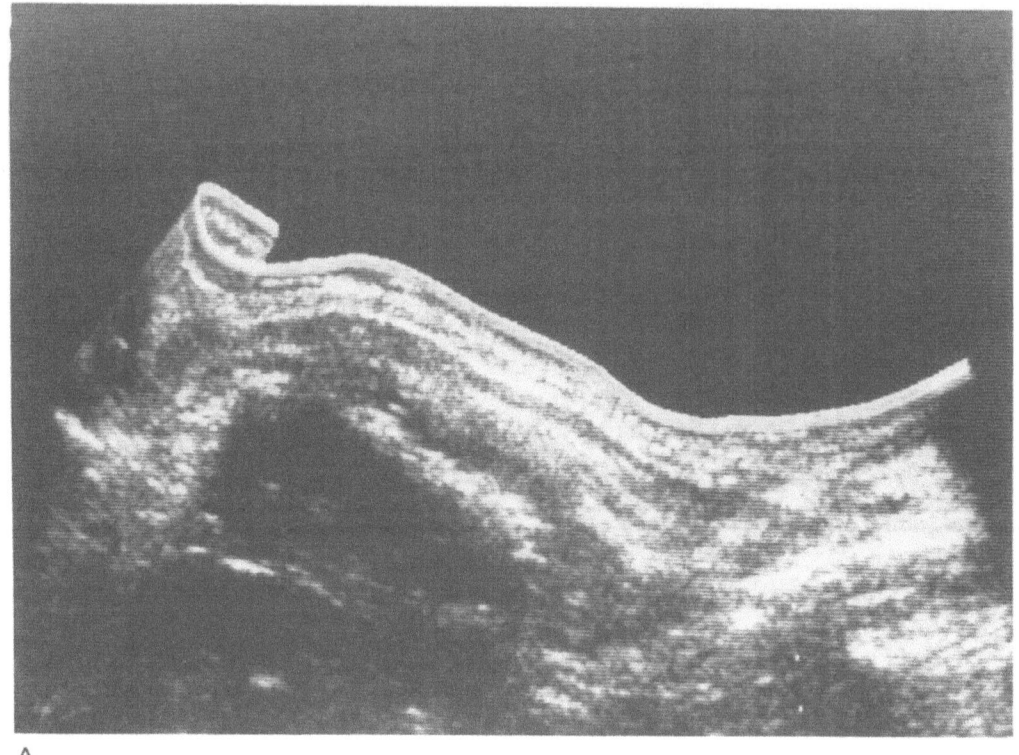

A

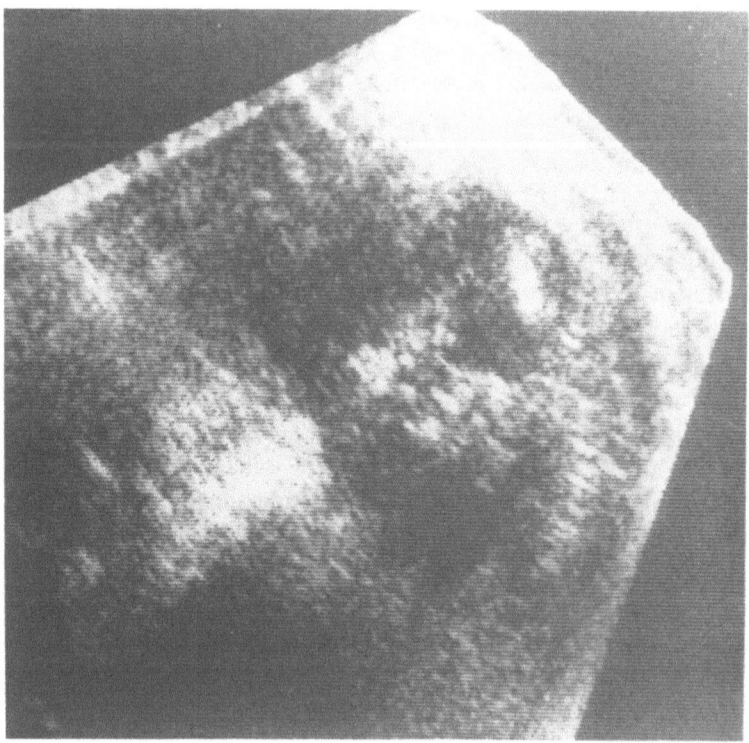

B

Fig. 14.1A and B. Ultrasound examination of the left upper abdomen: A: Longitudinal section shows a by oedema thickened, irregular, hypoechoic bowel wall. Note the central echogenic mucosa. B: Transverse section shows a by oedema thickened bowel wall (2 cm), with central echogenic colonic mucosa in the same patient.

15. DIFFERENTIAL DIAGNOSIS OF ISCHAEMIC COLITIS, ULCERATIVE COLITIS AND CROHN'S DISEASE OF THE COLON

15.1 Introduction

The diseases from which ischaemic colitis must be distinguished are diverticular disease, bacillary dysentery, amebiasis, campylobacter colitis, pseudomembranous colitis, tuberculous colitis, carcinoma, irradiation colitis and, especially, ulcerative colitis and Crohn's disease of the colon (Price, 1977).

The principle differential diagnostic criteria of ischaemic colitis versus ulcerative colitis and Crohn's disease are outlined in tables 15.1–15.5.

The major overlapping symptoms in ischaemic colitis, ulcerative colitis and Crohn's disease are diarrhoea with or without blood, abdominal pain, fever and weight loss.

Patients with Crohn's disease frequently have anal fissures and abscesses, indolent multiple ulcers of the perineum and a marked tendency to develop fistulas of the intestine. These signs are not found in ischaemic colitis (DeVroede, 1974).

Radiological and endoscopical examination can differentiate ischaemic colitis from other inflammatory bowel diseases, especially when the ischaemia is in the ulcerative phase. The laboratory findings are quite non specific. Leucocytosis with a shift to the left and elevation of the sedimentation rate are common in all three diseases.

15.2 Diagnostic features

The physician has two main diagnostic features by which he can distinguish ischaemic colitis from ulcerative colitis or Crohn's disease of the colon. These are the distribution and the character of the lesions.

15.2.1 Distribution of the lesions
In ischaemic colitis the lesions are most frequently found on the left side. Involvement of the rectum is uncommon (4%).

In *Crohn's disease of the colon* 'skip' lesions are predominantly right sided, with involvement of the small intestine and terminal ileum. The rectum is involved in almost 50% of cases.

In *ulcerative colitis* the lesions are predominantly left sided as in ischaemic colitis, but the rectum is more frequently involved (almost 100%).

In Crohn's disease diagnosis is more frequently made by barium enema examination, by which the disease can be detected in all parts of the colon by colonic narrowing, sinus tracts and mucosal abnormalities.

Segmental colitis of the left colon can be seen in all three diseases and therefore is not diagnostic. Segmental colitis of the transverse or right colon and 'skip' lesions of the colon or small intestine, however, are virtually diagnostic of Crohn's disease.

Antimesenteric sacculation, which can develop in a late stage of ischaemic colitis, is also a feature of mesenteric diverticular disease. However, diverticular disease with atypical localisation, might be suggestive of a post ischaemic colonic stenosis with secondary sacculation formation (van Dongen et al., 1982).

15.2.2 Character of the lesions

The asymmetrical ulceration around the circumference of the colonic wall characteristic of Crohn's disease is usually not found in ischaemic colitis.

Shallow and deep ulcers are more often seen in ulcerative colitis and Crohn's colitis than in ischaemic colitis.

Diffuse superficial ulcerations can be seen in both ischaemic colitis and ulcerative colitis.

Thrumbprinting, which is typical of ischaemic colitis, may also be seen in other conditions such as ulcerative colitis (Marshak and Lindner, 1973), Crohn's disease (DeVroede, 1974), amebiasis (Tchang, 1968; Hardy and Scullin, 1971) and schistosomiasis (Boley et al., 1963). A cobblestone appearance of the mucosa may be seen in the acute phase of ischaemic colitis and commonly in Crohn's disease.

Fissures, which appear predominantly in Crohn's disease, are uncommon in ulcerative col-

Table 15.1. Contrasts in the clinical features between ischaemic colitis, ulcerative colitis and Crohn's disease of the colon.

Clinical features	Ischaemic colitis	Ulcerative colitis	Crohn's disease of the colon
Age	80% > 50 yrs	20–30 yrs	20–50 yrs
Onset	Acute	Gradual, occasionnally rapid	Gradual
Diarrhoea	Bloody (mucosal slough)	Bloody ± mucus	Bloodless
Rectal bleeding	Rare	Common (95%)	Uncommon (50%)
Abdominal pain	Colicky	Uncommon, slight	Colicky (50%)
Anal lesion	No	Acute fissures (25%) abscess: (10%)	Chronic fissures (75%) anal fistula, chronic abscess
Colonic segments involved	Segmental, predominantly left sided (splenic flexure descending colon, sigmoid) sharp demarcation vital-non vital colon	Diffuse most frequently distal left colon (descending colon, sigmoid)	Segmental more right- than left-sided. (ascending colon, coecum, terminal ileum)
Rectum involved	4%	100%	50%
Prior cardiovascular disease	Common	No association	No association
Progress	Chronic 'non resolving' form	Exacerbation and remission	Chronic with acute ex acerbations

Table 15.2. Contrasts in the diagnostic features between ischaemic colitis, ulcerative colits and Crohn's disease of the colon.

Diagnostic features	Ischaemic colitis	Ulcerative colitis	Crohn's disease of the colon
Barium enema			
Segmental involvement	Common	Uncommon	Common, segments of disease with normal intervening mucosa
Continuity	Continuous	Continuous	Discontinuous, 'skip lesions'
Thumbprinting	Common in early phase	Rare	Uncommon
Transverse ridging	Common	No	No
Ulceration	Serpiginous, diffuse, superficial, cobblestone appearance	Granular, shallow, diffuse. no fissures	Deep, aphtoid, serpiginous, linear, cobblestone appearance, fissuring
Intramural barium	+	−	+
Tubular narrowing/ stricturing	+ (Late stage)	± (Late stage)	+
Sacculation	+	−	±
Loss of haustration	+ (Early and late stage)	+ (Early stage)	± (Incomplete loss)
Inflammatory polyposis	Never	Often, prominent and extensive	Seldom prominent and extensive
Shortening of colon	None (acute stage) only in stricturing stage	+ Due to muscle abnormality	+ Due to fibrosis

Table 15.3. Contrasts in the diagnostic features between ischaemic colitis, ulcerative colitis and Crohn's disease of the colon.

Diagnostic features	Ischaemic colitis	Ulcerative colitis	Crohn's disease of the colon
Endoscopy	Oedema, petechiae, suffusions, confluent.	Diffuse contactbleeding	Oedema, hyperaemia.
	haemorrhagic swelling of mucosa.	Blood, mucus, purulent secretion in lumen.	
		diffuse changes	discontinuous 'patchy' changes
	discrete, localized, serpiginous ulcers.	flat ulcerations	aphtoid, irregular ulcerations, surrounded by normal mucosa.
	pseudopolyps (bulbous protrusions)	pseudopolyps	'cobblestone appearance'
Rectoscopy	Normal in most cases	Often prominent and extensive ulcerations.	50% proctitis

Table 15.4. Contrasts in complications between ischaemic colitis ulcerative colitis and Crohn's disease of the colon.

Complications	Ischaemic colitis	Ulcerative colitis	Crohn's disease of the colon
Fistula/sinustracts	Never	Never	Not uncommon
Toxic dilation	Not uncommon	Common	Rare
Perforation	Common (In gangrenous phase)	Uncommon	Rare
Malignant degeneration	No association	Often	Rare

Table 15.5. Microscopical differences between ischaemic colitis, ulcerative colitis and Crohn's disease of the colon (modified after B.C. Horson, 1971).

Microscopical appearance	Ischaemic colitis	Ulcerative colitis	Crohn's disease of the colon
Pathological features			
Depth of inflammation	Mucosal/submucosal/transmural	Mucosal/submucosal	Transmural
Submucosa	Widened	Normal width or reduced	Widened
Crypt abscess	Common	Very common	Few
Sarcoid granulomas	Absent	Absent	Present (60%)
Goblet cells	Normal or slight reduction	Depletion	Normal or slight reduction
Fissuring	Not uncommon	Absent	Common
Precancerous epithelial changes	−	+	−
Submucosal oedema	+ (Acute phase)	Usually absent	+
Fibrosis	+ (Stricturing form)	−	ǀ
Haemosiderin laden macrophages	+	−	−
Intravascular platelet thrombi	+	−	−

itis and are absent in ischaemic colitis.

Much difficulty is experienced by pathologists in the differential diagnosis of inflammatory bowel disease, particularly between Crohn's disease, ulcerative colitis and ischaemic colitis. The pathological features of these three diseases are summarized in table 15.5. It must be emphasized, however, that none of these features alone is pathognomonic for a particular type of inflammation, except the pre-sence of granulomas in Crohn's disease and the 'haemosiderin laden macrophages' in ischaemic colitis.

There are no absolute differential diagnostic criteria to differentiate a stricturing form of ischaemic colitis from stricturing carcinoma, segmental stenosis in Crohn's disease, colonic strictures due to irradiation, retroperitoneal fibrosis and post strangulation strictures.

16. THERAPEUTIC METHODS FOR ISCHAEMIC COLITIS

16.1 Introduction

When considering the concept of ischaemic colitis one should not necessary think of it as a single definite disease entity. Two major categories have to be considered; acute spontaneous ischaemic colitis which is a multifactorial disease complex and ischaemic colitis secondary to angioplastic procedures e.g. aortic reconstructive surgery (chapter 4).

In both categories the ischaemia can be classified into the transient, stricturing, chronic 'non resolving' or gangrenous forms (chapter 5).

For effective treatment it is important to recognize the form of ischaemic colitis, because the therapeutic methods of choice are dependent upon the severity of ischaemia. Frequently, however, the symptoms regress without trace, the diagnosis being made retrospectively.

16.2 Non gangrenous ischaemic colitis

16.2.1 Transient form
Conservative treatment. Patients with a transient form of ischaemic colitis are best treated conservatively with:

- confinement to bed in a hospital;
- oral restriction and continual gastric aspiration;
- total parenteral nutrition;
  blood or plasma transfusions (in case of haemorrhagic shock, dehydration etc.);
- correction of acidosis;
- reequilibration of body water and electrolytes (potassium, magnesium);
- low molecular dextran 40 (Rheomacrodex®) to expand the intravascular volume and to reduce the viscosity of the blood;
- treatment of the main cause (i.e. cardiac arrhythmia, myocardial infarction etc.);
- polyvalent antibiotic treatment (erythromycin or neomycin) at high doses, may be useful in preventing microbial invasion and sepsis (Bernstein and Bernstein, 1963; Marston et al., 1966; De Dombal et al., 1969; Williams et al., 1969; Brown, 1972; Saegesser et al., 1981);
- clindamycin, lincomycin and tetracycline (which may cause diarrhoea) should be avoided

(Saegesser et al., 1981);

- oxygen therapy, depending upon blood oxygen levels in patients with tachycardia, dyspnoea etc.;
- if possible, corticosteroids should be avoided because they increase the possibility of colonic perforation and secondary infection;
- anticoagulant therapy is not recommended either in the acute stage when there is bleeding (Möller and Stjernvall, 1971) or in the later stages.

If the colon appears distended, it should be decompressed with nasogastric suction or a gastrostomy tube to prevent influx of fluid into the colon and the rectal tube irrigated with saline, since increased intralumenal pressure may further compromise the colonic blood supply. Because the transient form may progress to mural or transmural lesions under unfavourable conditions, the physician should be alert to deterioration of the condition of the patient.

Pulse rate, blood pressure and temperature should be monitored regularly. During the acute stage the abdomen should be re-examined frequently for aggravation of abdominal tenderness as a sign of impending peritonitis (Marcuson, 1972). In the absence of peritoneal signs, a barium enema and (serial) endoscopies should be performed as soon as possible to determine whether or not an operation is required.

If the condition worsens laboratory tests should indicate the development of metabolic disorders demonstrative of tissue necrosis (LDH, SGDT, SGPT, blood pH) (chapter 10). After such a course of conservative treatment the lesions may heal and the clinical condition of the patient improve within 10–14 days. If deterioration in the clinical course is indicated by increasing abdominal signs, fever and leucocytosis, or if the diarrhoea and/or bleeding persists for more than 2 weeks, irreversible damage almost certainly has occurred. There will be mural or transmural progression leading to the stricturing form, to the chronic 'non resolving' form or to transmural gangrene.

Surgical treatment. Surgery is only indicated, if there is progression to irreversible forms of ischaemic colitis.

16.2.2 Stricturing form

An asymptomatic patient with a stricture should be observed clinically as strictures may improve spontaneously after several months (Boley et al., 1978). Surgical treatment should only be considered if there are obstructive symptoms, persistent bleeding and diarrhoea.

The operation consists of excision of the affected bowel segment and restoration of the continuity by end-to-end anastomosis. Careful precautions should be taken to ensure an adequate blood supply to the resection-ends.

16.2.3 Chronic 'non resolving' form

In this chronic form of ischaemic colitis a resection of the involved colon is indicated preferably with restitution of intestinal continuity by primary anastomosis after a suitable period of observation and conservative treatment.

16.2.4 Ischaemic colitis secondary to colonic obstruction

When ischaemic colitis is caused by increased intralumenal pressure due to a distal colonic obstruction, the entire distended region of the colon may be affected. Decompression may be necessary if resection of the ischaemic bowel is contra-indicated. When the obstruction is relieved, the ischaemic colitis may prove to be transient and the patient may recover following intensive treatment, i.e. rehydration and administration of polyvalent antibiotics (chapter 16.2.1).

In the event of transmural ischaemic involvement resection of the entire gangrenous segment is indicated (Saegesser and Sandblom, 1975; Saegesser et al., 1981).

Careful inspection of the proximal colon, during surgery is at all times indicated in cases of stenosing colon lesions to exclude the existence of ischaemic colitis.

16.3 Gangrenous ischaemic colitis

16.3.1 Transmural gangrenous form

Progressive abdominal distension, blood gas deterioration, rise of serum alkaline phosphatase and amylase, metabolic acidosis and increasing peritoneal signs despite supportive therapy, are in-

MANAGEMENT OF ACUTE COLONIC NECROSIS

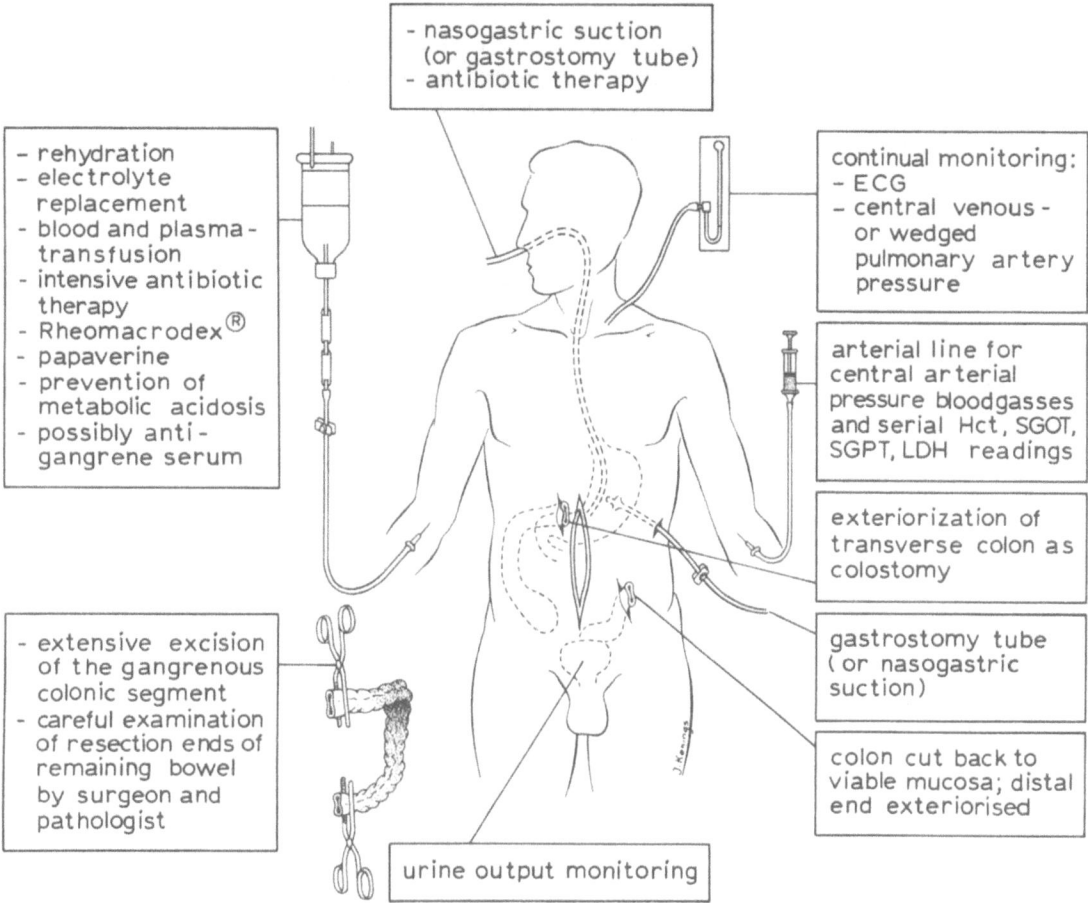

Fig. 16.1. (Modified after Marston et al., 1966).

dicative of the need for operative intervention, before the cause of the peritonitis has been confirmed.

Intensive care should be administered to the patient, before, during and after the operation. Careful monitoring is particularly important (Saegesser et al., 1981). Vigorous resuscitation with massive fluid replacements (transfusion of blood and plasma, rehydration or electrolyte replacement), intensive polyvalent antibiotic therapy and prevention or correction of metabolic acidosis are necessary (Fig. 16.1).

Alpha-blocking agents, such as phenoxybenzamine, together with papaverine, should be infused directly into the SMA-tree with the aid of a Seldinger catheter (Saegesser et al., 1981).

As soon as the circulation has been stabilized, laparotomy should follow with the aim of resection of the non viable bowel.

Factors which aggravate colonic ischaemia such as hypotension, low cardiac output, hypovolaemia, colonic distension and use of vasopressors (vasoactive amines, excessive digitalis) should be avoided before, during and after surgery. If a reduction of the digitalis level is contraindicated e.g. in aged cardiac patients, a continuous infusion of papaverine should be initiated to diminish the vasospastic reflexes of the peripheral splanchnic circulation (Saegesser et al., 1981).

Operative manipulation and anaesthesia can potentiate the splanchnic hypoperfusion (Boley et al., 1971; Williams, 1971).

These factors contribute to reactive vasospasm which may result in damaging ischaemic effects that may persist after re-establishment of blood flow to the bowel (Hayward et al., 1979).

In case of a clostridium infection, polyvalent antigasgangrene serum can be administered (20–40.000 IU) (Killingback and Williams, 1961).

When operation has to be delayed, any evidence of colonic dilatation should be treated with small bowel intubation, gastric suction or rectal tube (Fig. 16.1).

Surgical intervention should be undertaken as rapidly as possible, since resection of the gangrenous segment of the colon provides the only change of survival. Early operation can reduce the mortality – this is particularly true when the ischaemic colitis is caused by an embolic occlusion – 80% survival rates can be achieved (Bergan et al., 1969; Boley et al., 1971).

16.3.1.1 Surgical treatment

Bowel resection. There is a considerable divergence of opinions concerning the surgical technique.

Some authors (Windsberg, 1959; Glotzer et al., 1963; Hunt, 1976) suggest that in case of transmural colonic necrosis, only complete resection of ischaemic bowel with end-to-end anastomosis can be performed safely if the operation is carried out before perforation. The specimen should be opened immediately by the surgeon or by the pathologist, and examined carefully to survey the state of the mucosa. In case of ischaemic lesions at the point of transection an additional segment should be removed. It is not always easy to identify the extent of the process since the damage which is apparent in an early stage at the mucosal level is only revealed at the serosa a few hours later (Rausis et al., 1972; Saegesser et al., 1981). On laparotomy the serosal face of the colon may appear viable and healthy.

When the anastomosis is performed in an ischaemic segment of the colon leakage or stricture-formation may ensue necessitating reoperation.

Most authors have therefore suggested a colonic resection of the gangrenous colonic segment with exteriorization of the ends of the bowel (Hurwitz and Khafif, 1960; Killingback and Williams, 1961; Glotzer et al., 1963; Marston, 1971; Kaminski,

1973; Rosen et al., 1973; Heikkinen et al., 1974; Saegesser et al., 1979, 1981; Guivarc'H et al., 1982).

Re-establishment of continuity should be deferred for 6–8 weeks. The proximal end of the healthy colon should be exteriorized as a colostomy whilst the distal end should be attached to the lower end of the scar or brought out to the skin by a separate incision in the upper pubic or left iliac region (Saegesser, 1981) (Fig. 16.1).

If the gangrene extends as far as the ileocoecal valve, total colectomy and ileostomy are required. If the resection ends are free of ischaemia an ileorectal anastomosis can be performed, but it is preferable to create an ileostomy with re-establishment of continuity 6–8 weeks later (Saegesser et al., 1981).

Arterial reconstruction. Ottinger et al., (1972) recommend that when an ischaemic injury of the colon (of the occlusive form) is recognized, intraoperative management should consist not only of resection, but also of revascularization. As Marston (1964) pointed out, at laparotomy the surgeon should firstly examine the state of the mesenteric vessels to determine whether any arterial reconstruction is advisable. Every attempt then should be made to revascularize the colon prior to attempting a resection. Due to the nature and location of occlusion and associated diseases, the treatment can include embolectomy, endarteriectomy or a bypass operation. The persistence of pulsation in the marginal artery and the vasa recta indicates that there is no vascular obstruction, but this should not be considered as a proof of sufficient vascular perfusion (Saegesser et al., 1981).

Before a patent IMA is ligated in case of aortic aneurysmectomy, however, the integrity of the marginal artery, SMA and colour of the bowel wall have to be inspected; if doubt exists, the vessel must be reimplanted into the aortic prosthesis. To facilitate re-anastomosis of the IMA to the aortic graft, a cuff of aorta should be preserved (Descotes et al., 1963; Ottinger et al., 1972; Saegesser et al., 1972), particularly if this vessel is of large calibre, indicating that it is compensating for a partially obstructed SMA.

Most surgeons routinely reimplant a patent IMA in the bifurcation graft.

The backflow of the IMA should be evaluated. If backflow is pulsatile, perfusion via collaterals may be assumed to be adequate. If there is little backflow from the open distal vessel, reconstruction may be necessary. In case of thrombotic occlusion, revascularization by reimplantation of the IMA is not necessary because there will be a sufficient collateral circulation (Mavor et al., 1962; Ottinger et al., 1972; Ernst et al., 1976). If circulation through the SMA and the hypogastric vessels is impaired, reconstruction of the IMA is more likely to be necessary. Under these circumstances the IMA is usually dilated and can easily be implanted into a graft. At least one of the hypogastric arteries should be preserved.

If the iliac arteries are involved in an aortic aneurysm and have to be ligated, one of the limbs of the bifurcation graft can be implanted end to side in the external iliac artery, thus allowing retrograde flow to the hypogastric arteries (Papadopoulos et al., 1974).

If the coeliac artery and IMA are the site of partial occlusion, it is preferable to perform a bypass from the aorta to the SMA. The IMA under these circumstances is not large enough for reimplantation.

Postoperative complications.
- Through development of septicaemia and toxaemia, ischaemia of the bowel can progress and lead to death.
- The anastomosis can leak after a too limited resection of ischaemic bowel.
- Cardiac decompensation can occur due to circulatory disturbances, secondary to septicaemia.

16.3.1.2 Intra-operative flow measurements. Experimental studies and clinical experience have documented the unreliability of clinical parameters of viability in the ischaemic intestine during surgery, such as colour, peristalsis, arterial pulsation and bleeding from the cut edge of the bowel (Katz et al., 1974; Cooperman et al., 1978; Hayward et al., 1979; O'Donnell and Hobson, 1980).

Intra-operative flow measurements with Doppler ultrasound may be of some usefulness in providing more reliable information (Hobson et al., 1976).

16.3.1.3 Second look procedure. The purpose of the 'second look' is 'not just to allow a clear definition between dead and live bowel to take place, but also to allow time for the institution of supportive measures, which may render more of the bowel viable' (Shaw and Green, 1953; Schennach and Flora., 1972; Boley et al., 1978). Ottinger et al., (1972) believed the second look surgical approach to be of little value in the management of the ischaemic left colon, because conservation of colon length is not of high enough priority to justify a second operation.

At second look operation, normally 12–18 hours after the first one, the ischaemic damage will be more clearly delineated at that stage and viability of the anastomosis will usually be quite apparent. The second look procedure serves to detect progresssion of colonic necrosis (anastomotic leakage may be manifest only after 4–5 days). It is for this reason, that colonic resection with colostomy-ends is to be preferred to immediate end-to-end anastomosis.

The decision regarding the timing of a second operation must be made at the time of completion of the first laparotomy since signs and symptoms during the next 24 hours are unreliable.

If after a second look inspection a colonic re-resection is needed, a third look may be necessary to detect progressive gangrene of the bowel (Lubbers, 1983).

16.4 Literature review

In 1,024 patients reports in the literature (the articles used in this study are indicated in the references with a prefix ○), the therapeutic methods were described in detail for 645 patients (63%) (268 patients of the transient group, 75 patients of the stricturing group and 302 patients of the gangrenous group). In the reported articles we found a lack of information about certain problems, i.e. associated diseases, the exact localisation of the ischaemic segment, the duration of the illness before conservative and/or surgical treatment and the different forms of ischaemic colitis. Frequently no cause of death was mentioned, e.g. death due to the original disease (myocardial infarction, sepsis) or progression of the gangrene. Also whether or

70

not a second look operation was performed its effect was usually not mentioned.

Tables 16.1, 16.2 and 16.3 show the different therapeutic methods employed in the three different forms of ischaemic colitis, as described in these patients.

16.4.1 Transient form
In the *transient* form (table 16.1) 228 of the 268 (85%) patients, were treated conservatively. The survival rate was 90% in this group. Explorative laparotomy without colonic resection was performed in 14 cases with only one mortality.

A colonic resection with an end-to-end anastomosis was performed in 23 of the 268 patients (9%), because of suspicion that the ischaemic process was progressing into deeper layers.

Table 16.1. Results related to the different methods of treatment in 268 patients with transient ischaemic colitis (literature review, 1950–1982).

Methods of treatment	Result Death	Survival	Total number of patients
Conservative treatment	23	205	228
Colonic resection + end to end anastomosis	13	10	23
Colonic resection + colostomy	–	2	2
Colostomy; no colonic resection	1	–	1
Explorative laparotomy without colonic resection	1	13	14
Total number of patients	38	230	268

16.4.2 Stricturing form
In the *stricturing* form (table 16.2) in 49 of the 75 patients (65%) a colonic resection with end-to-end anastomosis was performed. The survival rate was 80% in this group. All 9 patients with primary decompression colostomy and colonic resection in a later stage survived. Thirteen of the 75 patients (17%) were treated conservatively. The survival rate in this group was 77%.

16.4.3 Gangrenous form
In the *gangrenous* form of ischaemic colitis (table

Table 16.2. Results related to the different methods of treatment in 75 patients with stricturing ischaemic colitis (literature review, 1950–1982).

Methods of treatment	Result Death	Survival	Total number of patients
Conservative treatment	3	10	13
Colonic resection + end to end anastomosis	10	39	49
Colonic resection + colostomy	–	9	9
Colostomy; no colonic resection	1	3	4
Total number of patients	14	61	75

16.3) 176 of the 302 patients (58%) underwent a colonic resection with an end-to-end anastomosis. The mortality was high (56%) in this group.

In 13 patients anastomotic leakage was mentioned. In 45 of the 302 patients (15%) a colonic resection with colostomy was performed. The survival rate in this group was 67%.

Conservative therapy was given in 62 of the 302 patients (21%); in this group the mortality was also high (79%). In these cases the diagnosis of ischaemic colitis had not been made prior to death.

Decompression colostomy without resection was performed in 15 of the 302 patients (5%). The survival rate in this group was 60%.

Table 16.3. Results related to the different methods of treatment in 302 patients with gangrenous ischaemic colitis (literature review, 1950–1982).

Methods of treatment	Result Death	Survival	Total number of patients
Conservative treatment	49	13	62
Colonic resection + end to end anastomosis	99*	77	176
Colonic resection + colostomy	15	30	45
Colostomy; no colonic resection	6	9	15
Explorative laparotomy without colonic resection	1	3	4
Total number of patients	170	132	302

* In 13 patients (7%) an anastomotic 'leakage' was mentioned.

PART II

CLINICAL STUDY: 199 PATIENTS WITH ISCHAEMIC COLITIS

17. AETIOLOGY OF ISCHAEMIC COLITIS

The analysis of our own patient material was based upon the study of 199 patients, (collected from 24 different hospitals in the Netherlands, during the period 1970–1980), in whom the diagnosis was made by radiological and/or endoscopical examination. Most cases were collected from the archives of pathology (autopsy material and/or surgically removed diseased tissue and biopsies). Later the relevant clinical data were added and the patient cases analysed.

17.1 Postoperative- versus spontaneous ischaemic colitis

Of the 199 patient-records studied, ischaemic colitis developed spontaneously in 156 patients (78%) (77 men and 79 women), and in 43 patients (22%) (29 men and 14 women) secondarily to a surgical procedure.

17.2 Incidence of different aetiopathogenic factors

The incidence of the different aetiopathogenic factors in our study is summarized in Fig. 17.1.

In 129 patients (65%) only 1 aetiopathogenic factor could be found, in 39 cases (20%) a combination of 2 or more factors was evident, and in 31 cases (15%) no aetiopathogenic factor was found.

Statistically, there is no significant difference in the distribution of the different aetiopathogenic factors between the sexes.

74

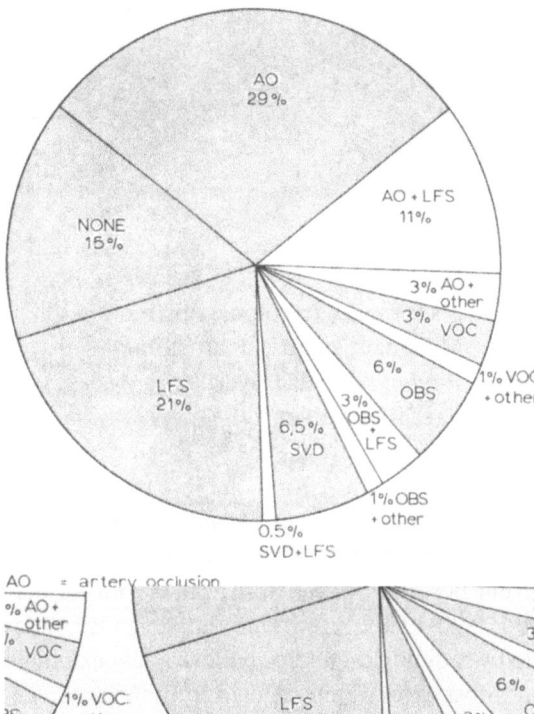

AO = artery occlusion

Fig. 17.1. The incidence of the different aetiopathogenic factors in our retrospective study of 199 patients.

17.2.1 Arterial occlusion

Arterial occlusion occurred in 43% of the cases (85 patients: 50 men and 35 women); in 29% it was the sole aetiopathogenic factor, in 11% it occurred in combination with a 'low flow' state and in 3% of cases in combination with one or more other causative factors.

17.2.2 Venous occlusion

Venous occlusion was present in 4% of the cases (10 patients: 7 men and 3 women); in 3% as the sole aetiopathogenic factor and in 1% of cases in combination with one or more additional aetiopathogenic factors.

17.2.3 'Low flow state'

A 'Low flow state' was present in 35.5% of the cases (74 patients: 38 men and 36 women), in 21% as the only aetiopathogenic factor; in 11% in combination with arterial occlusion and in 3.5% of the cases, in combination with one or more other aetiopathogenic factors.

17.2.4 Small vessel disease

Small vessel disease occurred in 7.5% of the cases (19 patients: 9 men and 10 women), in 6.5% as the sole aetiopathogenic factor, in 0.5% of cases in combination with a 'low flow state' and in 0.5% of cases in combination with other aetiopathogenic factors.

17.2.5 Colonic obstruction

Increased intralumenal pressure secondary to colonic obstruction was the cause of ischaemic colitis in 10% of the cases (31 patients: 18 men and 13 women), in 6% as the sole aetiopathogenic factor, in 3% in combination with 'low flow state' and in 1% in association with other aetiopathogenic factors.

17.3 Incidence of different aetiopathogenic factors in relation to incidence of different types of ischaemic colitis

17.3.1 Arterial occlusion

In table 17.1 the correlation between the incidence of the different forms of arterial occlusion and various types of ischaemic colitis is shown.

Occlusion of the main stem or branches of the SMA and/or IMA by either *thrombosis* or *emboli* was the most frequently found causative factor in the group of patients with transmural ischaemic colitis.

Occlusion of the IMA by an *abdominal aortic aneurysm* had led to transmural ischaemic colitis in 9 of the 11 patients.

An *aortic bifurcation prosthesis* operation leading to mucosal, mural and transmural ischaemic colitis was identified as the aetiopathogenic factor in 12% of the patients in whom arterial occlusion was diagnosed and in 5% of the total number of cases of ischaemic colitis studied. *Large vessel compression* due to haemorrhage was a rare finding (1%) in our patient material.

17.3.2 Venous occlusion

In table 17.2 the correlation between the different forms of venous occlusion and different types of ischaemic colitis is summarized.

Hypercoagulable states occurred in 4 patients with

Table 17.1. Correlation between the different forms of arterial occlusion and different types of ischaemic colitis.

Different types of ischaemic colitis	Mucosal form	Mural form	Mural form	Transmural form	Total number of patients
Arterial occlusion	Transient ischaemic colitis	Stricturing ischaemic colitis	Chronic 'non resolving' ischaemic colitis	Gangrenous ischaemic colitis ± perforation	
Thrombosis SMA	–	1	–	11	12
IMA	1	–	2	8	11
SMA + IMA	–	–	–	9	9
Embolus SMA	–	–	1	15	16
IMA	2	–	–	2	4
SMA + IMA	–	1	1	7	9
Abdominal aortic aneurysm	1	–	1	9	11
After aortic bifurcation prothesis	2	4	–	4	10
Intra abdominal compression	–	–	1	2	3
Total number of patients	6	6	6	67	85

Table 17.2. Correlation between the different forms of venous occlusion and different types of ischaemic colitis.

Different types of ischaemic colitis	Mucosal form	Mural form	Mural form	Transmural form	Total number of patients
Venous occlusion	Transient ischaemic colitis	Stricturing ischaemic colitis	Chronic 'non resolving' ischaemic colitis	Gangrenous ischaemic colitis ± perforation	
Hypercoagulable states	1	–	–	3	4
Carcinoma, leucaemia, lymfoma	–	–	1	1	2
Necrotizing pancreatitis	–	–	–	1	1
Intra abdominal compression	–	–	–	1	1
Porta thrombosis	1	–	–	1	2
Total number of patients	2	–	1	7	10

venous occlusion and subsequent ischaemic colitis (2 patients with polycythaemia vera rubra and 2 patients with essential thrombocytosis), *tumor infiltration* into mesenteric veins was the cause of venous occlusion in 2 cases of ischaemic colitis.

Necrotizing pancreatitis was seen in one patient with ischaemic colitis caused by venous occlusion. One case of *venous compression* due to haemorrhage and two cases of venous occlusion secondary to *porta thrombosis* were observed in our survey of patients with ischaemic colitis.

17.3.3 'Low flow state'
In table 17.3 the correlation between the various

causes of 'low flow' state and the different forms of ischaemic colitis is shown. *Septic shock, cardiopathy,* (congestive heart failure, myocardial infarction, cardiac arrhythmia) and *haemorrhage,* secondary to operation procedures or trauma were the most frequently found causes in this group, leading to ischaemic colitis, often of the transmural type.

In 2 patients *digitalis intoxication* was found. In one case transmural ischaemic colitis developed; in the other case, there was regeneration of normal colonic mucosa within 2 weeks following withdrawal of digitalis medication.

Dehydration occurred due to prolonged use of *di-*

Table 17.3. Correlation between the different forms of low flow state and the different types of ischaemic colitis.

Different types of ischaemic colitis	Mucosal form	Mural form	Mural form	Transmural form	Total number of patients
Low flow state	Transient ischaemic colitis	Stricturing ischaemic colitis	Chronic 'non resolving' ischaemic colitis	Gangrenous ischaemic colitis ± perforation	
Congestive heart failure	1	1	2	8	12
Myocardial infarction	1	–	–	5	6
Cardiac arrhythmia	4	2	1	7	14
Haemorrhage	–	1	2	7	10
Digitalis intoxication	1	–	–	1	2
Dehydration + diuretics	–	–	–	1	1
Dehydration	2	–	–	5	7
Septic shock	–	–	–	21	21
Massive pulmonary embolism	–	–	–	1	1
Total number of patients	9	4	5	56	74

uretics in 8 patients with ischaemic colitis.

Massive pulmonary embolus as a possible cause of transmural ischaemic colitis occurred only rarely in our patient material.

17.3.4 Small vessel disease
Table 17.4 shows the correlation between the different types of small vessel disease and different forms of ischaemic colitis.

Microangiopathy due to diabetes and/or hypertension, often in combination with 'low flow state' was most frequently found in our series.

Vasculitis of the mesenteric vessels due to systemic lupus erythematosus, periarteritis nodosa or rheumatoid arthritis could be found in 5 cases, in 4 cases leading to gangrenous ischaemic colitis and in 1 case to chronic 'non resolving' ischaemic colitis.

Of those patients with *irradiation vasculopathy,* 3 cases had undergone radiotherapy for a carcinoma of the bladder, 1 year, 3 years and 11 years previously.

In 1 case radiotherapy for an adenocarcinoma of the cervix had been carried out 5 years previously and in 1 case radiotherapy for adenocarcinoma of the rectum had been given 2 weeks previously.

Table 17.4. Correlation between the different forms of small vessel disease and the different types of ischaemic colitis.

Different types of ischaemic colitis	Mucosal form	Mural form	Mural form	Transmural form	Total number of patients
Small vessel disease	Transient ischaemic colitis	Stricturing ischaemic colitis	Chronic 'non resolving' ischaemic colitis	Gangrenous ischaemic colitis ± perforation	
Microangiopathy	–	1	–	5	6
Vasculitis	–	–	1	4	5
Irradiation vasculopathy	–	–	1	4	5
Amyloidosis	–	–	1	2	3
Total number of patients	–	1	3	15	19

Table 17.5. Correlation between the different forms of colonic obstruction and the different types of ischaemic colitis.

Increased intralumenal pressure secondary to colonic obstruction	Different types of ischaemic colitis	Mucosal form	Mural form	Mural form	Transmural form	Total number of patients
		Transient ischaemic colitis	Stricturing ischaemic colitis	Chronic 'non resolving' ischaemic colitis	Gangrenous ischaemic colitis ± perforation	
Benign stenosis (diverticular disease)		1	–	1	4	6
Malignant stenosis (carcinoma)		1	–	5	6	12
Faecal impaction		–	–	1	4	5
Total number of patients		2	–	7	14	23

In 3 cases *amyloidosis* was sufficiently severe to cause occlusion of small intestinal vessels; in combination with a 'low flow state' this had probably led to ischaemic colitis.

17.3.5 Increased intralumenal pressure secondary to colonic obstruction

Table 17.5 shows the correlation between the different types of obstruction and different forms of ischaemic colitis.

Twelve patients showed *malignant stenosis,* due to colonic adenocarcinoma. In 6 cases (50%) this had led to proximal gangrenous ischaemic colitis. In 5 of these 6 cases a perforation caused by transmural necrosis, was found. In 5 cases a chronic 'non resolving' ischaemic colitis developed due to a slight progression of stenosis over a longer period. Table 17.6 shows the patient-data from 12 cases of ischaemic colitis secondary to stenosing colonic carcinoma. In 8 cases (67%) ischaemic colitis proximal to malignancy of the sigmoid was found at laparotomy; in 1 of these cases the carcinoma was located in the rectum, in 1 case at the hepatic flexure and in 1 case there was a double carcinoma, located in the proximal part of the ascending- and in the transverse colon.

A normal colonic segment was present between

tumor and the proximal ischaemic bowel segment in 1 case (8%).

Six patients with ischaemic colitis showed *benign stenosis* of the colon due to *diverticular disease.* Table 17.7 shows data from 6 patients with ischaemic colitis associated with benign colonic obstruction, due to diverticular disease. In all patients the sigmoid was the location of the stenosing diverticular disease. In 3 cases (50%) stomal necrosis could be found. In 2 cases a normal non-ischaemic colonic segment was present between the benign stenosing process and the more proximal ischaemic bowel segment.

In 5 patients *faecal impaction* was found as the aetiopathogenic cause of ischaemic colitis.

Table 17.8 shows the data from these 5 patients. In 2 cases the right side of the colon was involved in the ischaemic process, due to more distal faecal impaction. In 2 cases the left side was involved, due to hard-stony scybala in the rectosigmoid region. In one of these, the combination of a small stenosing sigmoid carcinoma and stony barium scybala proximal to the carcinoma had led to total obstruction with secondary ischaemia of the transverse/descending colon and sigmoid.

CASE/ SEX	AGE	CLINICAL FEATURES	OPERATION	LOCALIZATION OF ISCHAEMIC COLITIS	LOCALIZATION OF COLONIC CARCINOMA	POST OPERATIVE COURSE	LEUCO'S	BARIUM ENEMA	PLAIN FILM	LOCALIZATION
♀	83	Bloody diarrhea, acute abdominal pain, peritonitis	I:double decompression transversostomy. II:1 day later: sigmoidresection, Hartmannprocedure, rectum closed, transversostomy	descending colon sigmoid	sigmoid	death stomal necrosis	18.000	+ CC no IC	–	
♀	74	Since 1 wk acute abdominal pain, nausea, vomiting, peritonitis (secondary to barium enema)	sigmoidresection Hartmannprocedure rectum closed, descending colostomy	transverse-, descending colon sigmoid	sigmoid	death	10.800	+ CC **	+ *	
♂	78	Abdominal pain, Bloody diarrhea.	Low anterior resection sigmoid, end-end anastomosis.	total colon+ terminal ileum	sigmoid	death stomal necrosis	8.800	+ CC no IC	–	
♀	79	Bloody diarrhea, Acute abdominal pain, nausea, ileus, peritonitis	I:Exteriorisation transverse colon, decompression-transversostomy. II:4 wks later: left-hemicolectomy, end-end anastomosis ascending colon/sigmoid	transverse colon (necrotizing)	splenic flexure	recovery	–	–	+ *	
♀	67	Since 1 day bloody diarrhea, acute abdominal pain	double decompression sigmoidostomy	total colon+ terminal ileum (necrotizing)	sigmoid	death	20.000	–	–	
♀	70	Since 1 day acute abdominal pain, nausea, vomiting, peritonitis	I:transverse colon resection,colostomy at ascending and descending colon II:2 months later: left hemicolectomy rectum closed. Hartmann procedure, ascending colostomy in situ.	transverse-, descending colon	sigmoid	recovery	11.000	+ CC no IC	–	

♀ 63	Bloody diarrhea, weight loss, ileus	Double decompression transverse-stomy. II: 1 month later: sigmoidresection, end-end anastomosis, closure transverso-stomy	transverse-descending colon, sigmoid	sigmoid	recovery	6.400 + Failed due to path	+ *
♀ 70	Since 2 days abdominal cramps, nausea, vomiting, diarrhea, ileus, peritonitis	I: ileocoecalresection, ligation; II: later ascending+transverse colectomy, ileotransverostomy; III: 4 days later: suturing perforation of ileum; anastomosis	rectum ascending colon	hepatic flexure	died acute second recovery	17.800 −	+ ***
♀ 73	Acute abdominal pain, ileus	sigmoidresection, Hartmann procedure; II: 6 days later: total colectomy + ileostomy; III: 3 months later ileosigmoidostomy	total colon (rectnot involved)	sigmoid	P.O.II colal normal P.O.II: recovery	20.200 + CC no IC	+ ***
♂ 85	Acute abdominal pain, ileus, peritonitis	left hemicolectomy, transverse-sigmoidostomy	transverse-descending colon sigmoid	sigmoid	death	23.400 +	+ ***
♀ 66	Abdominal cramps, nausea, melaena	recto-sigmoidresection, end-end anastomosis, II: 1 week later: decompression transverostomy	transverse-descending colon sigmoid	rectum	recovery	− + no CC no IC	−
♂ 84	Abdominal pain, nausea, vomiting, diarrhea	Right hemicolectomy, coeco-transversostomy + depacostomy	ascending, transverse colon	'double' carcinoma transverse colon	recovery	4.800 + CC no IC	−

IC = ischaemic colitis   * = colonic distension
CC = coloncarcinoma   ** = iatrogenic perforation
— = ileus   *** = ileus

Table 17.6. Data from 12 patients with ischaemic colitis secondary to stenosing or obstructing coloncarcinoma.

CASE/SEX	AGE	CLINICAL FEATURES	OPERATION	LOCALISATION OF ISCHAEMIC COLITIS	LOCALISATION OF BENIGN OBSTRUCTION	POST-OPERATIVE COURSE	LEUCO'S	BARIUM ENEMA	PLAIN FILM	LOCALISATION
♂	48	bloody diarrhea, abdominal pain	left hemicolectomy; transverse-sigmoidostomy	splenic flexure, descending colon, sigmoid	sigmoid	recovery	-	+ I.C. no obst.	-	
♀	63	colicky abdominal pain, nausea, vomiting, diarrhea	I:double transverse colostomy II:(after 3 ds) right hemicolec-tomy+ileostomy+transversostomy	descending-, transverse colon+congestion descending colon and sigmoid.	sigmoid	death anastomal necrosis	11.7	-	+***	
♀	70	abdominal pain, nausea, fever.	I:sigmoid+proximal rectum-resection (end-end) II:(6 ds later) relaparotomy: necrotic descending colon and half transverse colon resected; transversostomy, rectum closed.	transverse colon, splenic flexure, descending colon; sigmoid	sigmoid+ infiltration	death stomal necrosis	11.1	+ (diverticulitis-stenosis) no I.C.	-	
♀	91	rectal blood, nausea, vomiting, abdominal pain	left hemicolec-tomy + Hartmann procedure	splenic flexure, descending colon sigmoid (+perforation)	recto-sigmoid	death	12.3	-	+***	
♀	60	abdominal pain	left hemicolec-tomy + Hartmann procedure, descending colo-stomy; rectum closed	descending colon	sigmoid	recovery stomal necrosis	15.3	+ I.C. no sten.	-	
♂	61	abdominal pain, bloody diarrhea	conservative treatment	transverse colon, splenic flexure	sigmoid	death	15.4	-	+* I.C.	

obs= obstruction
sten= stenosis

*** = ileus
I.C = ischaemic colitis
+ = performed
- = not performed

= ischaemic colitis
= ischaemic colitis
= faecal impaction
- = obstruction due to diverticular disease

Table 17.7. Data from 6 patients with ischaemic colitis associated with benign colonic obstruction, due to diverticular disease.

CASE/ AGE/ SEX	CLINICAL FEATURES	OPERATION	LOCALISATION OF ISCHAEMIC COLITIS	LOCALISATION OF FAECAL IMPACTION	POST-OPERATIVE COURSE	LEUCO'S	BARIUM ENEMA	PLAIN FILM	LOCALISATION
♀ 79	Ileus	Ileocecal resection; (ileal-) perforation; ileostomy and transversostomy	Ascending and proximal transverse colon	coprostasis descending colon and recto-sigmoid	death, sigmoid anamn.	26.9	–	+	
♂ 78	Abdominal pain, rectal blood, nausea, vomiting	Conservative treatment	caecum	coprostasis colon	death	7.3	no i.c. (color. no sten. perfor)	+ (color. perfor)	
♂ 76	Abdominal pain, to deface, blood, diarrhoea, nausea, vomiting	recto-sigmoid resection	sigmoid	coprostasis recto-sigmoid	death	–	–	*** (perfor)	
♂ 85	Rectal blood, vomiting	double colostomy sigmoid	transverse colon, splenic flexure descending colon, sigmoid	stony barium sequels after repetitive bariumenemas (3x) in descending-sigmoidcolon+ slight stenosing sigmoidcarcinoma	death	–	+ (failed 3x)	+ ***	
♂ 83	Cramp abdominal pain, bloody diarrhoea, nausea, vomiting	sigmoidresection + descending colostomy + rectum closed	total colon	coprostasis distal colon	death	13.0	–	+ ***	

obs= obstruction
sten= stenosis

*** = ileus
I.C = ischaemic colitis
+ = performed
– = not performed

▨ = ischaemic colitis
▥ = faecal impaction
+ = performed
– = obstruction due to diverticular disease

Table 17.8. Data from 5 patients with ischaemic colitis associated with benign colonic obstruction, due to faecal impaction.

18. CLASSIFICATION AND DEFINITIONS OF THE DIFFERENT FORMS OF ISCHAEMIC COLITIS

18.1 *Different forms of ischaemic colitis*

18.2 *Definitions*
  18.2.1 transient (mucosal) ischaemic colitis
  18.2.2 chronic 'non resolving' (mural) ischaemic colitis
  18.2.3 Stricturing (mural) ischaemic colitis
  18.2.4 Gangrenous (transmural) ischaemic colitis

18.3 *Incidence*
  18.3.1 Non gangrenous group
  Transient (mucosal) form
  Chronic 'non resolving' (mural) form
  Stricturing (mural) form
  18.3.2 Gangrenous group
  Gangrenous (transmural) form with perforation
  Gangrenous (transmural) form without perforation

18.1 Different forms of ischaemic colitis

In our retrospective study of 199 patients with ischaemic colitis, we used a combination of the clinical classification after Marston et al., (1966) and of a histological classification, based on the depth of ischaemia in the colon wall, as proposed by Swerdlow et al., 1981. (Fig. 18.1). In this revised classification mucosal colonic ischaemia is equivalent to the transient clinical form of ischaemic colitis; mural colonic ischaemia may lead to the stricturing form or to the chronic 'non resolving' form of ischaemic colitis and transmural colonic ischaemia is equivalent to gangrenous ischaemic colitis.

18.2 Definitions

18.2.1 Transient (mucosal) ischaemic colitis
The *(acute) transient (mucosal) form* of ischaemic colitis can be defined as a form which involves reversible morphological mucosal colonic changes. A sufficient collateral circulation allows complete regeneration and complete structural and functional recovery within 1–2 weeks.

18.2.2 Chronic 'non resolving' (mural) ischaemic colitis

18.2.3 Stricturing (mural) ischaemic colitis
The chronic 'non resolving' form of ischaemic colitis and the (subacute or chronic) stricturing (mural) form of ischaemic colitis can be defined as forms which involve irreversible morphological mural changes, ulceration and varying degrees of fibrosis leading to either persisting ulcerative colitis or to tubular stenosis.

The collateral blood supply is sufficient to prevent progression to transmural ischaemia, but damage is too deep to be complete.

18.2.4 Gangrenous (transmural) ischaemic colitis
The *gangrenous (transmural) form* of ischaemic colitis can be defined as a massive tissue necrosis involving the entire wall with a secondary demarcating inflammatory reaction.

18.3 Incidence

18.3.1 Non gangrenous group
In the *non gangrenous group* of ischaemic colitis the transient (mucosal) form of ischaemic colitis was found in 35 patients (17.5%) (17 men and 18 women).

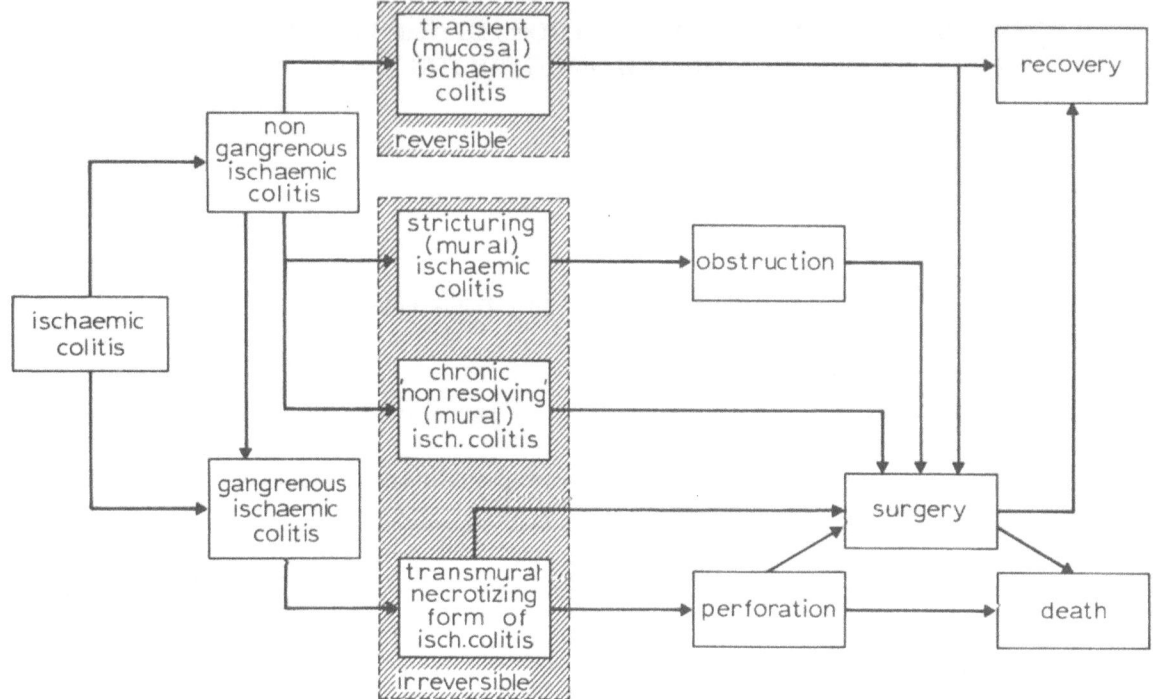

Fig. 18.1. Different forms of ischaemic colitis.

The chronic 'non resolving' (mural) form was present in 18 cases (9%) (7 men and 11 women).

The stricturing (mural) form of ischaemic colitis was detected in 15 cases (7.5%) (9 men and 6 women).

18.3.2 Gangrenous group

In the *gangrenous group* of ischaemic colitis colonic transmural gangrene had led to perforation in 26 patients (13%) (13 men and 13 women). No perforation occurred in 105 patients (53%).

19. VARIATIONS IN THE INCIDENCE OF ISCHAEMIC COLITIS WITH AGE AND SEX OF THE PATIENT

19.1 *Variations in the incidence of ischaemic colitis with age and sex of the 199 patients studied*

19.2 *Variations in the frequency of occurrence of the different forms of ischaemic colitis with the age and sex of the patient*

19.3 *Age and aetiopathogenic factors*

19.1 Variations in the incidence of ischaemic colitis with age and sex of the 199 patients studied

Most of the 199 patients studied with ischaemic colitis (166 patients = 81% in this group) were between the 6th and 9th decade with a mean of 72.8 years (see Figs. 19.1, 19.2). The difference between the number of men and the number of women in this group is statistically insignificant (p = 0.24). The mean age of the total group was 69.1 years.

The difference in age between men and women studied in the total group was statistically significant (p = 0.028) according to the X^2 test. The age of the female patients was somewhat higher than the age of the men. Only 2 patients in our series were below 30 years of age, a 20 year old girl and a 29 year old man, both with transient 'evanescent' colitis. The sex distribution was 106 men and 93 women (1.14 : 1).

19.2 Variations in the frequency of occurrence of the different forms of ischaemic colitis with the age and sex of the patient

The age- and sex distribution of the different forms of the non gangrenous and gangrenous group of ischaemic colitis is summarized in figures 19.3–19.7.

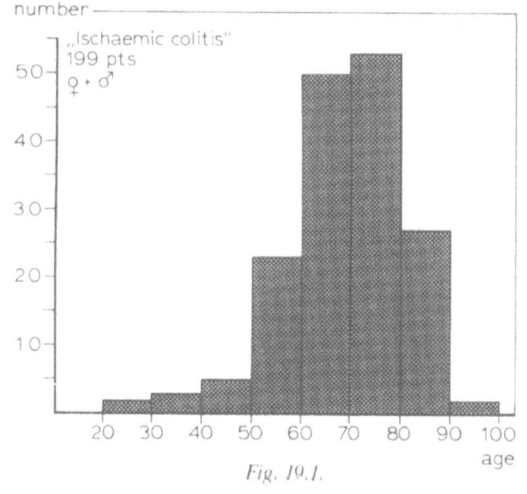

Fig. 19.1.

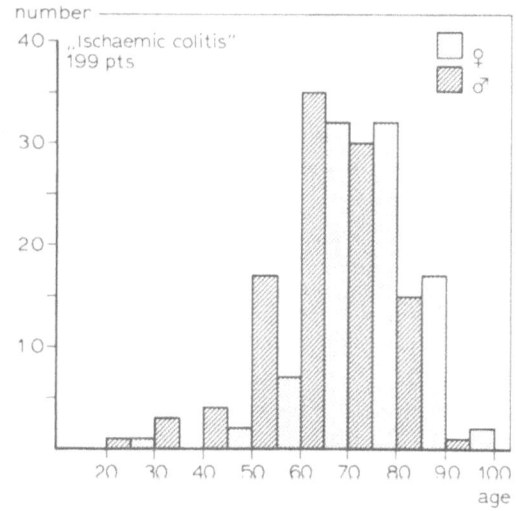

Fig. 19.2.

Fig. 19.1–19.2. Age and sex distribution of 199 patients with ischaemic colitis.

86

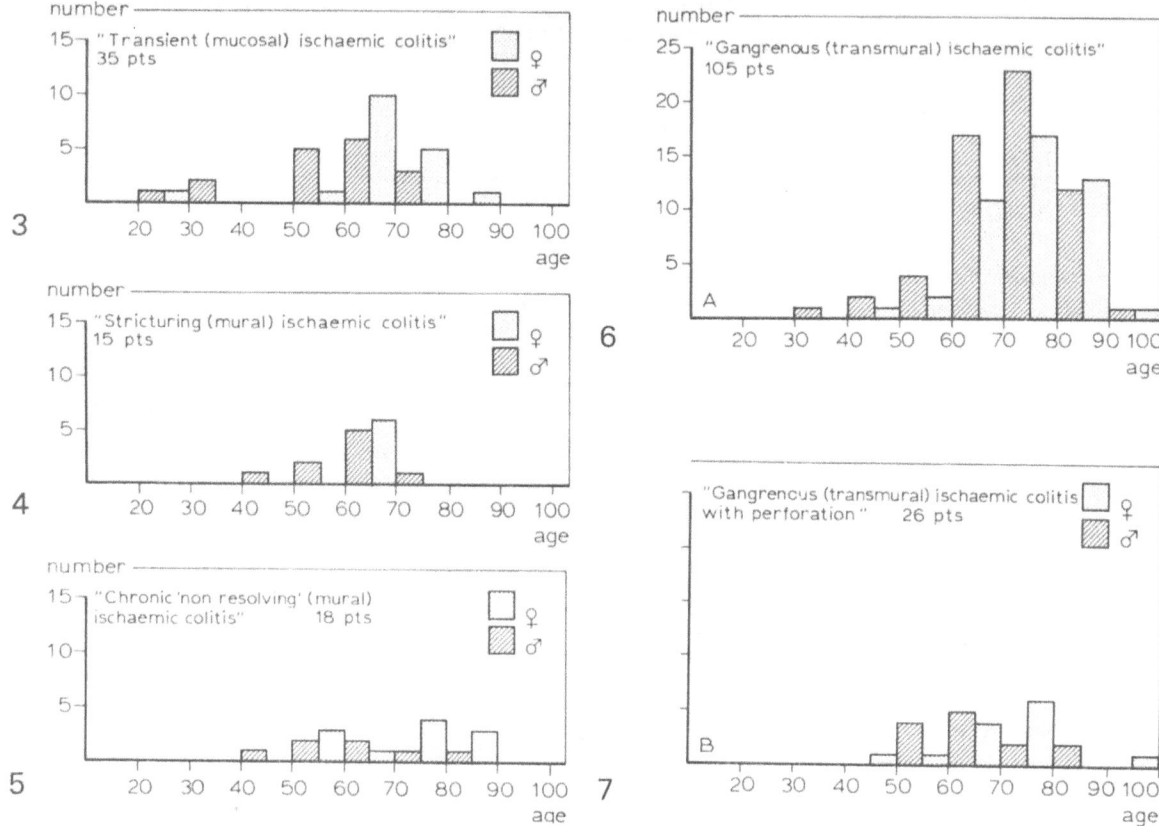

Fig. 19.3–19.7. Age and sex distribution of 199 patients with ischaemic colitis.

19.3 Age and aetiopathogenic factor

In order to discover whether there was any statistically significant difference between the average age of patients falling into different aetiopathogenic groups, the X^2 test was applied.

The difference in the average age of patients with major aetiopathogenic factors such as arterial occlusion, venous occlusion, small vessel disease or increased intralumenal pressure secondary to colonic obstruction (or some combinations of these) and the average age of patients with other aetiopathogenic factors, but without any of the principle factors mentioned above, was not statistically significant (p = 0.10, resp. p = 0.17, p = 0.67, p = 0.23). The difference between the average age of patients with a 'low flow state' (alone or in combination with one or several of the principle aetiopathogenic factors, mentioned above) and that of patients with other aetiopathogenic factors without a 'low flow state' was statistically significant (p = 0.002): patients with a 'low flow state' were older than patients not suffering from this condition.

The difference between the average age of patients in whom no aetiopathogenic factor was detected and that of patients with one or more aetiopathogenic factors was statistically significant (p = 0.0001): patients without known aetiopathogenic factors were older than the patients in whom one or more aetiopathogenic factors were found.

20. ASSOCIATED DISEASES

Table 20.1 represents the different diseases, associated with the ischaemic colonic damage, occurring in 11 patients below 50 years of age and in 188 patients above 50 years of age. In the 11 cases in our series where the patients were below 50 years of age, in 3 patients only (27%) could a single predisposing factor be found.

In the 188 cases in our series where the patients were above 50 years of age, 120 cases presented with one (99 patients) or more (21 patients) associated diseases.

The combination of hypertension with diabetes was most frequently found in this older group (15 cases, 8%). Hypertension was present in 34 patients (17%) either alone (14 patients) (7%) or in combination with other diseases (20 patients) (10%).

Cardiac arrhythmia occurred in 13 patients (7%), either alone (6 patients) (3.5%), or in combination with hypertension and/or diabetes (7 patients) (3.5%), predisposing to serious arteriosclerotic disease.

Table 20.1. Associated diseases in ischaemic colitis occurring in 11 patients below 50 years of age and in 188 patients above 50 years of age.

Age Associated diseases	<50 yrs	≥50 yrs	Total number of patients
No associated diseases	8	68	76
Rheumatoid arthritis	–	12	12
Thrombosis/embolism	–	4	4
Cerebrovascular accident	–	5	5
Claudication	–	2	2
Cardiac valve replacement	1	4	5
Radiotherapy for malignancy	–	5	5
Myocardial infarction	1	25	26
Pectoral angina	–	6	6
Cardiac arrhythmia	–	6	6
Hypertension	–	14	14
Diabetes	1	16	17
Hypertension + myocardial infarction + diabetes	–	9	9
Hypertension + cardiac arrhythmia	–	1	1
Hypertension + cardiac arrhythmia + diabetes	–	6	6
Myocardial infarction + rheumatoid arthritis	–	1	1
Hypertension + rheumatoid arthritis		2	2
Hypertension + myocardial infarction	–	2	2
Total number of patients	11	188	199

21. CLINICAL PRESENTATION

21.1 *Clinical symptoms and different forms of ischaemic colitis*

21.2 *Physical signs and different forms of ischaemic colitis*

21.1 Clinical symptoms and different forms of ischaemic colitis

Table 21.1 represents the frequency of observation of various clinical symptoms in our series of 199 patients with ischaemic colitis. *Abdominal pain, rectal blood* and *diarrhoea* were the most frequent and constant signs of ischaemic colitis.

Nausea/vomiting was present in 45% of the patients. *Tenesmus* has not been described in this study, because it was often not mentioned in patient reports. Within the transient (mucosal) group rectal bloodloss (89%) and diarrhoea (60%) were most frequently found. Within the stricturing (mural) group diarrhoea (93%) and rectal blood

loss (86%) occurred most frequently. Within the chronic 'non resolving' group rectal bleeding (56%) and diarrhoea (56%) were most frequently encountered. In the gangrenous (transmural) form abdominal pain (80%) was the most frequently found sign with rectal blood loss in 44%, diarrhoea in 44%, and nausea/vomiting in 47% of the cases.

21.2 Physical signs and different forms of ischaemic colitis

Table 21.2 represents the correlation between physical signs and different forms of ischaemic colitis in our series of 199 patients. No physical signs were present in 21% of our patients with ischaemic colitis. In 12% of the patients the gangrenous (transmural) ischaemic colitis was silent and no abnormality could be detected on physical examination. Ileus signs were found in 21% of our cases.

In 131 patients with the gangrenous (transmural) form of ischaemic colitis, distension (38%), per-

Table 21.1. Correlation between the clinical symptoms and different types of ischaemic colitis in our series of 199 patients.

Different types of ischaemic colitis	Mucosal form	Mural form	Mural form	Transmural form	Total number of patients
Clinical symptoms	Transient ischaemic colitis	Stricturing ischaemic colitis	Chronic 'non resolving' ischaemic colitis	Gangrenous ischaemic colitis ± perforation	
Total number of patients	35	15	18	131	199
Abdominal pain	16 (46%)	9 (60%)	6 (33%)	105 (80%)	136 (68%)
Rectal bloodloss	31 (89%)	13 (87%)	10 (56%)	58 (44%)	112 (56%)
Diarrhoea	21 (60%)	14 (93%)	10 (56%)	58 (44%)	103 (52%)
Nausea/vomitus	14 (40%)	7 (47%)	7 (39%)	61 (47%)	89 (45%)

itoneal tenderness (40%) and pressure pain (33%) were the most frequently found clinical signs; in 68 patients with non gangrenous ischaemic colitis pressure pain alone was the most frequently presenting symptom.

Distension (58%), peritoneal tenderness (60%) and pressure pain (50%) were most frequently encountered within the group of transmural gangrenous ischaemic colitis. The other signs occurred with equal frequency throughout the other groups of ischaemic colitis.

Table 21.2. Correlation between the physical signs and different types of ischaemic colitis in our series of 199 patients.

Different types of ischaemic colitis	Submucosal form	Mural form	Mural form	Transmural form	Total number of patients
Physical signs	Transient ischaemic colitis	Stricturing ischaemic colitis	Chronic 'non resolving' ischaemic colitis	Gangrenous ischaemic colitis ± perforation	
Total number of patients	35	15	18	131	199
Normal	8 (23%)	5 (33%)	4 (22%)	24 (18%)	41 (21%)
Distension	4 (11%)	5 (33%)	4 (22%)	76 (58%)	89 (45%)
Peritoneal tenderness	1 (3%)	6 (40%)	4 (22%)	79 (60%)	90 (46%)
Pressure pain	23 (66%)	9 (60%)	5 (28%)	66 (50%)	103 (52%)
Ileus	1 (3%)	5 (33%)	2 (11%)	33 (25%)	41 (21%)

22. ANATOMICAL DISTRIBUTION OF ISCHAEMIC COLITIS

22.1 Localisation of ischaemic colonic lesions

In our patient material of 199 patients with ischaemic colitis the ischaemic lesions were predominantly found in the left side (62%), with the highest incidence in the descending colon (25%) and sigmoid (22%). We found a higher percentage of right sided colonic ischaemia (34%) in our series than in the literature (23%) (see chapter 9).

Not only the right side of the colon, but also the terminal ileum was involved in the ischaemic process in 15% of our cases, indicating occlusion of a large branch of the SMA as causative factor.

In 7% of the patients transmural gangrene of the whole colon, including the terminal ileum, occurred after occlusion of both mesenteric arteries. Rectal ischaemia involvement was found in only 4% of our cases.

The distribution and the length of the colon involved in our patients with ischaemic colitis are summarized in Fig. 22.1 with a detailed breakdown in Fig. 22.2.

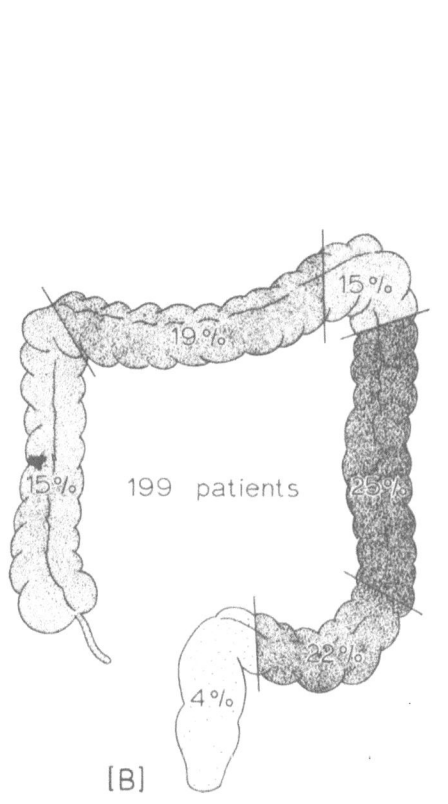

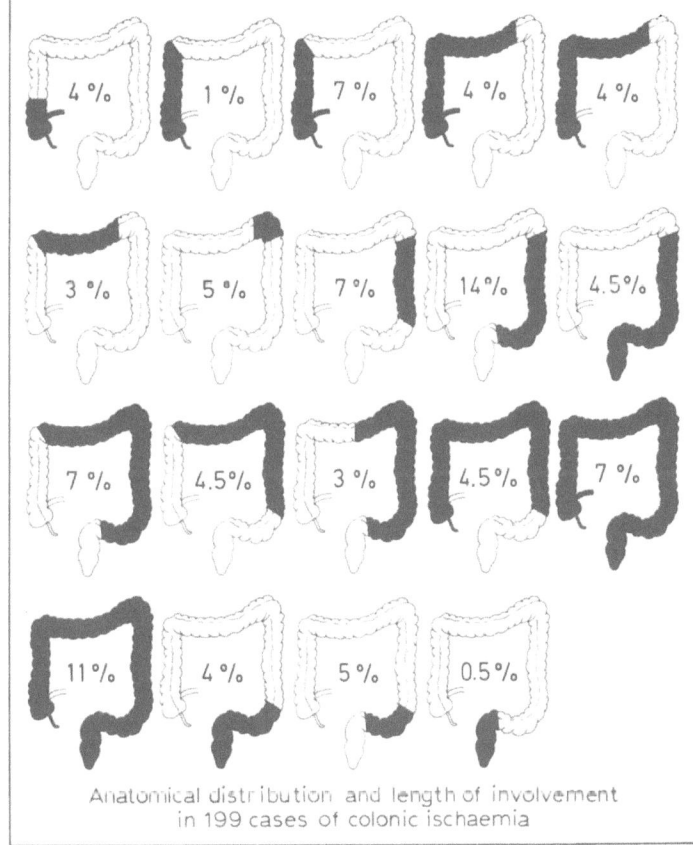

Fig. 22.1. Anatomical distribution of ischaemic colitis in 199 patients (our material).

Fig. 22.2. Detailed breakdown of Fig. 23.1.

22.2 Anatomical distribution and aetiopathogenic factors

As a result of embolism of the main branch of the SMA right sided ischaemia (14%) has been most frequently found. In case of occlusion of the IMA left sided ischaemia (46%) has been most frequently found.

Right sided colonic ischaemia was more usually the consequence of distal colonic obstruction (4%).

23. LABORATORY INVESTIGATIONS*

23.1 *Leucocyte (WBC) count*

23.2 *Erythrocyte sedimentation rate (ESR)*

23.3 *Stoolcultures*

23.4 *Bloodcultures*

23.5 *Guajac test*

23.1 Leucocyte (WBC) count

A leucocyte count was performed in 169 of the 199 patients (85%).

The count was normal ($\leq 10,8 \times 19^9 L$) in 24% and elevated in 76% of the cases. No count was

carried out in 30 of the 199 patients (15%).

Table 23.1 shows the WBC elevations in relation to the different forms of ischaemic colitis.

The leucocyte count was elevated in 66% of the cases with mucosal colonic necrosis; in 66% of the cases with mural colonic necrosis and in 81% of the cases with transmural colonic necrosis.

23.2 Erythrocyte sedimentation rate (ESR)

The erythrocyte sedimentation rate was assessed in 161 of the 199 patients. In 12% of the cases the ESR was normal (≤ 20 mm in 1 hr.; Westergren method) and in 88% of the cases was elevated.

No ESR test was performed in 38 of the 199 patients (19%). Table 23.1 shows the ESR eleva-

Table 23.1. Correlation between (preoperative) WBCC and ESR values and the different types of ischaemic colitis.

Laboratory investigations	Different types of ischaemic colitis	Mucosal form — Transient ischaemic colitis	Mural form — Stricturing ischaemic colitis	Mural form — Chronic 'non resolving' ischaemic colitis	Transmural form — Gangrenous ischaemic colitis ± perforation	Total number of patients
Leucocyte count (WBCC)	Elevated	19 (66%)	8 (67%)	11 (65%)	90 (81%)	128
	normal	10	4	6	21	41
	not done	6	3	1	20	30
Erythrocyte sedimentation rate (ESR)	Elevated	26 (84%)	14 (100%)	17 (100%)	85 (86%)	142
	Normal	5	–	–	14	19
	Not done	4	1	1	32	38
Total number of patients		35	15	18	131	199

* All laboratory values are from preoperative investigations.

tion in relation to the different forms of ischaemic colitis.

The ESR was elevated in 84% of the cases with mucosal colonic necrosis; in 100% of the cases with mural colonic necrosis and in 86% of the cases with transmural colonic necrosis.

23.3 Stoolcultures

In our series of 199 patients stoolcultures were taken in 51 cases. In only 4 (8%) of these patients were the cultures positive for gram negative organisms.

23.4 Bloodcultures

Bloodcultures were taken in 60 cases. In 21 of the 60 cases (35%) the cultures were positive and in 39 of the 60 cases (65%) negative.

23.5 Guajac test

The Guajac test for occult blood was positive in 59 of the 70 cases (84%) in which the test was done.

24. RADIOLOGICAL ASPECTS IN DIAGNOSIS OF ISCHAEMIC COLITIS

24.1 *Barium enema*
    24.1.1 Number, time and findings of per-
formed barium enema
    24.1.2 Radiological signs and stage of isch-
aemic colitis

24.2 *Repeat barium enema*

24.3 *Angiography*
    24.3.1 Number of angiographies and findings
    24.3.2 Pathological angiographical findings
and distribution of the colonic ischaemia

24.1 Barium enema

24.1.1 Number, time and findings of performed barium enema

In the radiological material from our series of 199
patients with ischaemic colitis there were 75 (first)
barium enemas (38%).

Fifty-one (first) barium enemas were performed

during the first week, 7 in the second week and 17
after two weeks following onset of symptoms.

The barium enema was normal in 9 patients; a
benign or malignant stenosis was found in 6 cases;
dilatation in 1 case, a benign/malignant stenosis
with proximal dilatation in 1 case. In 58 cases
(77%) the results were indicative of ischaemic colitis. In 5 of these 58 cases a distal colonic carcinoma
was observed.

24.1.2 Radiological signs and stage of ischaemic colitis

Table 24.1 shows the correlation between the different radiological signs and the time interval between onset of symptoms and time of performing
the first barium enema.

'Thumbprinting', ulceration, loss of haustration
and narrowing due to spasm were most frequently
present in the early stage of ischaemia (1–7 days).

Intramural gas was seen in only 2 cases (6%). In
the second week all signs, except the presence of
intramural gas and stricturing could be found.

Table 24.1. Correlation between the different radiological features and the time interval between onset of symptoms and the time of performing the barium enema in 58 patients with ischaemic colitis.

Time interval between onset of symptoms and the time of performing a barium enema	1–7 days	8–14 days	>14 days	Total number of patients
Radiological features				
Number of barium enemas	35	7	16	58
Thumbprinting	26	3	4	33
Transverse ridging	7	4	–	11
Ulceration	16	4	8	28
Sacculation	–	2	12	14
Intramural gas	2	–	–	2
Spasm	10	3	–	13
Stricturing/tubular narrowing	–	–	10	10
Loss of haustration	14	4	12	30

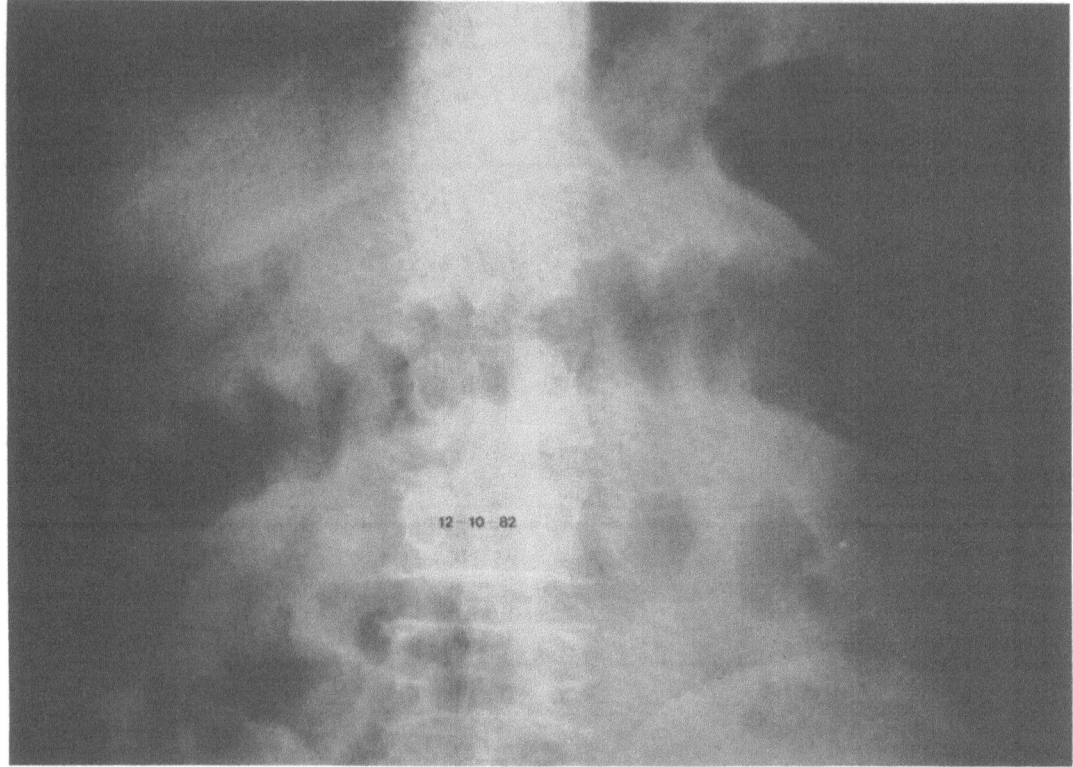

Fig. 24.1. Plain film of the abdomen in an early stage of ischaemic colitis. Multiple thumbprints are evident on the transverse colon.

After 2 weeks stricturing, ulceration and loss of haustration were most frequently found. Sacculations were found in 2 patients in the second week and in 12 patients on the barium enema after 1–3 months (75%). In table 11.1, the frequency of the different radiological signs associated with ischaemic colitis as reported in the literature and as found in our series, is compared.

Thumbprinting and ulceration were most frequently encountered, in both the literature and in our own series. There was a similar frequency of occurrence of tubular narrowing and/or stricturing, both in our own series and in the reports found in the literature.

However, we found a lower percentage of loss of haustration in our cases than has been reported elsewhere. Transverse ridging occurred in 19% of the cases in which a barium enema had been performed.

24.2 Repeat barium enema

In 30 non-operated patients from the 58 patients with positive radiological evidence for ischaemic colitis on the first barium enema, a repeat barium enema was performed.

In 3 patients the enema was performed within 2 weeks, in 12 within 2 weeks–1 month, in 3 cases between 1–3 months and in 12 cases after 3 months.

In 6 patients the radiological appearance of the colon remained unchanged after 3 months of conservative therapy. These patients were classified as having a chronic 'non resolving' ischaemic colitis. In 24 patients the colonic ischaemia had improved following conservative treatment.

24.3 Angiography

24.3.1 Number of angiographies and findings
Angiography (aortography with or without selective studies), was performed in 33 (17%) of 199

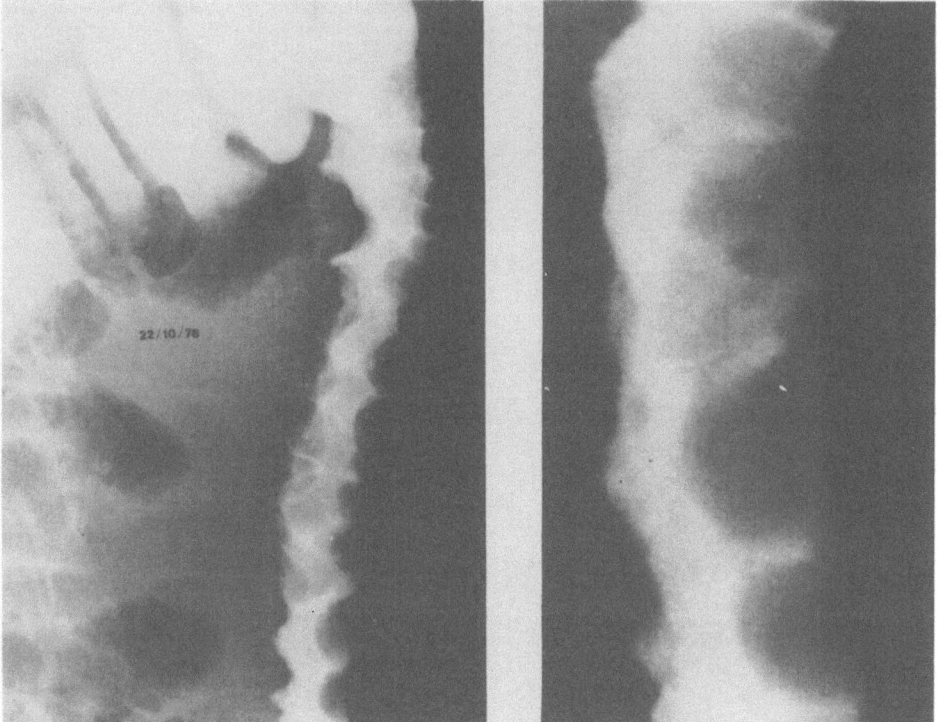

A

B

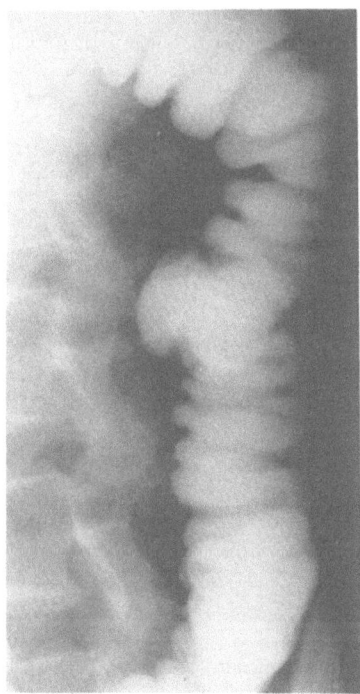

C

Fig. 24.2. (A) Early stage of transient ischaemic colitis with multiple translucent, oval or rounded filling defects extending into the lumen in the filled phase of a barium enema in the descending colon. (B) Magnification of the pseudopolyps taken from another film of the barium enema in the same patient. (C) Repeat barium enema in the same patient 3 weeks after a course of conservative treatment, shows a normal descending colon.

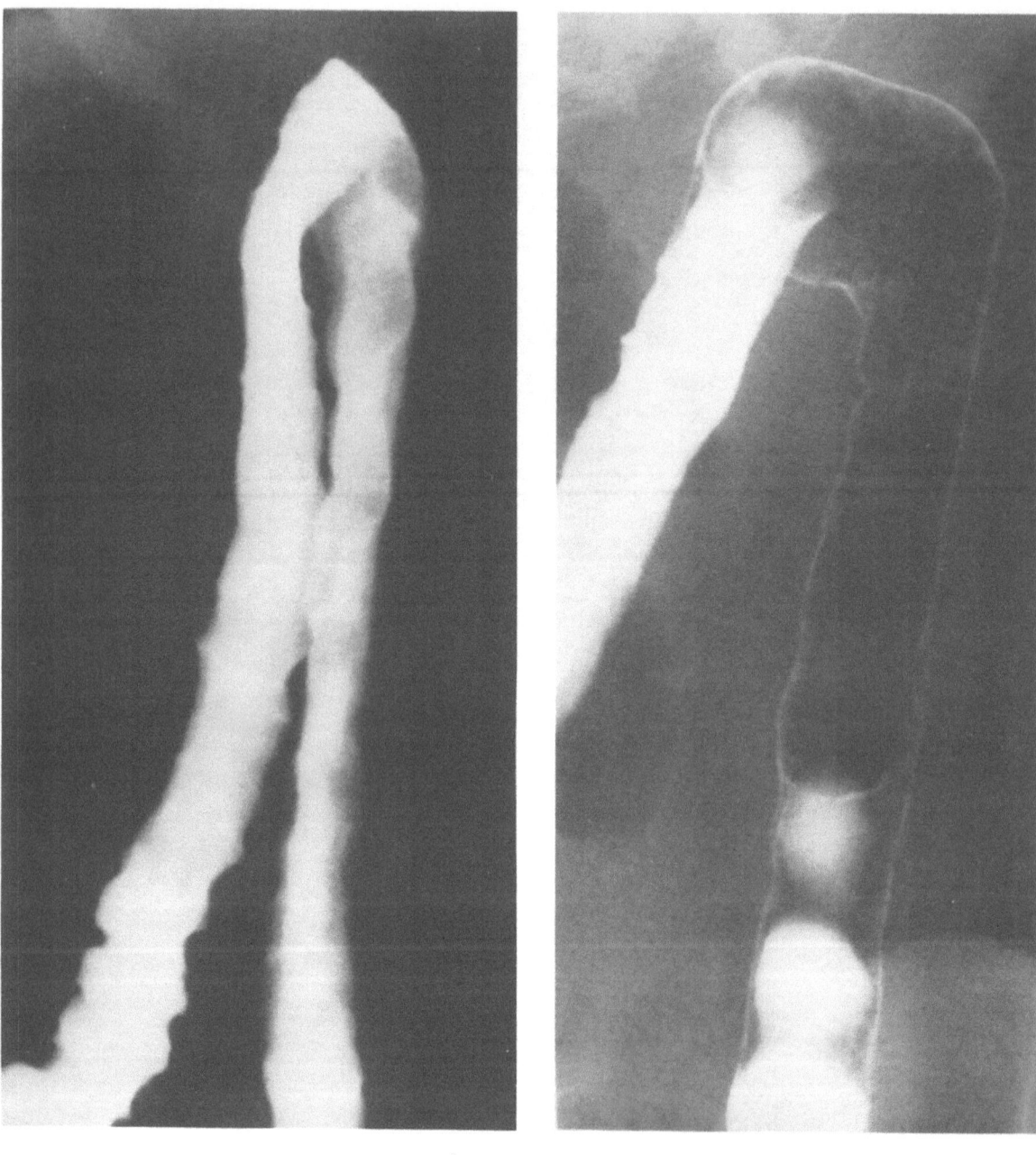

A

B

Fig. 24.3A. Thumbprinting in the region of the splenic flexure, seen during filling stage of barium enema.
Fig. 24.3B. Obliteration of thumbprinting with air-insufflation. Overlying mucosa normal.

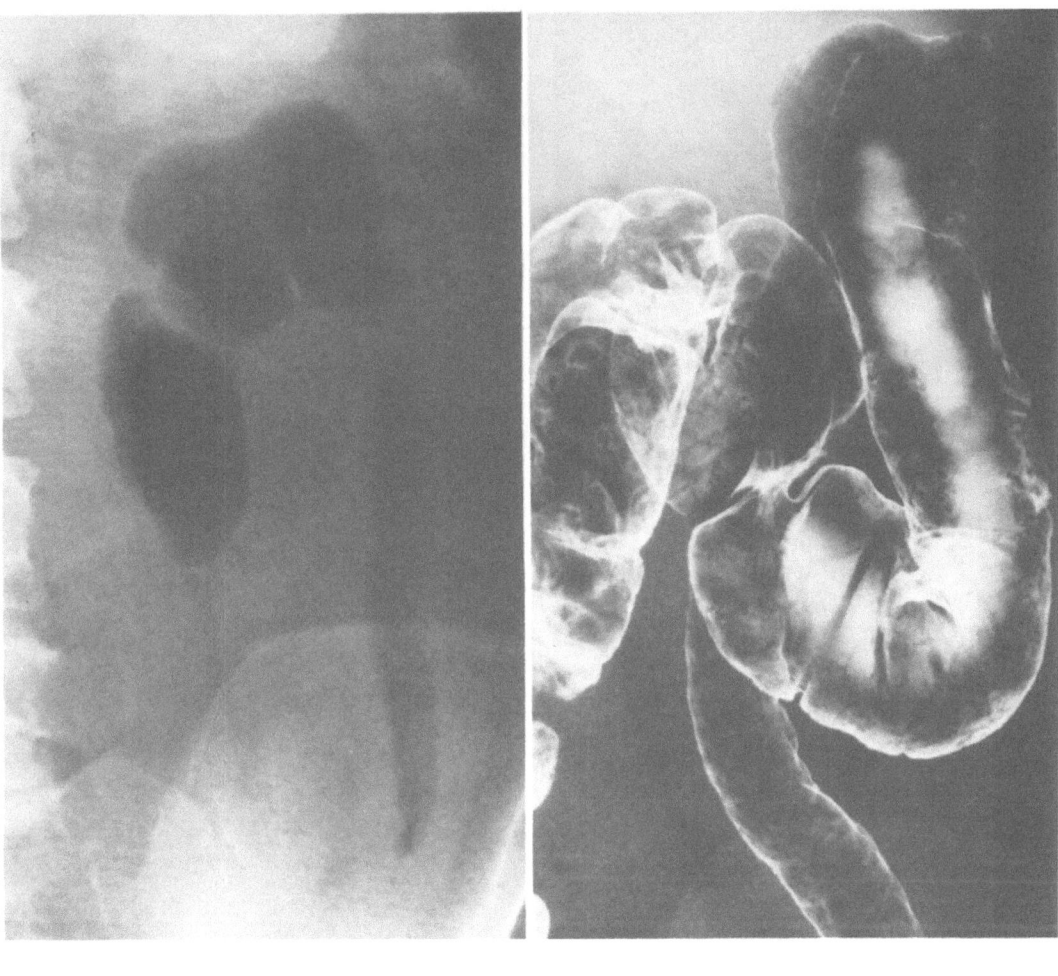

A   B

Fig. 24.4A. Plain abdominal radiograph. Thumbprinting in the descending colon.
Fig. 24.4B. Barium enema, loss of thumbprinting with air insufflation. Overlying mucosa not ulcerated.

patients with ischaemic colitis in our series.

In 7 patients only generalized atherosclerosis of aorta and mesenteric vessels without occlusion or stenosis was found. The main stem or branches of the SMA were occluded in 1 case, the IMA in 8 cases and both mesenteric vessels in 1 case, all occlusions being due to atherosclerosis or thrombosis. A stenosis of both mesenteric arteries had occurred in 4 patients. Lesions of the iliac arteries and abdominal aortic aneurysm were present in 8 patients. The angiographic findings were normal in 4 patients.

24.3.2 Pathological angiographical findings and distribution of the colonic ischaemia
The correlation between pathological angiographical findings and localisation of the ischaemic colonic segment is shown in table 24.2.

In generalized atherosclerosis the whole colon can be involved in the ischaemic process although lesions are most frequently found in the descending colon and sigmoid.

In 1 case with occlusion of the SMA ischaemic involvement of the splenic flexure only was found. In 8 cases with occlusion of the IMA the descending colon and sigmoid were the most frequently observed locations of ischaemic colitis.

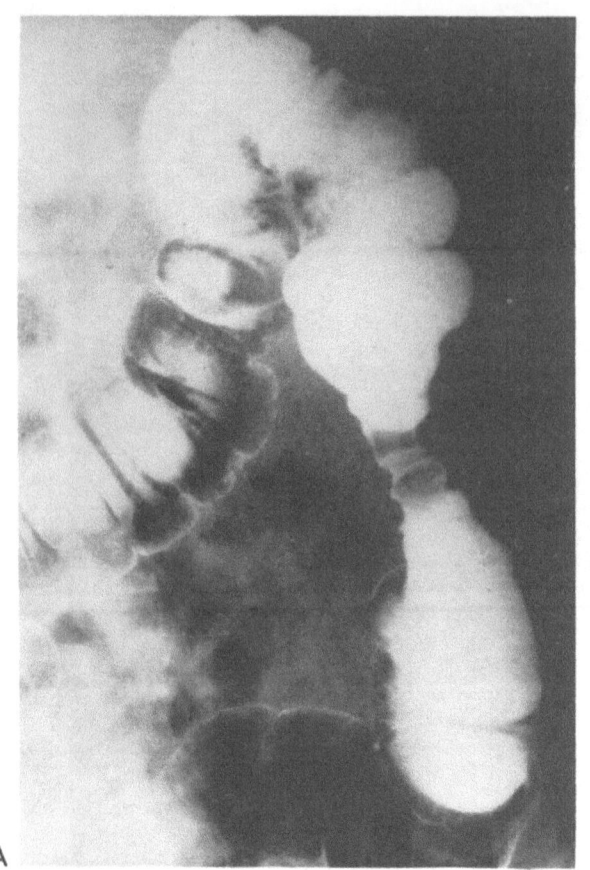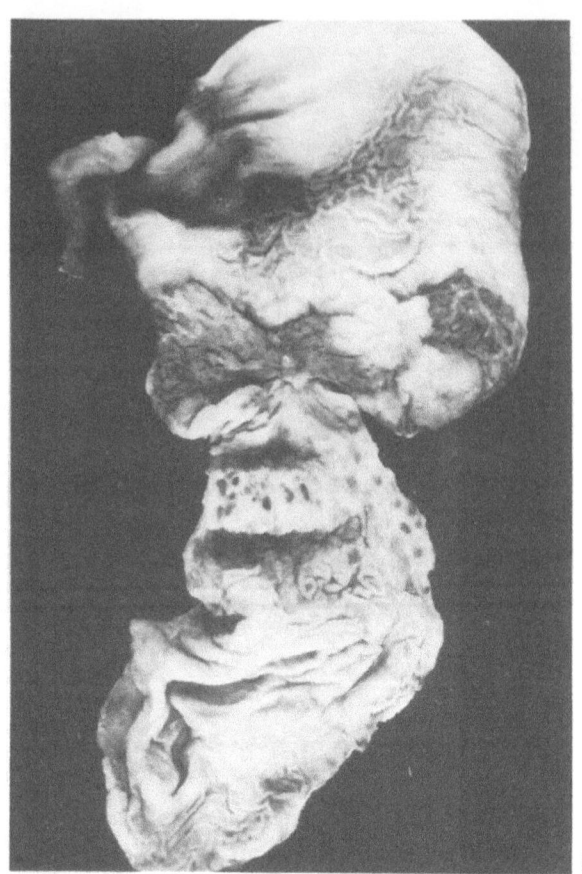

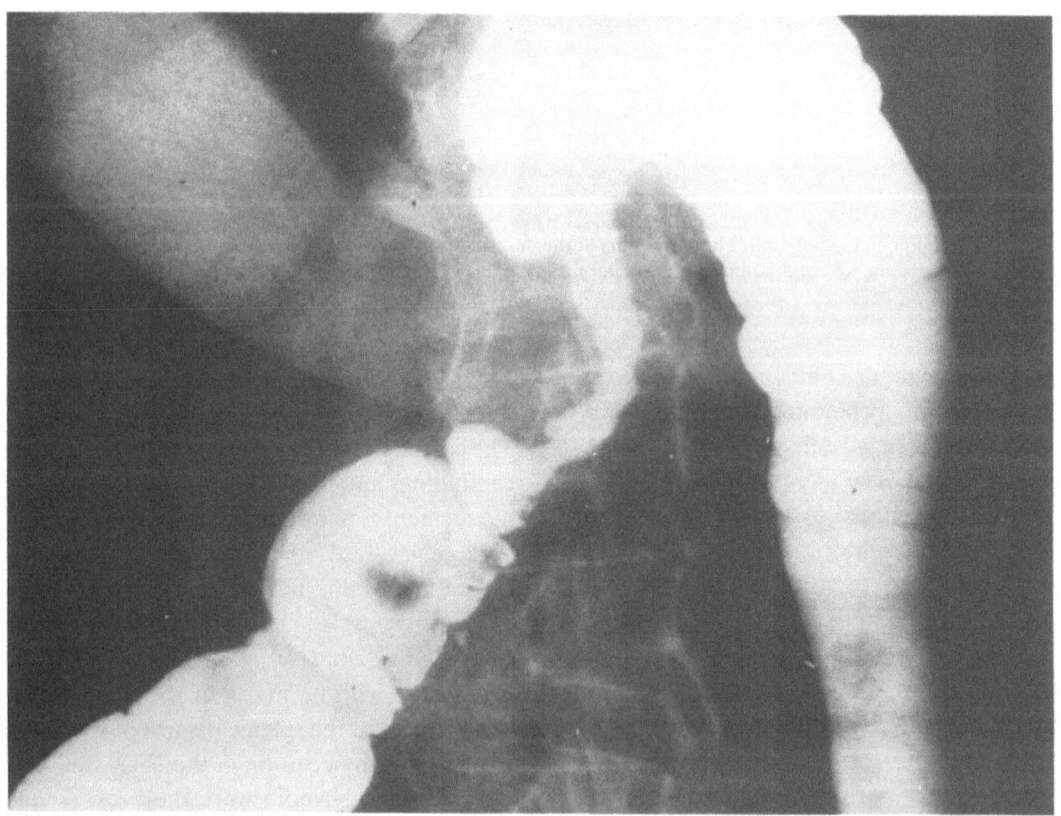

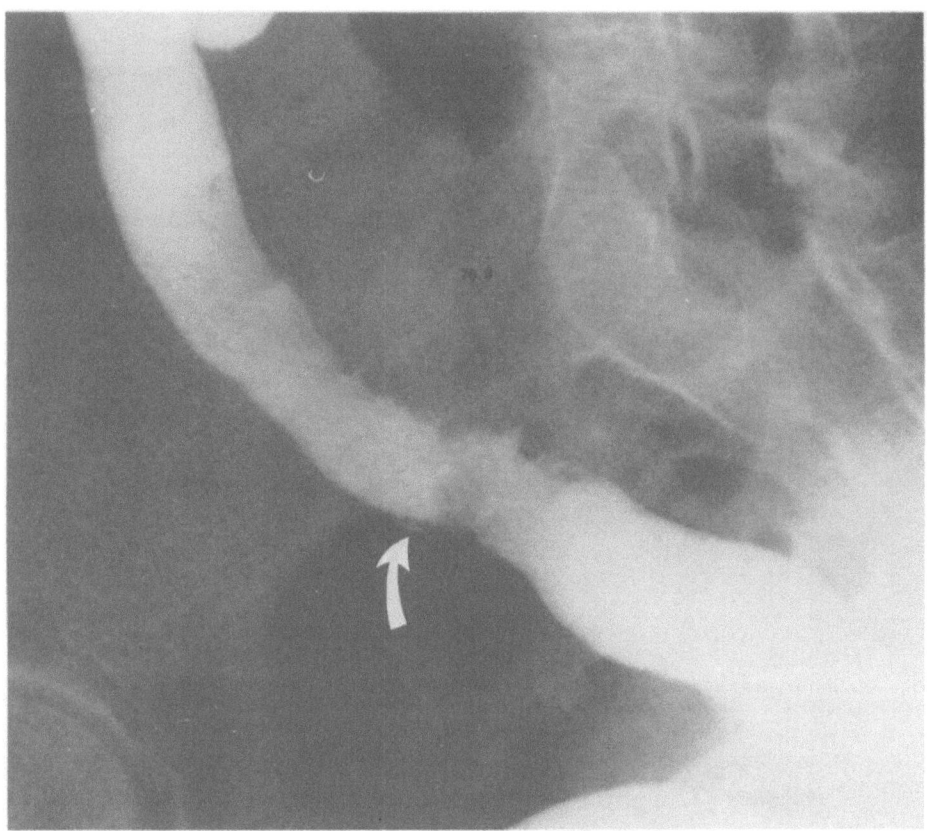

Fig. 24.7. Ischaemic colitis of the sigmoid colon in which the severely damaged submucosa has been lifted up, allowing submucosal diffusion of the barium: this is visualized as linear aggregations of barium (see arrow).

Occlusion of both the SMA and the IMA led to ischaemic involvement of the transverse colon, the splenic flexure and the descending colon in 1 case.

In 4 cases with stenosis of both the SMA and the IMA the splenic flexure, descending colon and sigmoid were the most frequently occurring sites of colonic ischaemia. In patients having lesion of the iliac arteries or abdominal aortic aneurysm, the ascending colon, the transverse colon and the sigmoid were most frequently involved in ischaemic damage.

Table 24.2. Correlation between pathological angiographic findings and different localisations of ischaemic colitis in 33 patients.

Pathological angiographic findings	Localisation of ischaemic colitis	Ascending colon	Transverse colon	Splenic flexure	Descending colon	Sigmoid	Rectum
Generalized atherosclerosis		2	2	2	4	6	2
Occlusion SMA		–	–	1	–	–	–
Occlusion IMA		1	4	4	7	8	–
Occlusion SMA + IMA		–	1	1	1	–	–
Stenosis SMA + IMA		1	2	3	3	3	–
Peripheral vascular lesions		3	4	2	2	4	1

Fig. 24.5. (A) Gradual merging of the narrowed proximal descending colon into the normal adjacent colon; this observation is referred to as 'funneling'; (B) Resected specimen of the same patient shows more widespread ischaemic damage. The stricturing is shorter than in the initially involved segment.

Fig. 24.6. Sharply demarcated merging of the narrowed ischaemic distal transverse colon into the normal adjacent colon in a female patient, 2 months after the acute onset of symptoms indicative of ischaemic colits.

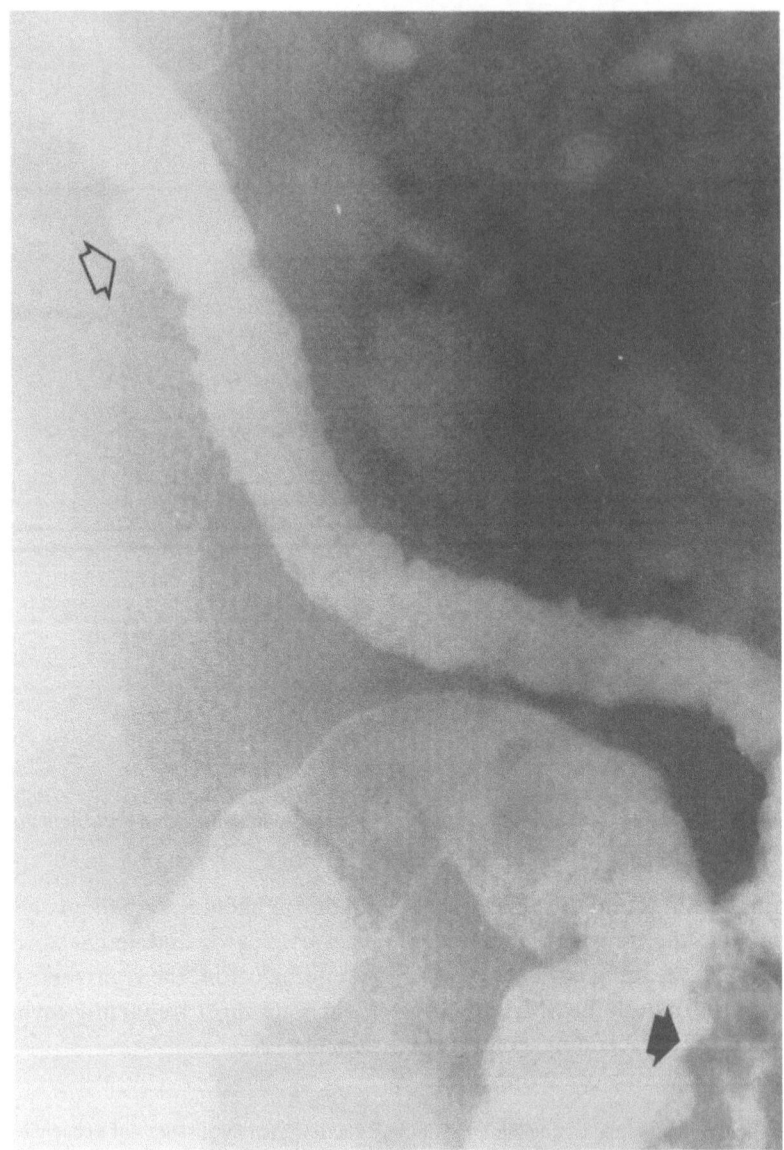

Fig. 24.8. Female patient, 78 years of age, with ischaemic colitis of the left colon proximal to an annular carcinoma of the sigmoid. A double decompression transversostomy had been performed. Barium enema administered via a distal transverse colostomy shows 'dissection of barium' within the damaged mucosa of the ischaemic segment of the descending colon (white arrow). Note the stricturing process in the sigmoid (black arrow).

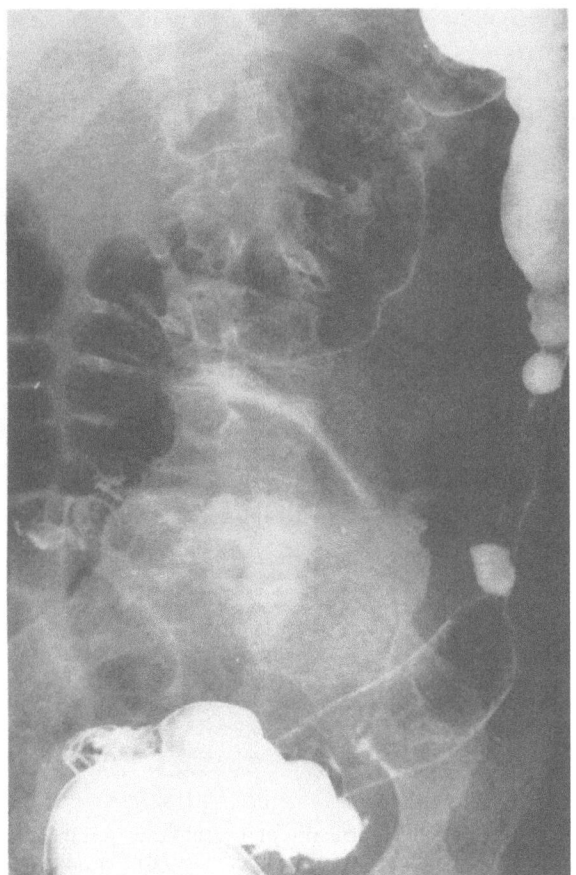

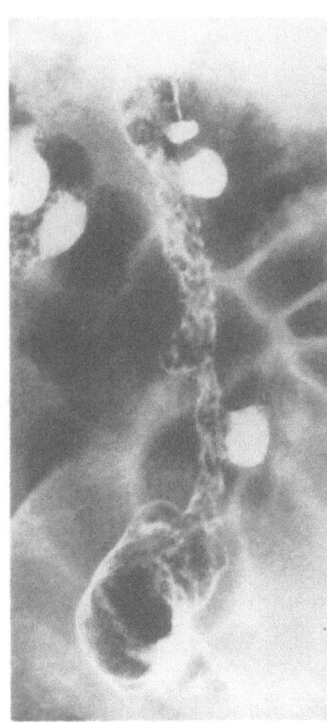

Fig. 24.9(A/B). Multiple shallow, wide mouthed outpouchings or pseudodiverticula of the descending colonic wall on the anti-mesenteric side, 4 months after the first symptoms, which were suggestive for ischaemic colitis.

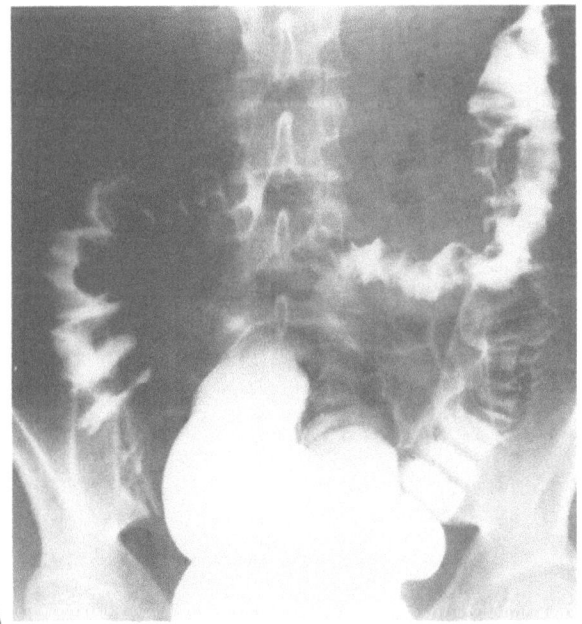

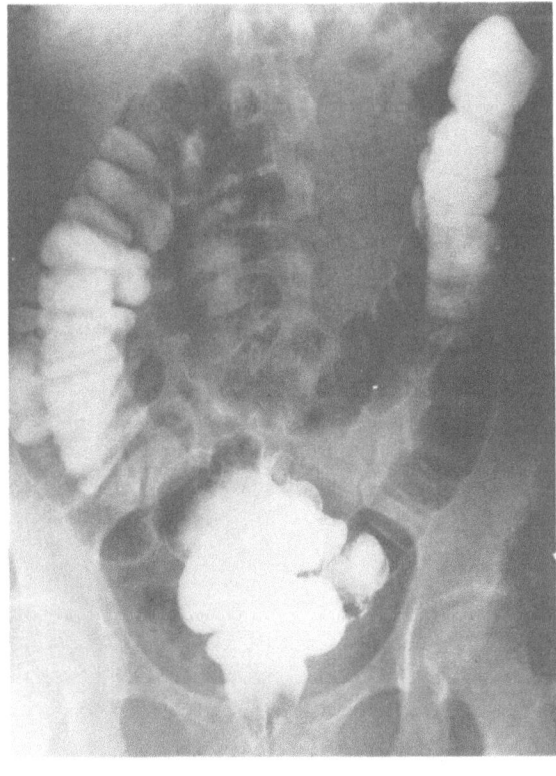

Fig. 24.10. (A) 'Evanescent ischaemic colitis' of the ascending-, transverse- and descending colon in a young 18 years old female. (B) A repeat double contrast barium enema in the same patient, 3 weeks after conservative treatment, showed a normal colon without any sequelae.

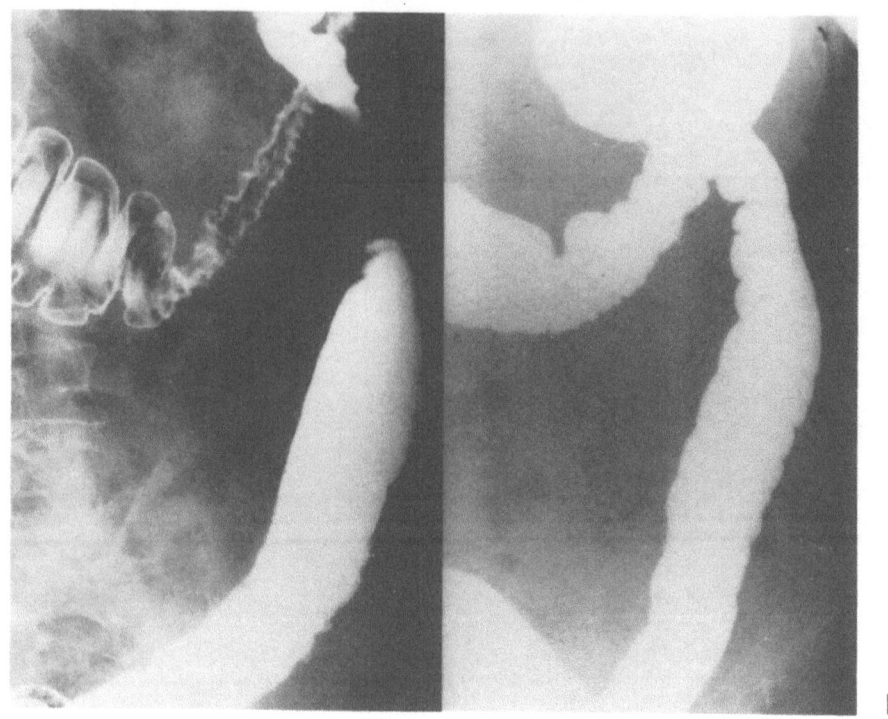

A   B

Fig. 24.11. (A) Progressive stage of transient ischaemic colitis with 'ragged saw tooth irregularity' of the (sub)mucosa at the distal transverse colon, splenic flexure and proximal descending colon, as a result of diffuse superficial ulceration. (B) Repeat barium enema in the same patient, 5 weeks after conservative treatment. The colon mucosa is normalized.

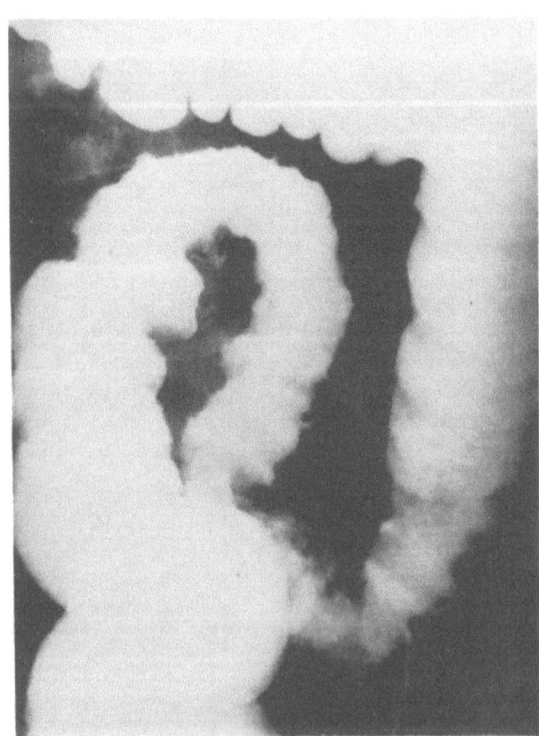

Fig. 24.12. Fine ulcerations at the sigmoid colon, 2 weeks after this patient presented with acute onset of symptoms, suspect for ischaemic colitis. Endoscopy and biopsies were positive for colonic ischaemia.

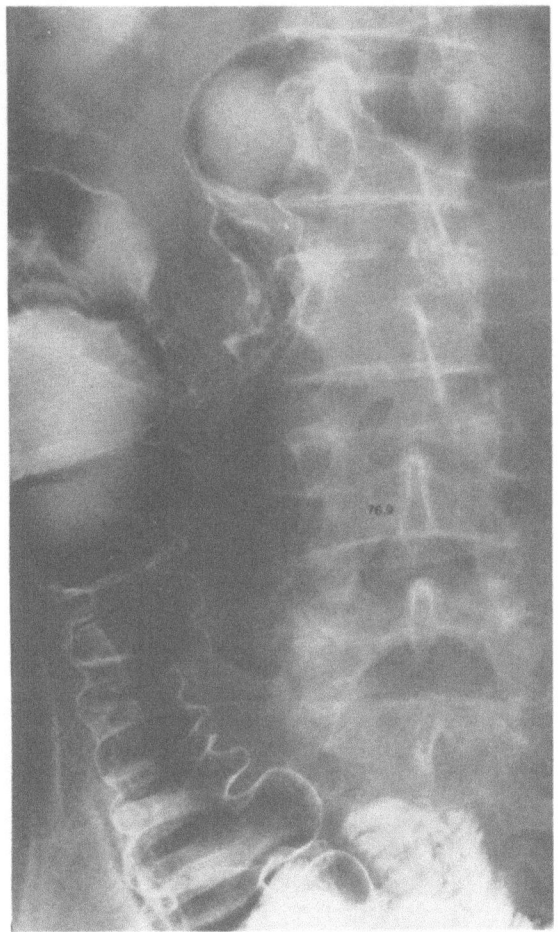

A

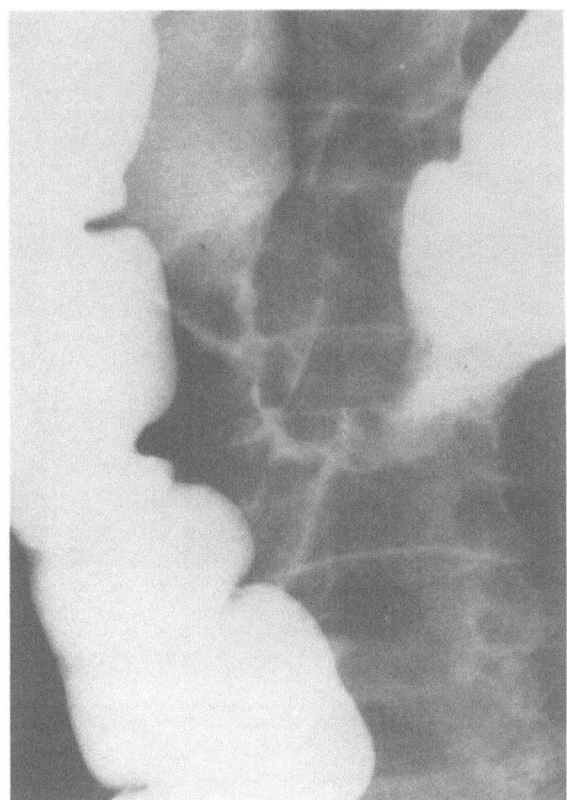

B

Fig. 24.13. (A) Early stage of transient right-sided colonic ischaemia of unknown aetiopathogenic origin. Thumbprinting and
narrowing due to spasm can be seen at the hepatic flexure and
proximal transverse colon. (B) Magnification of the ischaemic
segment in the filled phase.

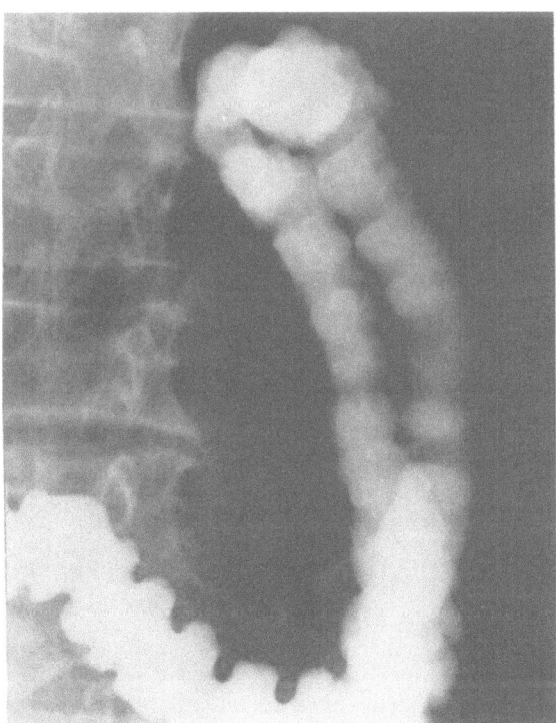

Fig. 24.14. 'Transverse ridging' at the distal transverse colon,
the splenic flexure and the proximal descending colon, due to
deep transverse contractions, running perpendicular to the colonic axis.

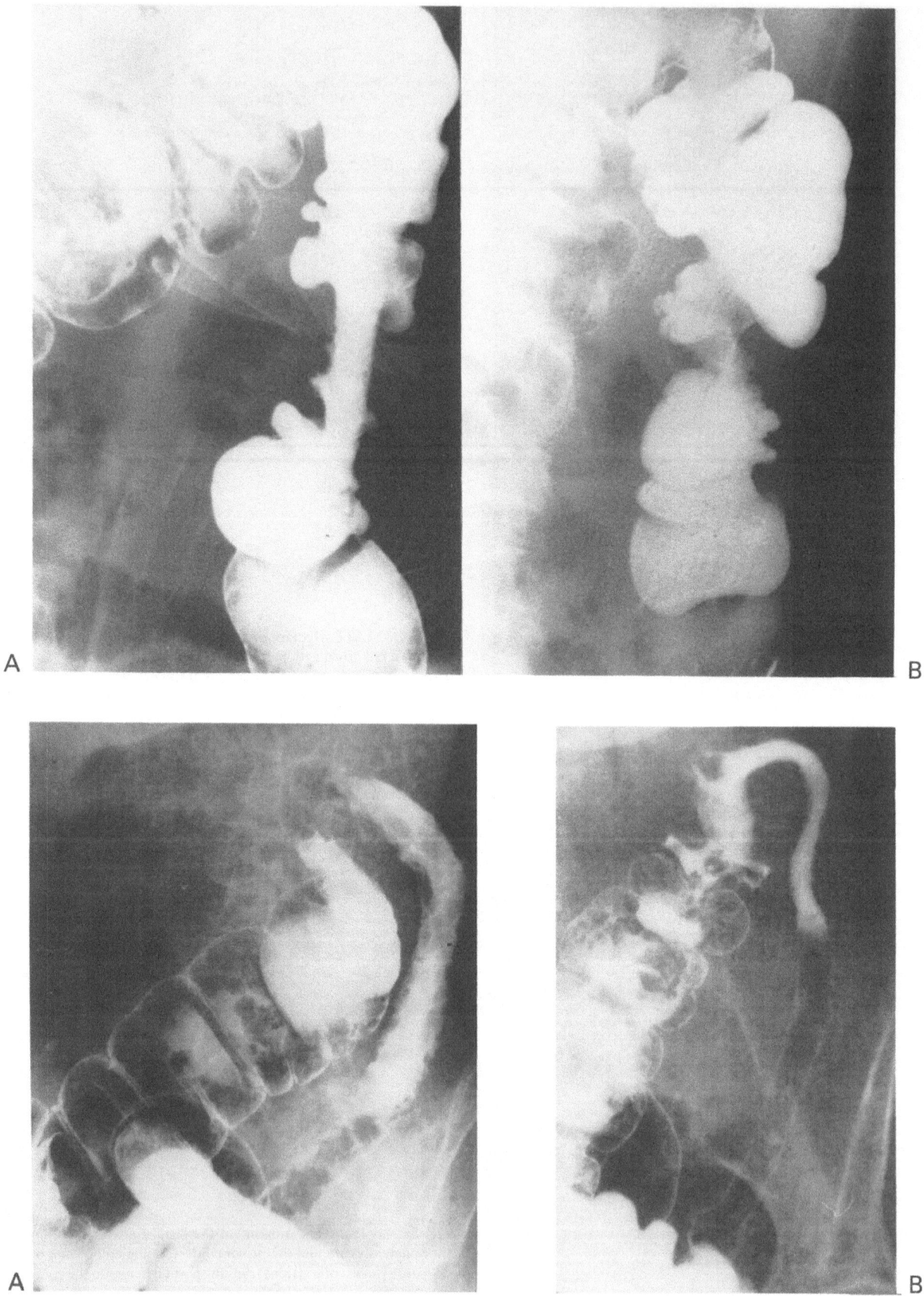

A

B

A

B

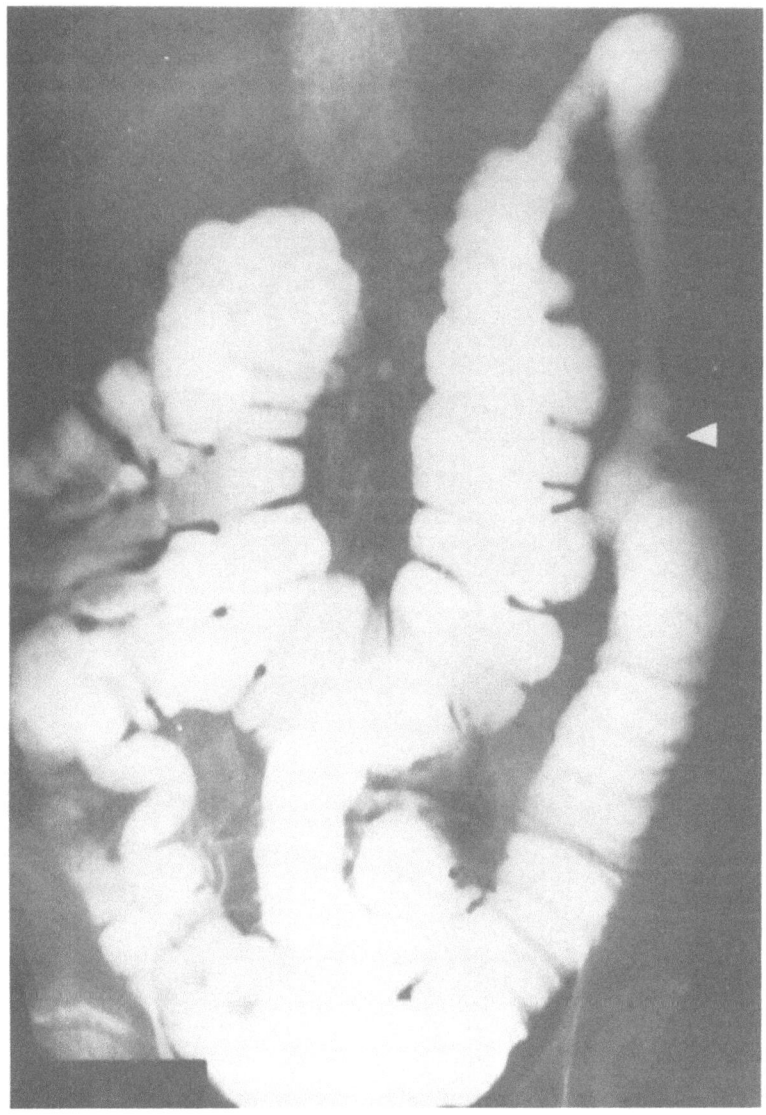

Fig. 24.17. Tubular narrowing of the splenic flexure and proximal descending colon with onset of sacculae formation on the antimesenteric side (see white arrow), 3 months after the acute onset of the ischaemic colonic episode.

Fig. 24.15. (A) Ischaemic stricture at the proximal descending colon, 4 weeks after acute onset of abdominal crampy pain, nausea, vomiting and rectal bleeding. (B) Follow-up double contrast barium enema in the same patient performed 6 months after a course of conservative treatment, shows stricturing at the proximal descending colon. Clinically there were no indications of dilatation and/or obstruction.

Fig. 24.16. (A) Barium enema in an early stage of ischaemic colitis, shows multiple thumbprints and narrowing due to spasm at the splenic flexure and descending colon. (B) Tubular narrowing and stricturing as final stages of ischaemic colitis, due to progressive fibrosis and (sub)mucosal reorganisation, can develop 3 weeks to 12 months after the onset of colon ischaemia. Repeat double contrast barium enema in the same patient, performed 4 weeks after conservative treatment, shows tubular narrowing at the splenic flexure and descending colon.

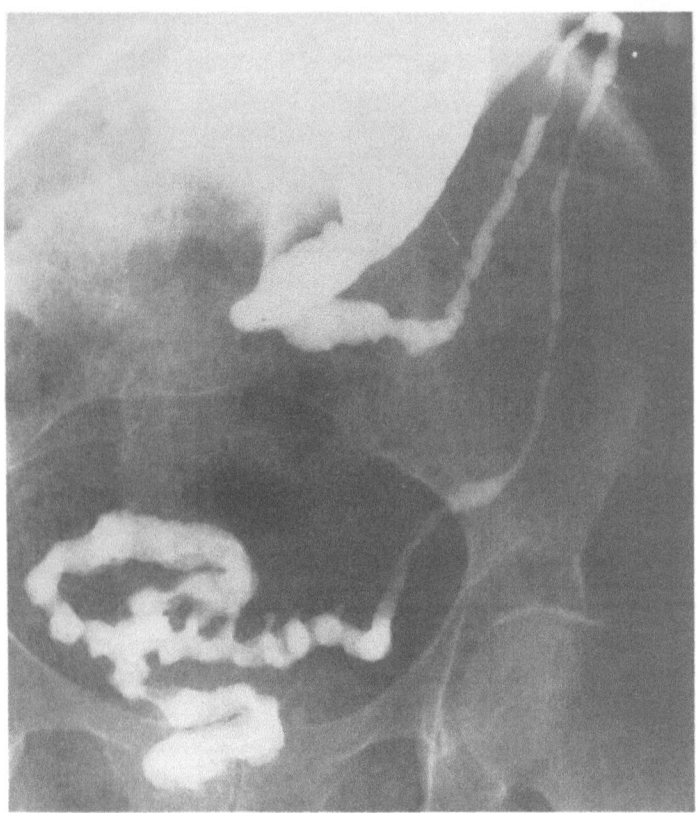

Fig. 24.18. Late stage of chronic 'non resolving' ischaemic colitis visualized after anterograde introduction of contrast agent via distal colostomy at the transverse colon.

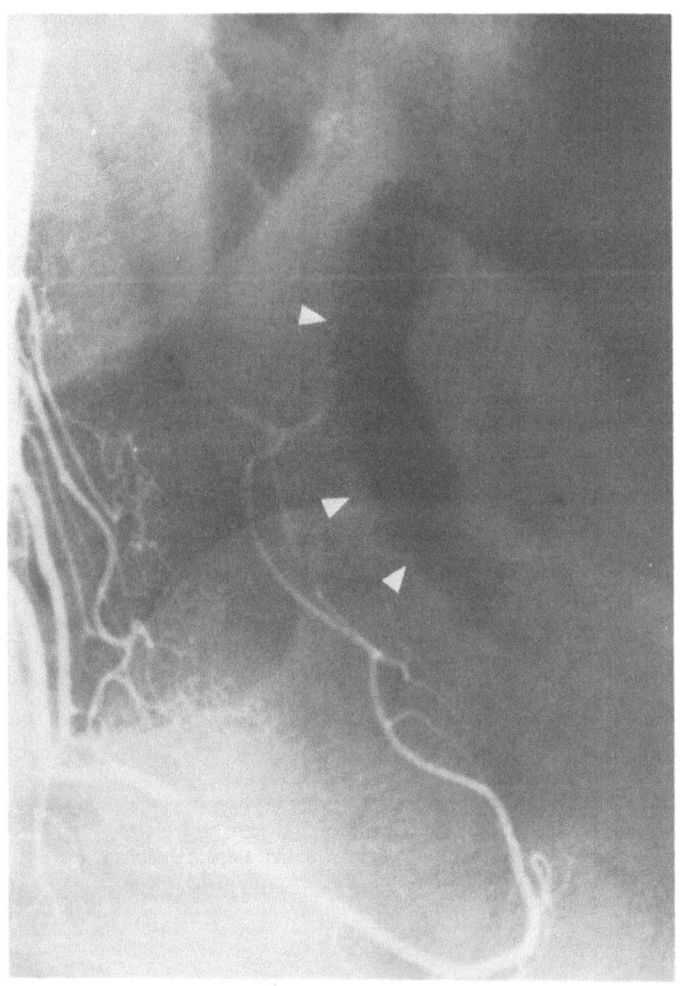

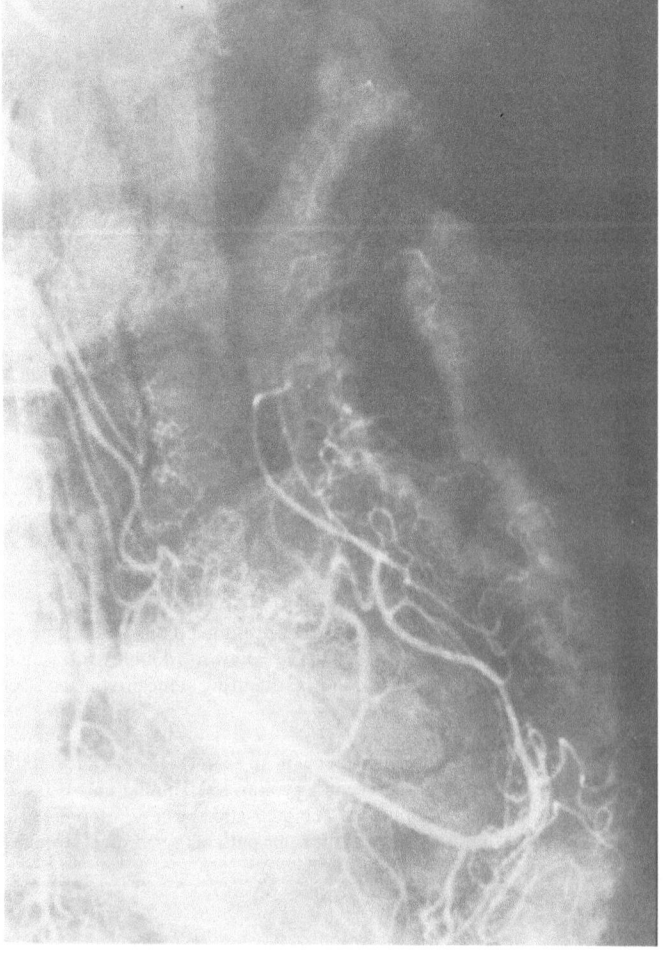

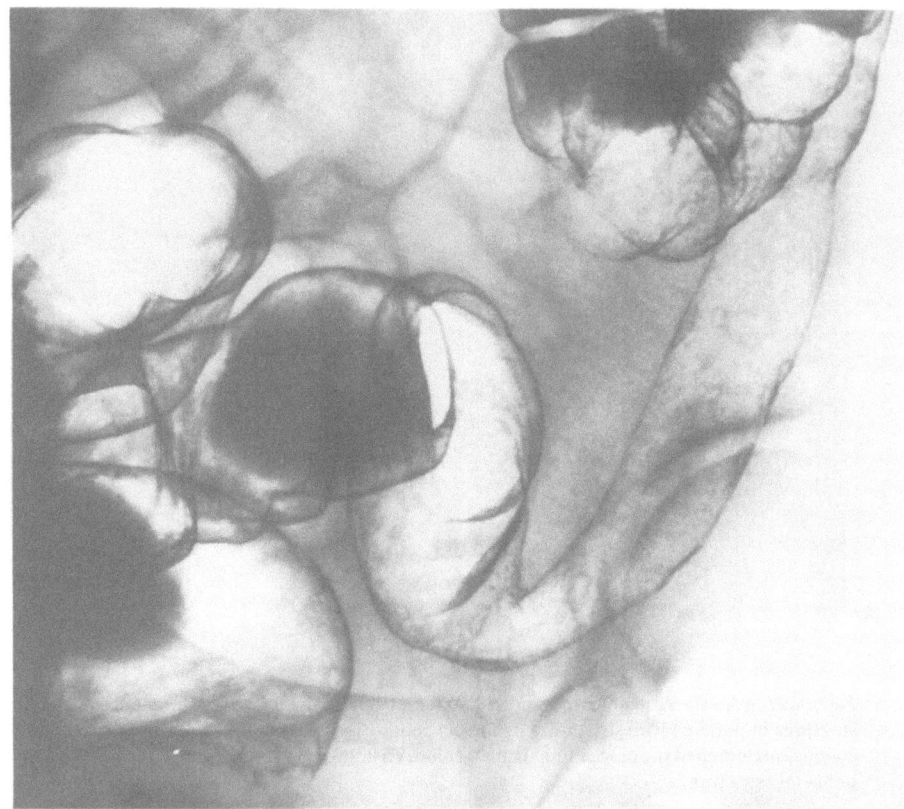

Fig. 24.20. Ischaemic colitis in a 54-year-old female who had a sudden onset of abdominal pain and rectal bleeding. A supine double contrast view shows narrowing of the distal descending colon and granularity of the mucosa suggestive of the colonic surface covered with regenerated epithelia. The histological section was reported as showing occlusion of an arteriole under the subserosal layer.

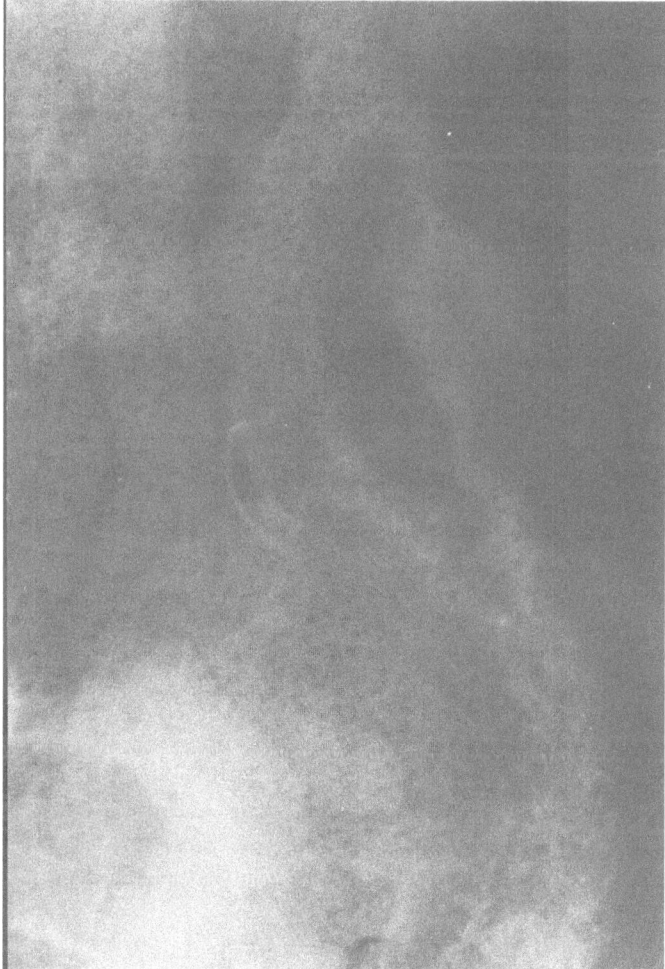

Fig. 24.19. (A, B, C) Arteriography in the early stage of colonic ischaemia usually does not show arterial or venous occlusion, but rather a paradoxical hypervascularity of the bowel wall and early venous opacification, as shown in this case. Note the thumbprints in the descending colon (see arrow heads).

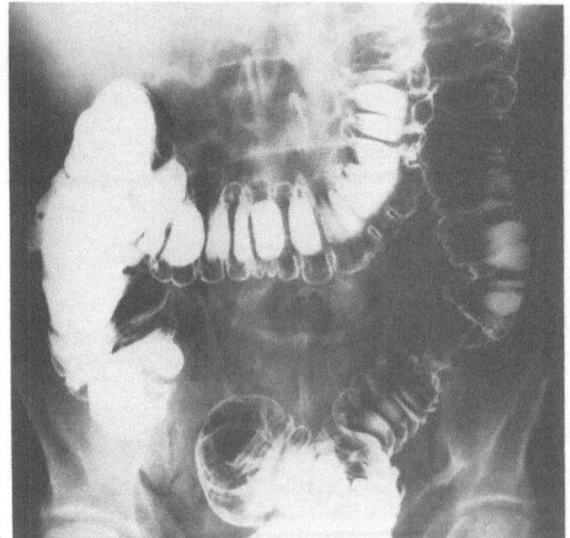
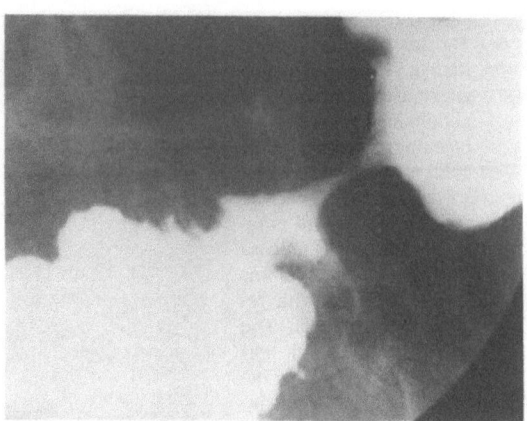

Fig. 24.21. (A+B) A major problem that may not be resolved by barium enema examination is the precise identification of strictures in patients with stricturing ischaemic colitis. This patient had been operated upon following a provisional diagnosis of colonic carcinoma of the descending sigmoid colon. Histological examination of the resected colon specimen revealed a benign post-ischaemic stricture.

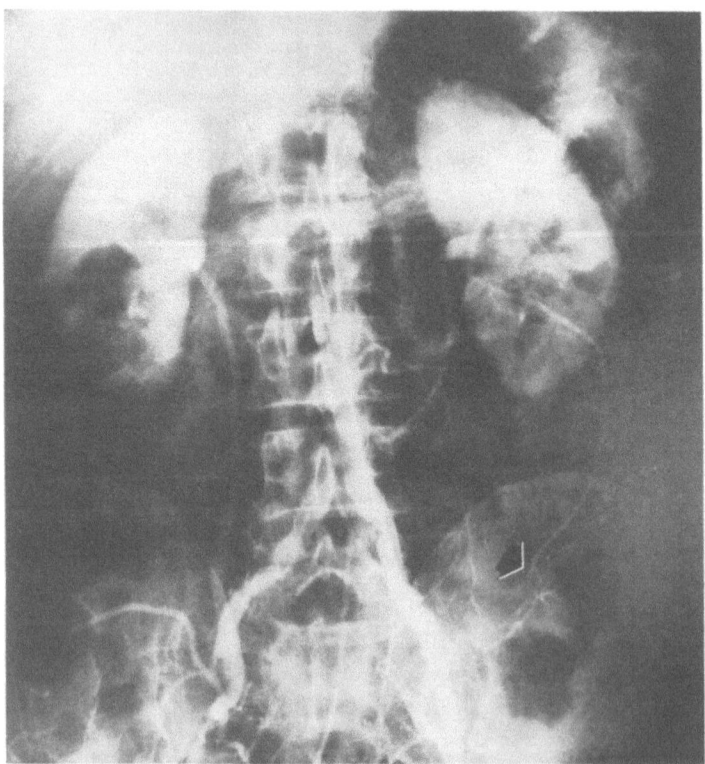

Fig. 24.22. Angiography in the same patient shows generalized atherosclerosis, occlusion of both right iliac arteries and a thrombotic occlusion in the distal course of the colosigmoid artery (see arrow).

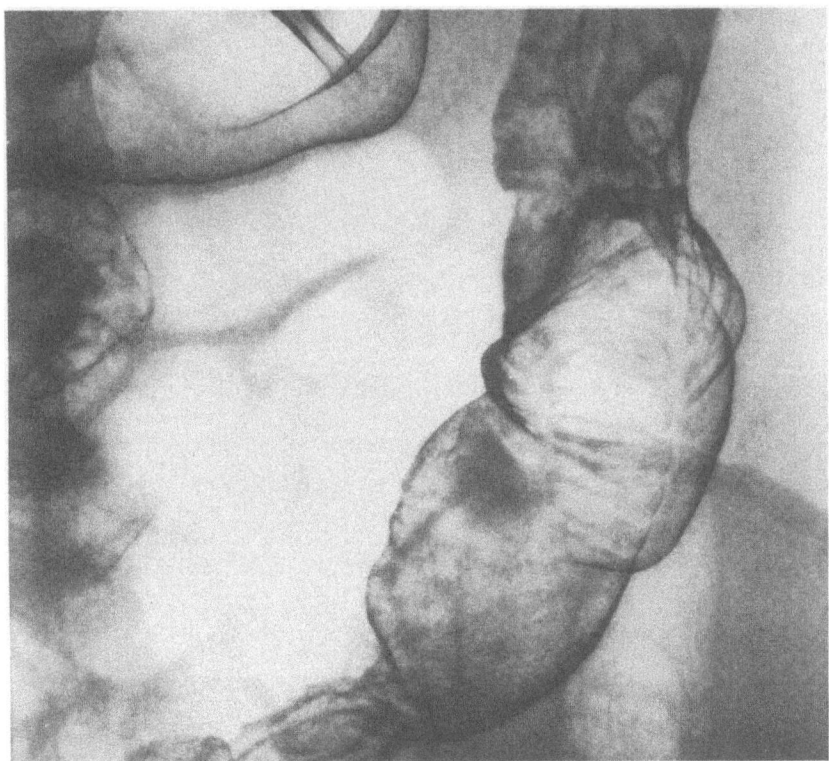

Fig. 24.23. Ischaemic colitis in a 45-year-old female who had rectal bleeding and abdominal pain 2 months prior to the barium enema examination. A supine double contrast view shows a faint linear ulceration with radiating mucosal folds in the sigmoid colon.

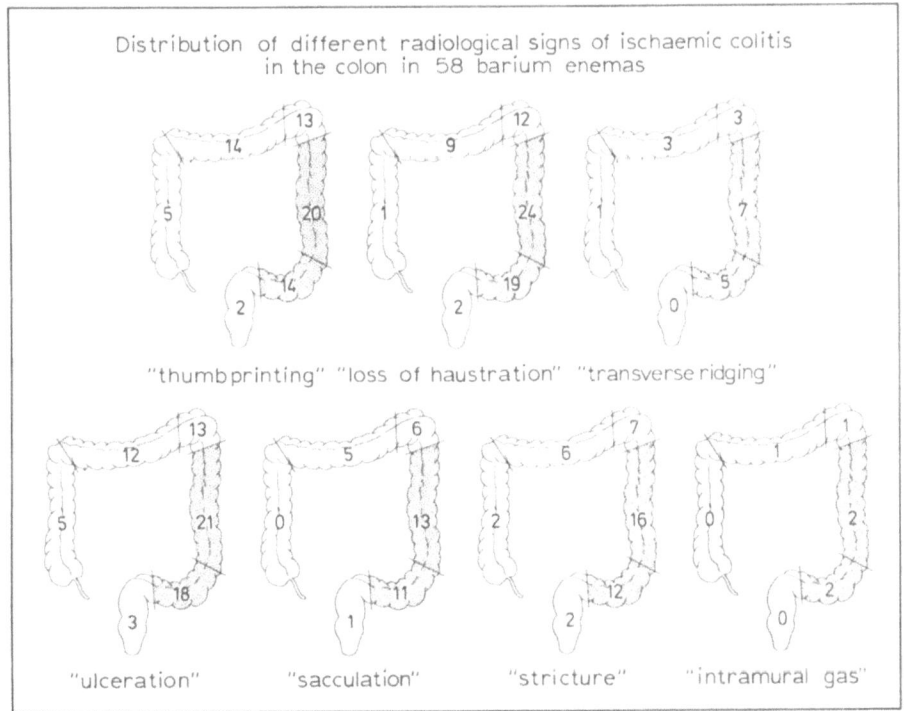

Fig. 24.24. Colonic distribution of different radiological signs of ischaemic colitis at the time of the barium enema: The distribution of the different radiological signs of ischaemic colitis in 58 barium enemas is shown in Fig. 24.24. All signs were most frequently found on the left side, e.g. the descending colon and sigmoid.

25. ENDOSCOPY IN DIAGNOSIS OF ISCHAEMIC COLITIS

25.1 *Number of endoscopies*

25.2 *Endoscopical features and time of performing endoscopy*
  Oedema/harmorrhage (bulbous protrusions)
  Ulceration
  Reepithelialisation
  Spasm
  Tubular narrowing and/or stricturing
  Sacculation

25.3 *Correlation between features revealed by endoscopy and different forms of ischaemic colitis*

25.4 *The anatomical distribution of features observed at endoscopy which were considered to be diagnostic for ischaemic colitis*

25.5 *Repeat colonoscopy*

25.1 Number of endoscoples

In our retrospective study of 199 patients a colonoscopy was performed in 39 patients (20%) (20 men and 19 women). No correlation could be made between the endoscopical and radiological features of ischaemic colitis in most cases because the time interval between the barium enemas and the colonoscopies was too long.

25.2 Endoscopical features and time of performing endoscopy

Table 25.1 represents the correlation between the different endoscopical features and the time interval between the onset of symptoms and the time of performing the colonoscopy. In 16 cases the endoscopy was performed in the first week, in 3 cases in the second week, and in 20 cases more than 2 weeks after the onset of symptoms.

Oedema, haemorrhage (bulbous protrusions) were found in 88% of cases in which endoscopy has been performed in the first week, in 67% where endoscopy was performed in the second week and in 25% where endoscopy was performed 2 weeks after onset of symptoms.

Table 25.1. Correlation between different features of ischaemic colitis revealed by endoscopy and the time interval between the onset of symptoms and time of performing a colonoscopy.

Endoscopical features \ Time interval between onset of symptoms and endoscopy	1–7 days	8–14 days	>14 days	Total number of patients
Number of endoscopies	16	3	20	39
Oedema - haemorrhage (bulbous protrusions)	14	2	5	21
Ulceration ± haemorrhage	4	3	14	21
Reepithelialisation	3	2	8	13
Spasm	3	–	–	3
Tubular narrowing/stricturing	–	–	7	7
Sacculation	–	–	2	2

114

→

Fig. 25. 1a Bleeding from the more proximal colonic segment, due to ischaemic damage. 1b Coarse nodular bloody elevations (corresponding to 'thumbprinting') due to extensive mucosal and submucosal bleeding during the early phase of ischaemic damage. 2a Abrupt transition from normal intestinal mucosa to extensively ulcerated large intestine. Extensive sloughing of the mucosal lining has occurred due to ischaemic damage. 2b Tiny haemorrhagic mucosal blebs surrounded by superficial sloughing of the mucosa. 3a Area of superficial ulceration with tiny remaining mucosal islands; reepithelialisation will start from such remaining healthy mucosa. 3b The superficial ulcerations are irregular serpiginous in shape and are surrounded initially by oedematous friable mucosa. 4a Characteristic extensive superficial ulceration due to ischaemic damage. Note that part of the circumference is lined with mucosa of normal appearance. 4b Small remaining mucosal island in the center of a large ulceration during early reepithelialisation. 5 Later stage of colonic ischaemia. Tiny mucosal sprouts become visible in a previously completely ulcerated area, indicating the process of reepithelialisation and repair. 6 Early stricturing after ischaemic damage with obvious remaining ulceration. 7 Detail of ischaemic stricture with ulceration limited to the narrowed zone. 8 Late scarring with intersecting fine whitish lines.

Ulceration with or without haemorrhage was present in 25% of first week endoscopies; in 66% of second week endoscopies and in 70% endoscopies performed after 2 weeks.

Reepithelialisation had occurred in 19% of endoscopies carried out in the first week, in 60% of those performed in the second week, and in 70% of those performed 2 weeks after onset of symptoms.

Spasm was found in 19% of the cases in which endoscopy was performed in the first week.

Tubular narrowing and/or stricturing had occurred in 35% of cases in which endoscopy was performed after 2 weeks.

In 2 patients endoscopy was performed after 2 weeks and showed shallow 'diverticular-like' outpouchings of the colonic wall, which were con-sidered to be synonymous with the *sacculations* observed by radiography.

25.3 Correlation between features revealed by endoscopy and different forms of ischaemic colitis

Table 25.2 shows the correlation between the features of ischaemic colitis as revealed at endoscopy and the different forms of ischaemic colitis in 39 patient. 20 endoscopies were performed in the transient (mucosal) group; 8 in each of the stricturing (mural) group and the chronic (mural) 'non resolving' ischaemic colitis group and 3 in the gangrenous (transmural) group.
Oedema/haemorrhage (bulbous protrusions) and ulceration were most frequently found in the transient (mucosal) group (80% and 60% of the cases respectively), while ulceration and reepithelialisation were most commonly seen in chronic (mural)

Table 25.2. Correlation between features of ischaemic colitis revealed by endoscopy and the different types of ischaemic colitis in 39 patients.

Different types of ischaemic colitis	Mucosal form	Mural form	Mural form	Transmural form	Total number of patients
Endoscopical features	Transient ischaemic colitis	Stricturing ischaemic colitis	Chronic 'non resolving' ischaemic colitis	Gangrenous ischaemic colitis ± perforation	
Total number of endoscopies	20	8	8	3	39
Oedema - haemorrhage (bulbous protrusions)	16	3	–	2	21
Ulceration ± haemorrhage	12	3	6	–	21
Reepithelialisation	3	5	5	–	13
Spasm	3	–	–	–	3
Tubular narrowing stricturing	–	6	–	1	7
Sacculation	–	2	–	–	2

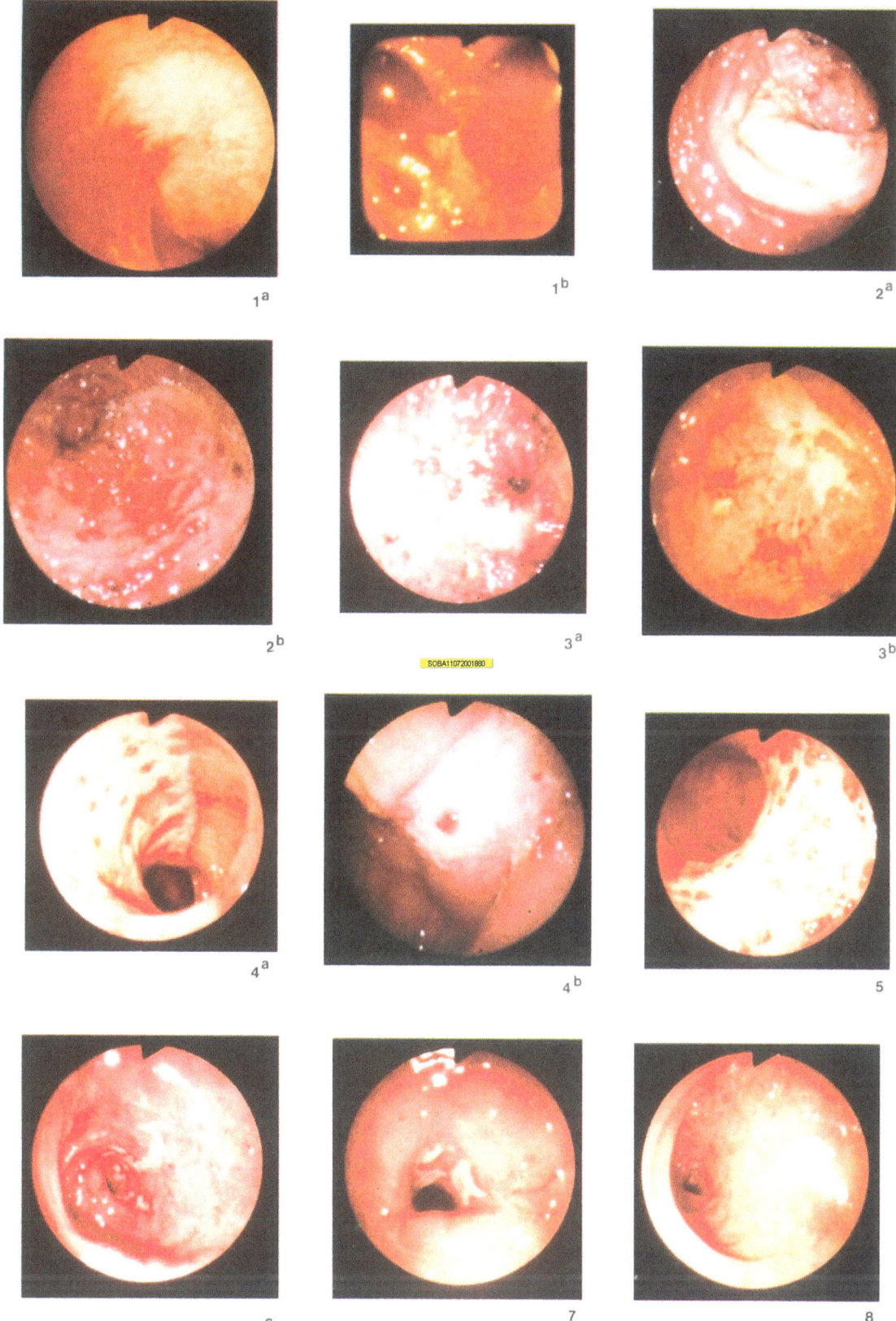

116

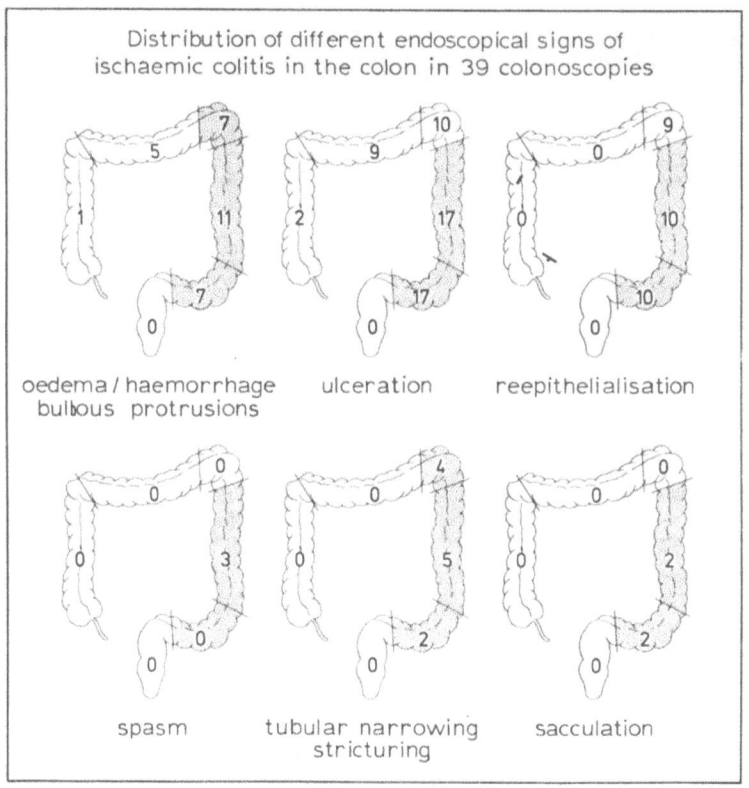

Fig. 25.9.

'non resolving' ischaemic colitis, (75% and 63% of the cases respectively).

In 6 cases (75%) a tubular narrowing or stricture was observed endoscopically in the stricturing mural form.

25.4 The anatomical distribution of features observed at endoscopy which were considered to be diagnostic for ischaemic colitis

Although in a retrospective study it is difficult to describe the distribution of the lesions observed at colonoscopy – frequently because of a lack of detailed description – it seemed useful to construct a map, to show the distribution of different signs of ischaemic colitis in the colon in 39 well documented colonoscopies. Figure 25.9 shows that most lesions observed at endoscopy were located in the left half of the colon; this corresponds with observations made following the performance of barium enemas as described in chapter 24.

25.5 Repeat colonoscopy

In 26 cases a follow-up colonoscopy, following conservative treatment, was performed (14 men and 12 women); 8 were carried out within 2 weeks of the first colonoscopy, 4 between 2 weeks–1 month, 6 between 1–3 months, and 8 3 months following the first colonoscopy. In 6 patients the second endoscopy revealed that the ischaemic colonic damage was unchanged when compared with the observations at first colonoscopy, the ischaemic damage was diminished in 19 patients, and had become more severe in 1 patient.

26. HISTOPATHOLOGY OF ISCHAEMIC COLITIS

26.1 Introduction

Because of increasing interest in inflammatory diseases of the large bowel, histopathology has attained more importance in its diagnosis and management.

The clinician faced with the differential diagnosis between ulcerative colitis and other inflammatory conditions of the colon, in particular Crohn's disease and ischaemic colitis, will rely increasingly on the expert interpretation of colonic histopathological material.

Especially the chronic 'non resolving' form of ischaemic colitis may mimick other chronic ulcerative conditions of the colon. In several instances such lesions had been interpreted as ulcerative- or granulomatous colitis, which resulted in inappropriate therapy being given to the patient.

Our selection procedure (51% of our material came from autopsy studies) tends to skew the patient representation into the more severe end of the spectrum of ischaemic colitis. However, this in-depth study of these more severe cases will hopefully improve our understanding of this illness and lead to a better patient management.

26.2 Histopathological material.

The histological material was collected from various hospitals in the Netherlands as shown in table 26.1.

Histological examination was performed on 82 resected colon specimens (96 laparotomies: in 14 cases no colonic resection had been performed): 108 autopsy studies (of the 127 patients who died, autopsy had been refused in 19 cases) and 32 biopsies (Table 26.2).

In 53 cases the colonic resection had been performed within 1–7 days following the onset of clinical symptoms; in 9 patients the colon had been resected between the 8th and the 14th day and in 20 cases after more than 2 weeks. In 46 cases the autopsy had been performed between 1–7 days after the onset of clinical symptoms; in 14 cases between the 8th and the 14th day and in 48 cases after 2 weeks. Biopsies were taken in the first week after the onset of clinical symptoms in 13 cases;

118

Table 26.1. Number of patients with (histologically checked) ischaemic colitis and the different hospitals of origin.

Rotterdam, the Netherlands	*	**	Amsterdam, the Netherlands	*	**
Sint Franciscus Gasthuis	52	52	Academic Medical Centre		
'Eudokia' Hospital	12	12	(Wilhelmina Gasthuis, Binnengasthuis)	25	22
Bergweg Hospital	20	20	Academic Hospital		
Academic Hospital 'Dijkzigt'	8	7	Free University (AZVU)	19	18
'Van Dam-Bethesda Hospital	4	4	Stichting Hospital 'Amstelveen'	2	–
'Zuider' Hospital	3	–	Burgerhospital	2	–
			Prinsengrachthospital	1	–
			Andreas Hospital	4	4
			Onze Lieve Vrouwen Gasthuis	4	–
	99	95		57	44

Delft, the Netherlands	*	**	Other different hospitals in the Netherlands	*	**
O.N. Gasthuis	3	3	Academic Hospital 'Utrecht' (AZU)	3	–
Bethelhospital	3	3	St. Elisabeth Gasthuis, Haarlem	4	2
St. Hippolytus Hospital	4	4	St. Radboud University Hospital, Nijmegen	4	3
	10	10	Canisius-Wilhelmina Hospital, Nijmegen	3	2
Belgium	*	**	St. Elisabeth Hospital, Amersfoort	2	–
St. Raphaël Hospital, Leuven	3	–	Medical Centre, Alkmaar	1	–
			Academic university Hospital, Leiden (AZL)	12	9
			Academic University Hospital, Groningen (AZG)	1	–
				30	16

* = Number of patients with ischaemic colitis.
** = Number of patients with histologically checked ischaemic colitis.

between the 8th and the 14th day in 1 case and after 14 days in 12 cases. In 6 cases a control biopsy was available.

In our group of 199 patients 35 patients presented with transient (mucosal) ischaemic colitis and from 14 of these histology was available (2 colonic resections and 12 colonic biopsies). The 2 colonic resections had been performed for obstructive lesions distal to the mucosal ischaemia. Fifteen of our patients presented with the stricturing (mural) form of ischaemic colitis and from 7 of these histology was available (6 colonic resections/autopsy and 8 biopsies). Eighteen of our patients presented with the chronic 'non resolving' (mural) form of ischaemic colitis. In all these cases histology was available (16 colonic resections and 8 biopsies). In 131 of our patients the gangrenous (transmural) ischaemic colitis occurred: histology was available from 126 of these patients (60 colonic resections, 3 biopsies and 99 autopsy studies). The biopsies were performed at a time when there was no clinical evidence for a gangrenous bowel.

Table 26.2. Histological material of our studies of 199 patients with ischaemic colitis.

Histological material:		
Colonic resections		82
Autopsies		108
Biopsies		32

Stages of colonic ischaemia	Number of patients	Number of histologically checked patients
Acute ischaemia		
Transient ischaemia	35	14
Gangrenous ischaemia	131	126
Chronic ischaemia		
Chronic 'non resolving' ischaemia	18	18
Chronic ulcerative colitis with stricture formation	15	7
Total number of patients	199	165

26.3 Depth- and surface extension of the ischaemic lesion

For the microscopical evaluation of the histological specimens (from autopsy and resection studies) we used the histological classification of Swerdlow et al., (1981) – which is based solely on the depth of colonic necrosis i.e. mucosal, mural and transmural ischaemia.

In all cases of transient ischaemic colitis damage was limited to the mucosa; in all cases of stricturing ischaemic colitis and chronic 'non resolving' ischaemic colitis it was mural and in all cases of gangrenous ischaemic colitis transmural. No correlation between various aetiopathogenic factors and depth of ischaemic lesions could be established.

If the causative factor persists, then the ischaemic damage progresses and the ischaemic lesion may extend from the mucosa into deeper layers or to adjacent bowel segments. A combination of ischaemic lesions of varying severity and depth may be found in the same colonic segment.

The distribution of ischaemic lesions may be multifocal, segmental or massive distribution. Table 26.3 shows the correlation between the surface extension and histological depth of the ischaemic lesion.

26.4 Ischaemic or haemorrhagic colonic necrosis

Depending on the rapidity of onset, the type and extent of vascular occlusion and the quality of the collateral circulation, colonic necrosis may have a pale ischaemic-or a congested red haemorrhagic appearance depending on whether extravasation of blood has taken place in the tissues. 6 of our patients with acute mucosal lesions were of the haemorrhagic type, whilst in 8 patients early ischaemic necrosis was present.

Transmural haemorrhagic necrosis occurred in 28 cases against 98 cases of the ischaemic form.

The haemorrhagic type can be expected to occur in patients with venous occlusion or with slowly developing occlusive and non-occlusive ischaemic lesions, but no clear correlation could be established with the various types of aetiopathogenic factors in our material.

26.5 Autopsy findings

In 18 cases ischaemic colitis was an unexpected finding, probably occurring as a consequence of hypotension before death. Very early microscopical changes of (sub)mucosal ischaemia of the colon were present in the postmortem studies in 11 of these 18 cases.

Surprisingly however, in 7 patients, transmural gangrenous ischaemic colitis was found, which had passed completely undetected clinically.

26.6 Macroscopical- and microscopical appearance in ischaemic colitis

26.6.1 Introduction
As expected, the histological findings in our patient material did not differ from the earlier description by Morson (1971) and Whitehead (1972, 1976). We made a selection of the most representative mac-

Table 26.3. Correlation between the surface area, affected by the ischaemic colonic lesion and histological depths of ischaemic colitis.

Depth of ischaemic colitis Surface extension of ischaemic colitis	Mucosal Ischaemic colitis	Mural Ischaemic colitis	Transmural Ischaemic colitis ± perforation	Total number of patients
Multifocal extension	4	6	7	1/
Segmental extension	10	19	55	84
Massive extension	–	–	64	64
Total number of patients	14	25	126	165

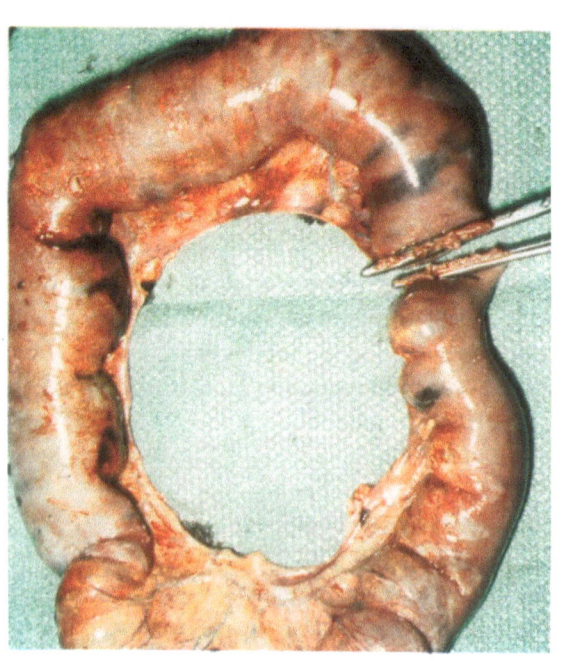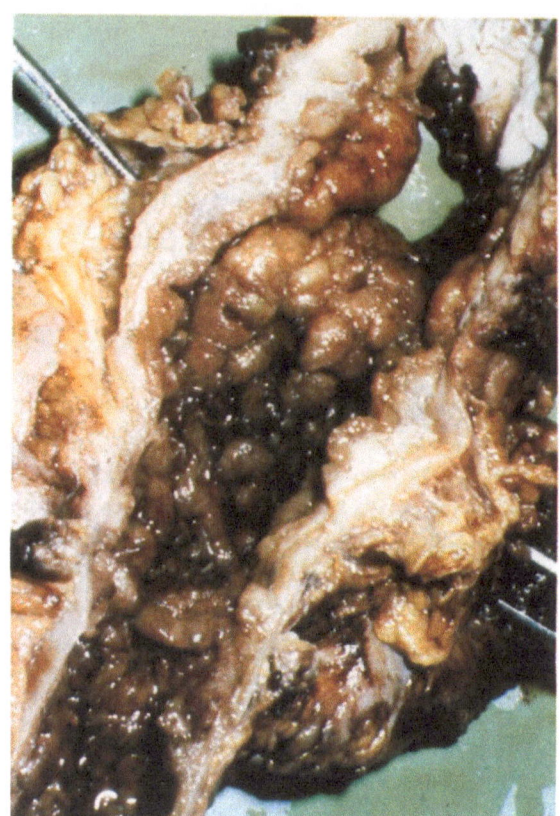

Fig.1　　Fig. 2

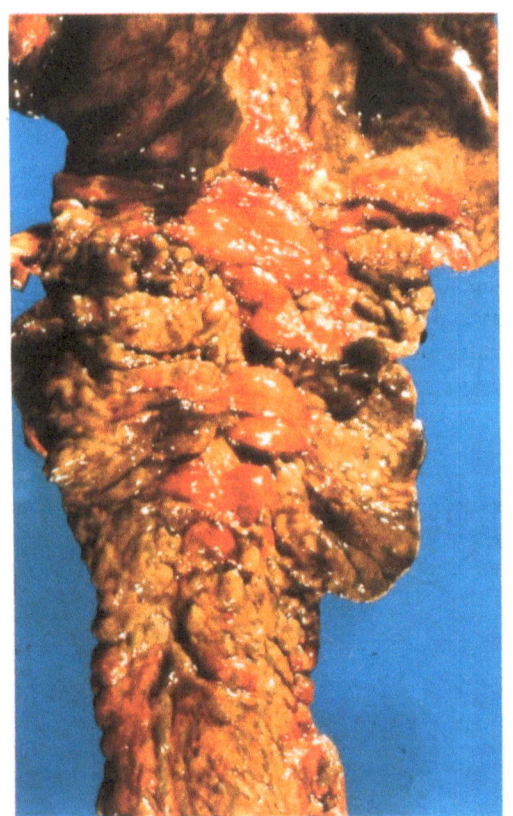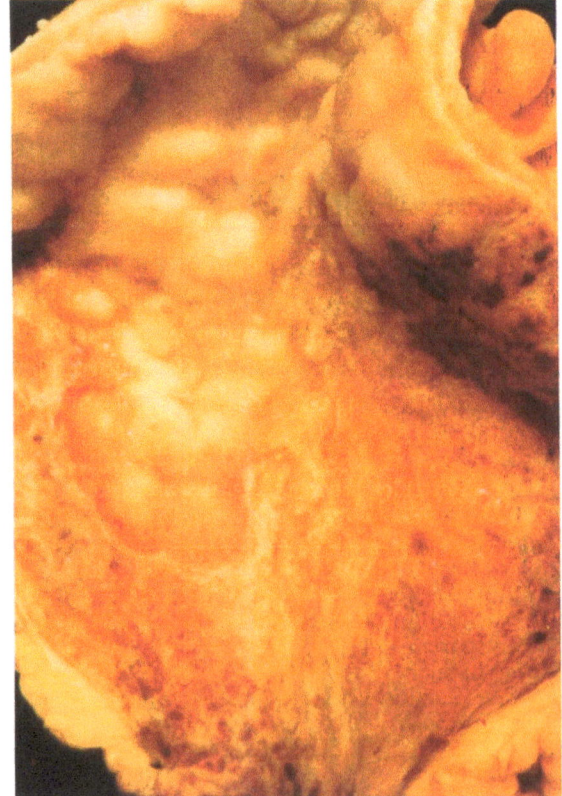

Fig. 3　　Fig. 4

Fig. 26.1. Resected colonic specimen with acute transmural ischaemia. The wall is greyish green with specks of haemorrhagic fibrin visible on the serosa.

Fig. 26.2. Haemorrhagic swollen mucosa. Parts of the mucosa are black due to fixation in formaldehyde.

Fig. 26.3. Greenish necrosis of colonic mucosa before the stage of sloughing.

Fig. 26.4. Reparative phase of chronic ulcerative ischaemic colitis; the ulcerations have sharp margins.

roscopical and microscopical photographs of the different stages of the ischaemic colonic process in our patient material (see Figs. 26.1–45).

26.6.2 Macroscopical appearance
Macroscopical features of ischaemic colitis are shown in Fig. 26.1 – 4.

26.6.3 Microscopical appearance

26.6.3.1 Early phase. Very early mucosal changes comprise vasodilation, haemorrhage and oedema, necrosis of surface and crypt epithelium. Figure 26.5, 6, 7 show a spectrum of early changes in which a wedge-shaped necrosis and distended crypts filled with mucus can be seen. The surface epithelium has disappeared, there is a superficial layer of fibrin and granulocytes, crypt epithelium is desintegrating, the lamina propria is distended by haemorrhage, oedema and cell debris. The capillaries contain numerous thrombi (pseudomembranous type of early ischaemic colitis).

Early mucosal ischaemia in which the structural appearance of the mucosa is more or less preserved is shown in Fig. 26.8. There is necrosis of the superficial epithelium, of crypts and of the lamina propria. The capillaries are filled with thrombi. Polymorphonuclear leucocytes infiltrate the mucosa and start to form a demarcation zone towards still vital tissue layers.

Lysis of red cells and a progressive loss of structures lend a ghostlike appearance to the mucosa (Fig. 26.9). The granulocytic demarcation zone is more pronounced and is frequently situated in the muscularis mucosae in rather mild cases.

Bacterial colonisation may be evident on the surface (Fig. 26.10).

Characteristic thumbprint lesions (26.11, 12, 13) arise when necrosis affects the mucosa and part of the submucosa which becomes greatly widened by oedema and haemorrhage. There is extensive granulocytic infiltration and the submucosal vessels are widely dilated; many contain thrombi. A demarcating wall of polymorphonuclears divide the necrotic layer from the still vital tissue below. Depending on the virulence of the bacterial flora phlegmonous inflammatory conditions may sometimes develop (Fig. 26.14) in which intramural gasformation may occur.

The muscularis and also the autonomous neurologic tissues are much more resistant to ischaemia than the mucosa, but also become damaged when the ischaemia is more severe and of longer duration.

In extreme conditions transmural necrosis will occur (Fig. 26.15, 16). In the pale ischaemic type of such lesions the wall of the colon is frequently much thinner than normal due to collapse of tissue when no oedema or haemorrhage is present.

26.6.3.2 Ulcerative phase
(Sub)acute stage. Sloughing of the necrotic mucosa may start between 24–48 hours following the ischaemic insult (Whitehead, 1976). Granulocytes are replaced by an infiltration of plasma cells, lymphocytes and macrophages. There is a marked proliferation of blood capillaries (Fig. 26.17, 18, 19) and hyperplastic neurogenic structures may be evident (Fig. 26–20).

The ulcer base may have a flat surface or may form wedge-shaped penetrations into the submucosa or into the muscularis propria (Fig. 26.21), and will undermine the edge of the undamaged adjacent mucosa (Fig. 26.22).

Chronic stage. Depending on the depth of the ischaemic damage and on the duration of the ischaemic insult, complete restoration to normal or permanent morphologic changes will ensue. In the latter case the cellularity of the inflammatory reaction

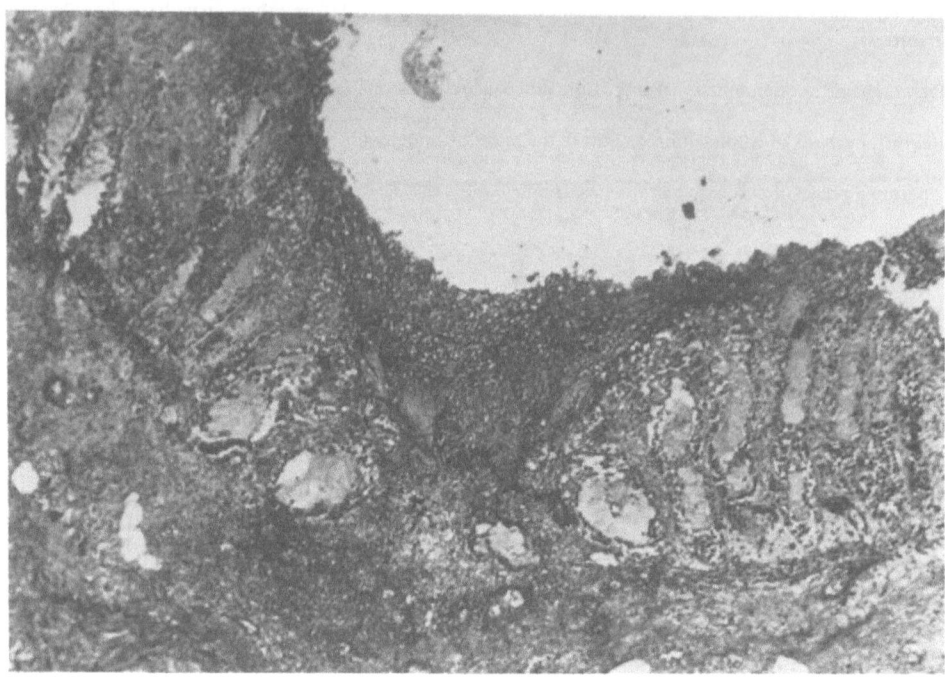

Fig. 26.5. Early mucosal necrosis and wedge-shaped ulceration (HA × 48).

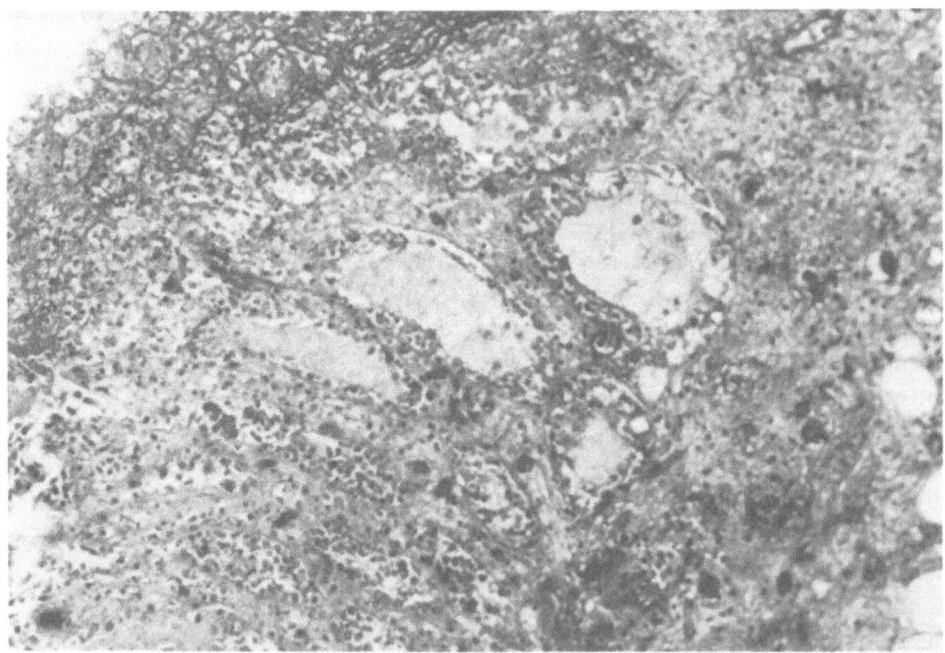

Fig. 26.6. Detail of fig. 26.5. The surface (left upper part of figure) is covered by fibrin and leucocytes. The mucosal crypts are distended by mucus; the crypt epithelial cells are necrotic or swollen and desintegrating. The lamina propria shows necrosis, haemorrhage and infiltration by disintegrating polymorphonuclears; fibrin thrombi are present in capillaries (HA × 120).

123

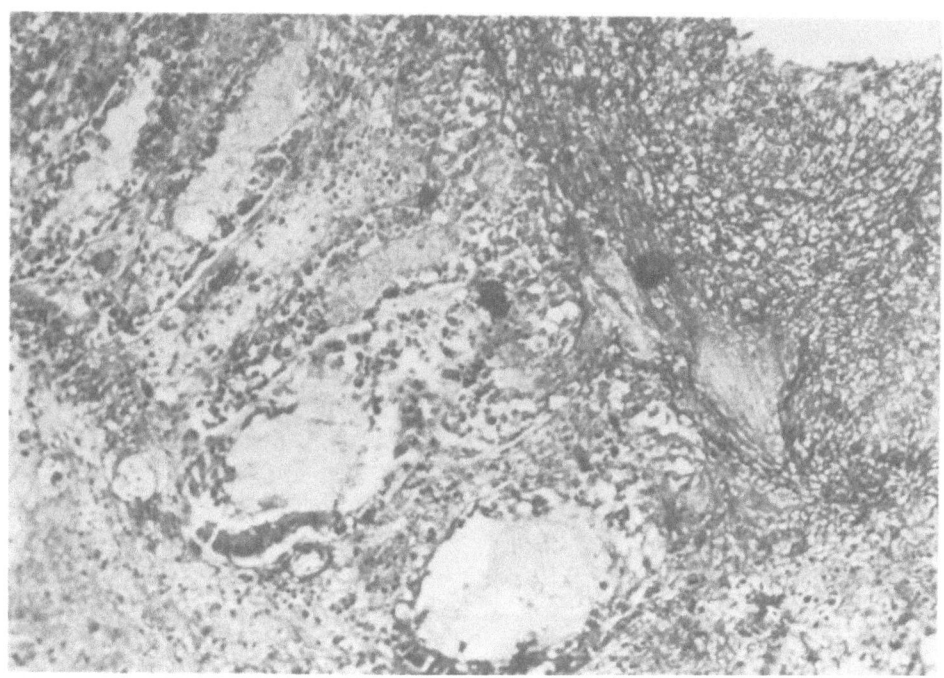

Fig. 26.7. Detail of fig. 26.5. Pseudomembranous type of early ischaemic mucosal lesion (HA × 300).

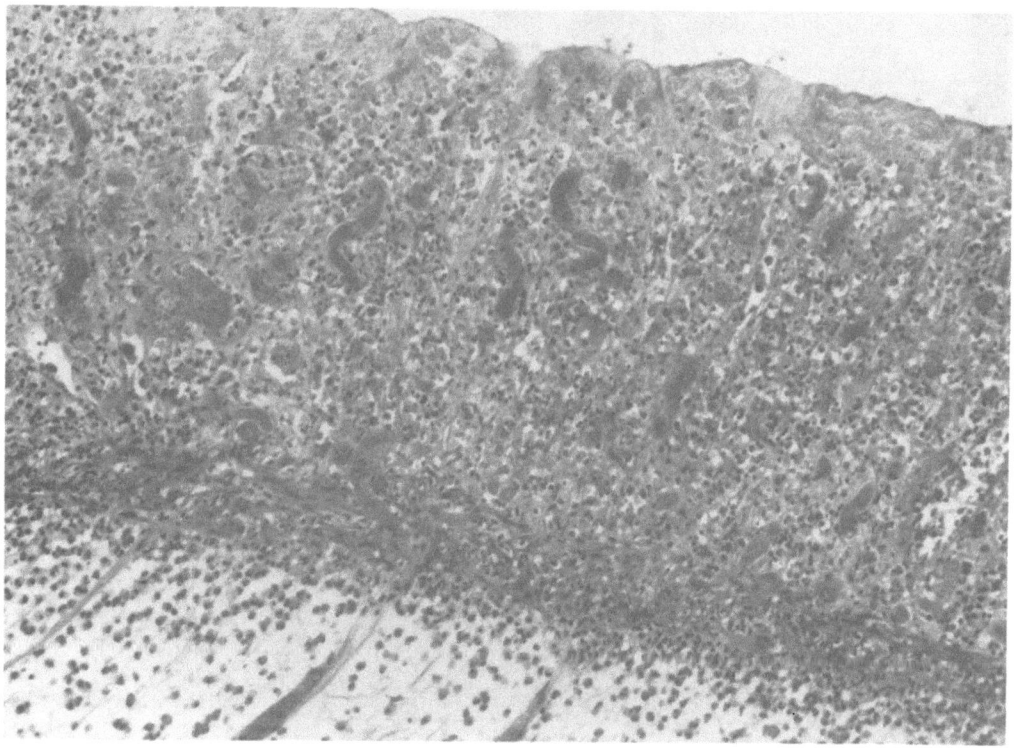

Fig. 26.8. Early ischaemic mucosal necrosis. Numerous fibrin thrombi are visible in the mucosal vessels (HA × 120).

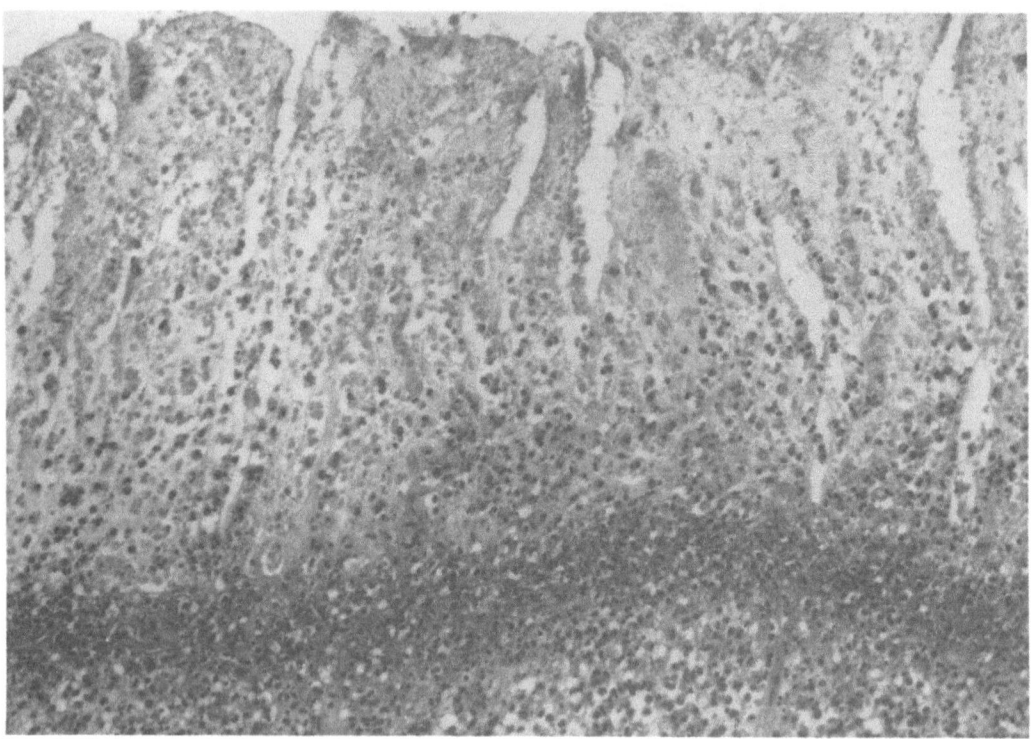

Fig. 26.9. Ischaemic necrosis of the mucosa; leucocytic demarcation along the muscularis mucosae (HA × 120).

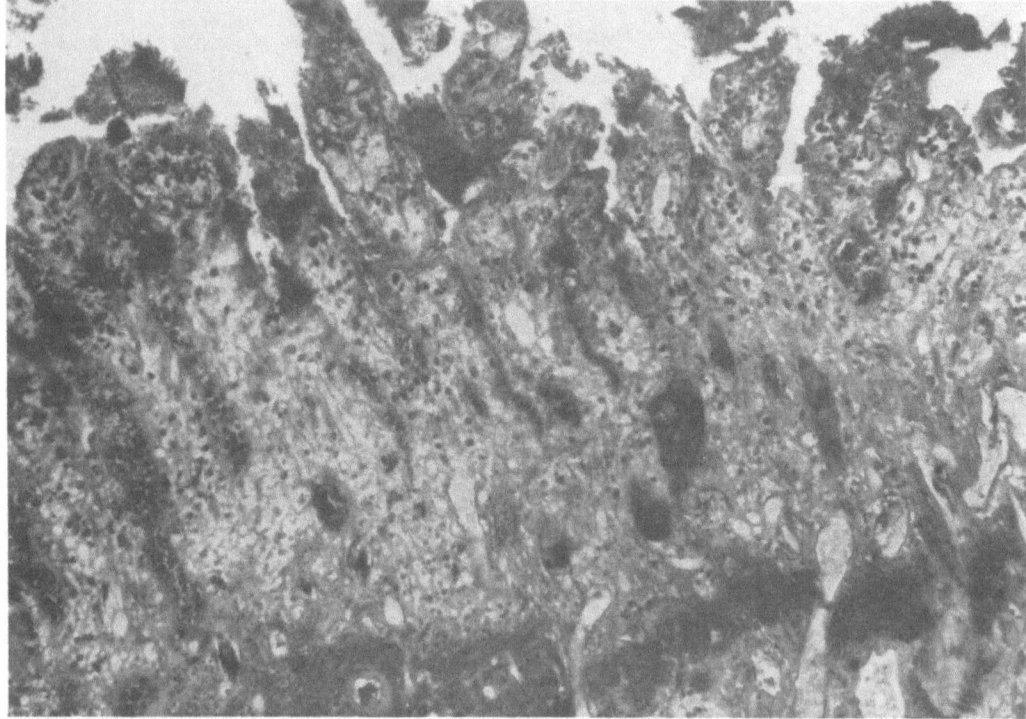

Fig. 26.10. Ischaemic necrosis of the mucosa; ghostlike crypts and remnants of thrombi are clearly seen. There is also superficial bacterial growth present (HA × 120).

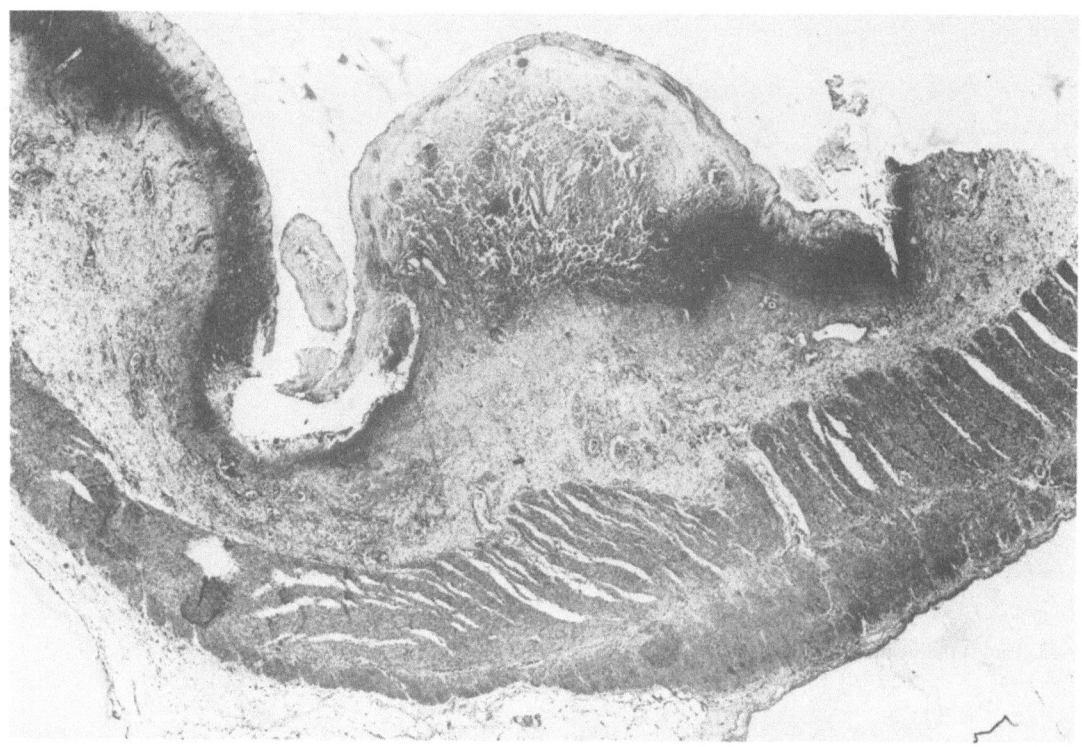

Fig. 26.11. Thumbprint lesion. Acute ischaemic necrosis of the mucosa and part of the submucosa with demarcating granulocytic infiltrate in the submucosa. Note widening of the submucosa by oedema and ghostlike crypt remnants in the mucosa (HA × 10).

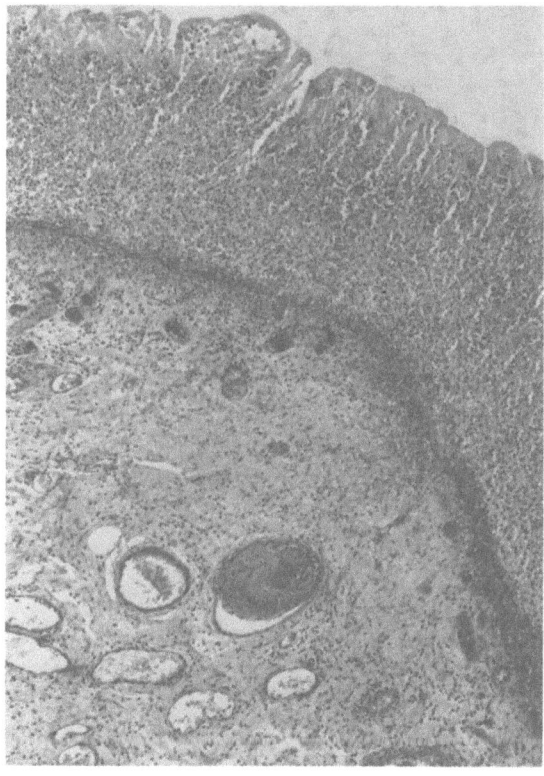

Fig. 26.12. Detail of a thumbprint lesion. Acute ischaemic necrosis of the mucosa, oedema and vasodilatation and leucocytic infiltration in the submucosa. Thrombi in submucosal vessels (HA × 48).

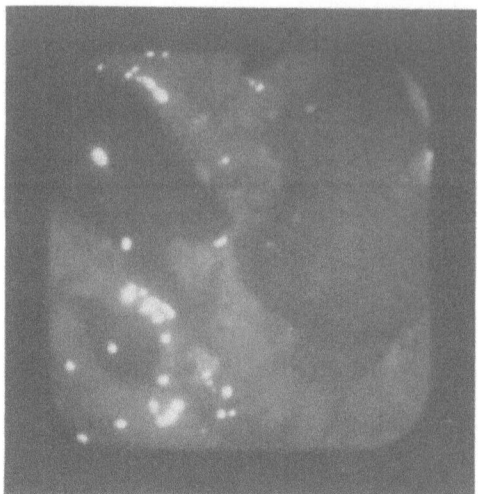

Fig. 26.13. Endoscopical aspect of thumbprint lesions (bulbous protrusions).

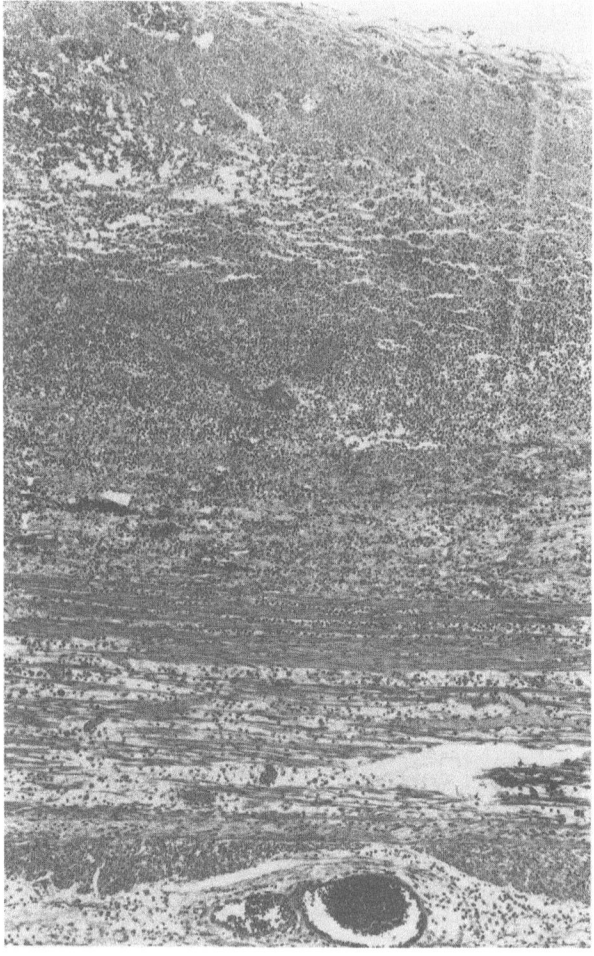

Fig. 26.14. Acute transmural necrosis of colonic wall secondary to vasculitis. Note desintegration of inner muscularis propria and extensive infiltration of polymorphonuclears. The lumen is at the upper part of the photograph (HA × 48).

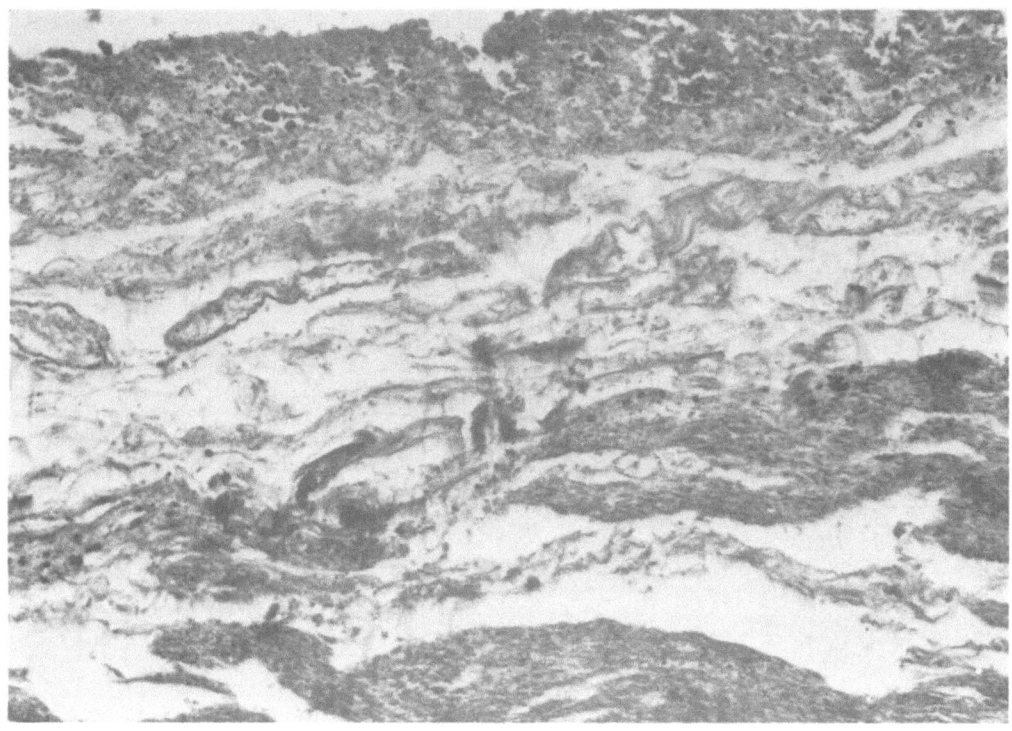

Fig. 26.15. Ischaemic transmural necrosis without polymorphonuclear infiltrate (HA × 48).

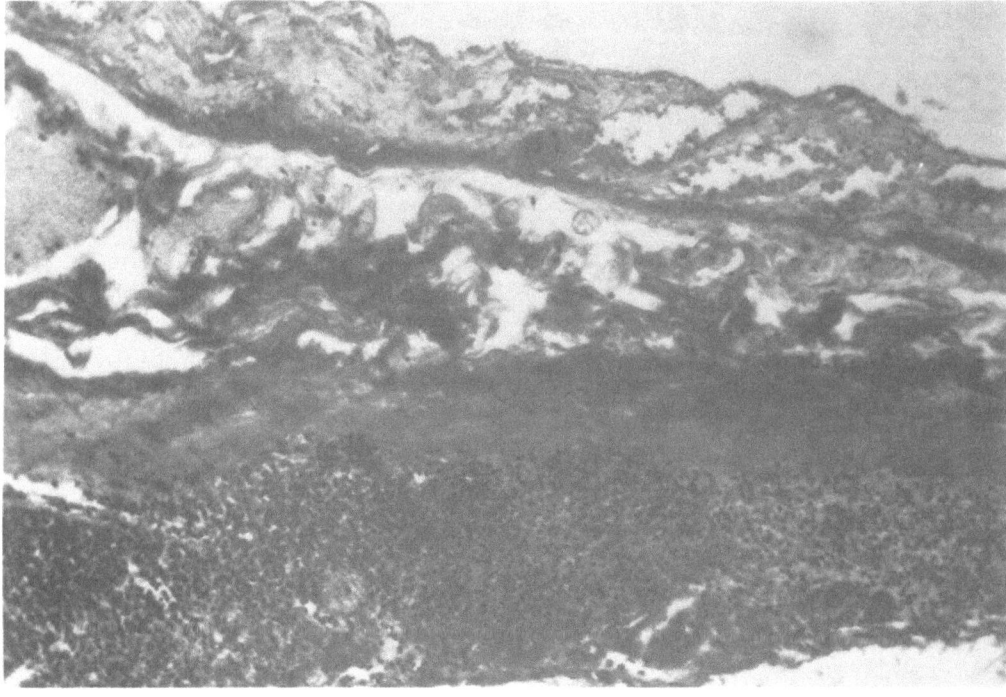

Fig. 26.16. Transmural necrosis with demarcating granulocytic infiltration of the serosa. The colonic wall is much thinner than normal (HA × 48).

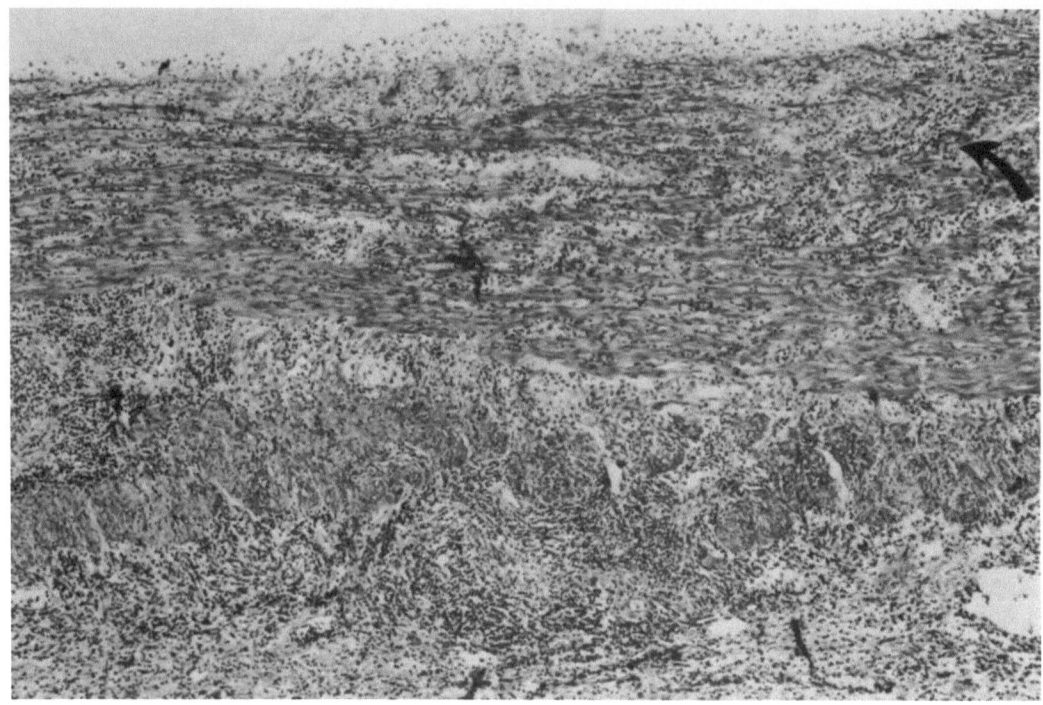

Fig. 26.17. Transmural inflammation under ulcerating surface (top of picture), after sloughing of ñecrotic mucosa and part of submucosa. The inner layer of the muscularis is partly destroyed (see arrow) (HA × 48).

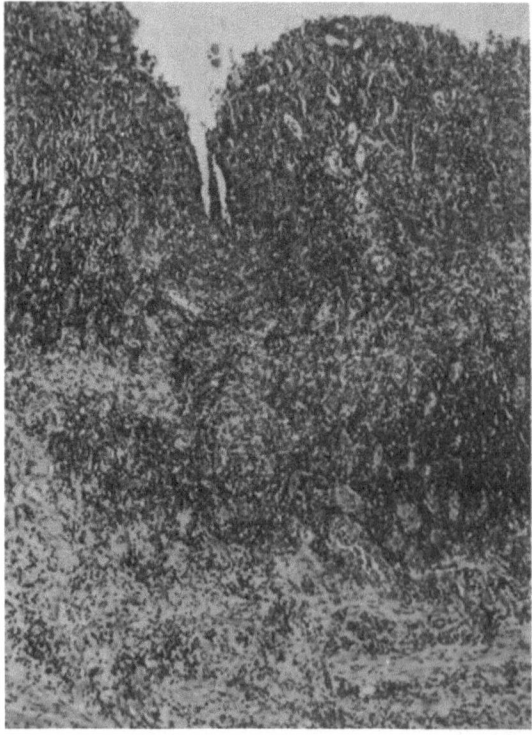

Fig. 26.18. Subchronic ulceration. The ulcer base contains a dense mononuclear infiltrate (HA × 48).

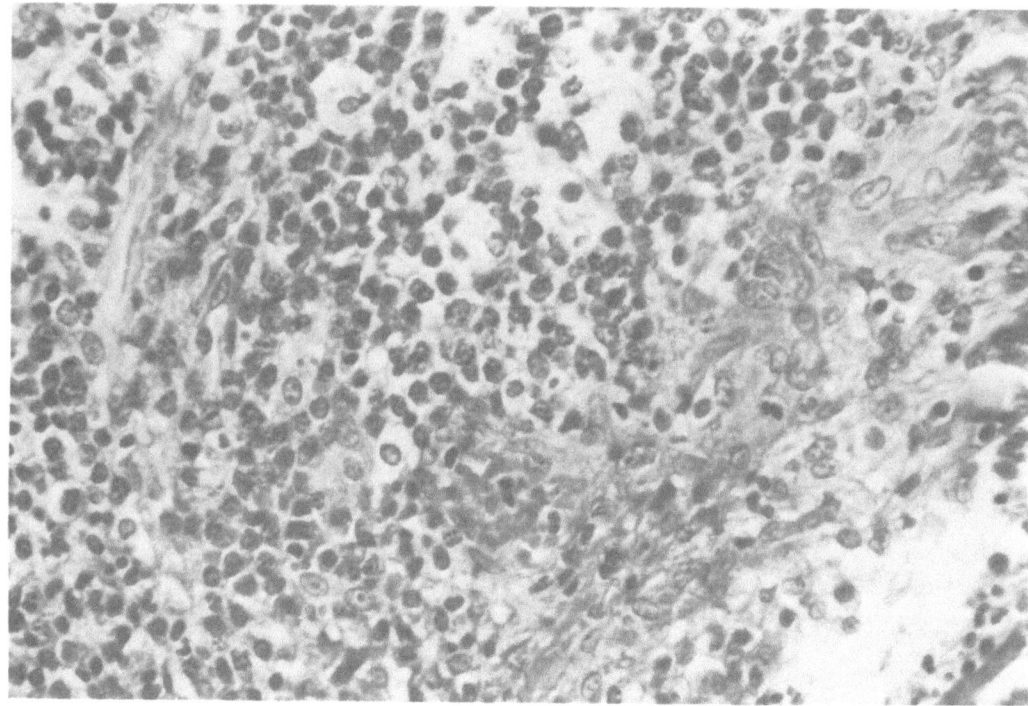

Fig. 26.19. Ulcer base; sheets of proliferating endothelial cells forming capillary sprouts. Mitosis on the right (HA × 300)

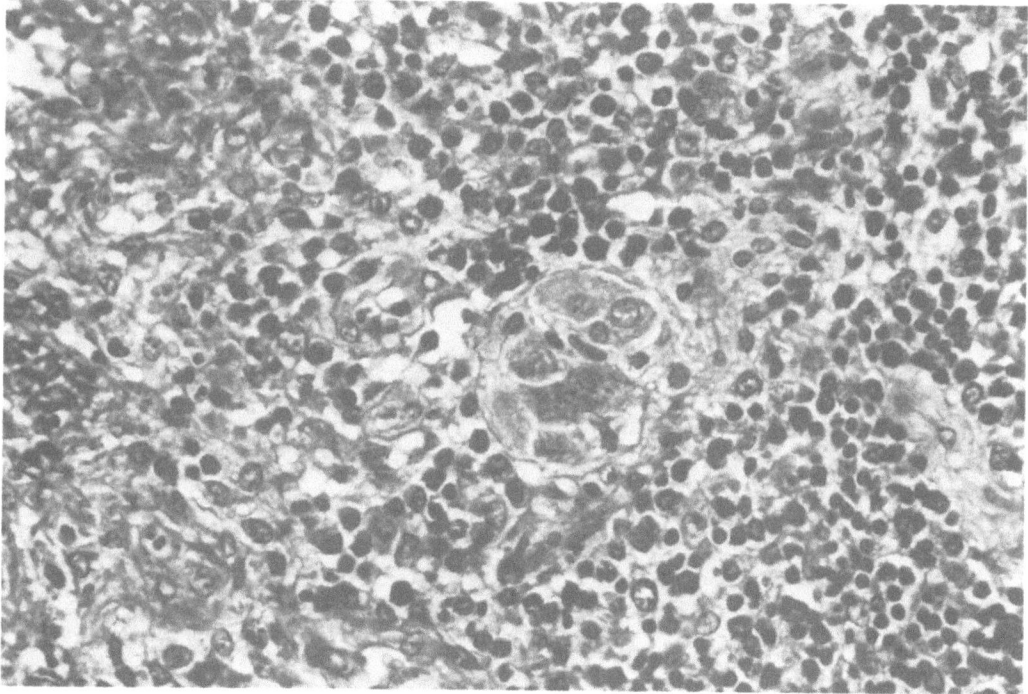

Fig. 26.20. Dense mononuclear infiltrate in ulcer base, comprising lymphocytes, plasmacells and histiocytes. Note proliferation of capillaries with swollen endothelial cells and hyperplastic neural structures of Meissner plexus (HA × 300).

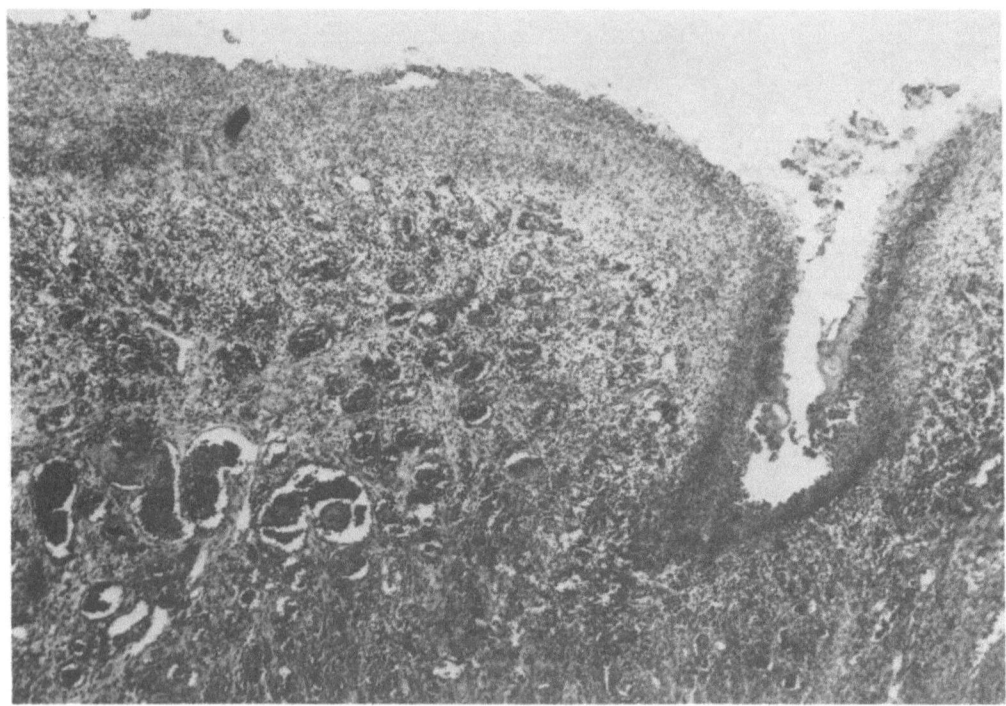

Fig. 26.21. Wedge-like ulcer penetrates inner muscularis (HA × 48).

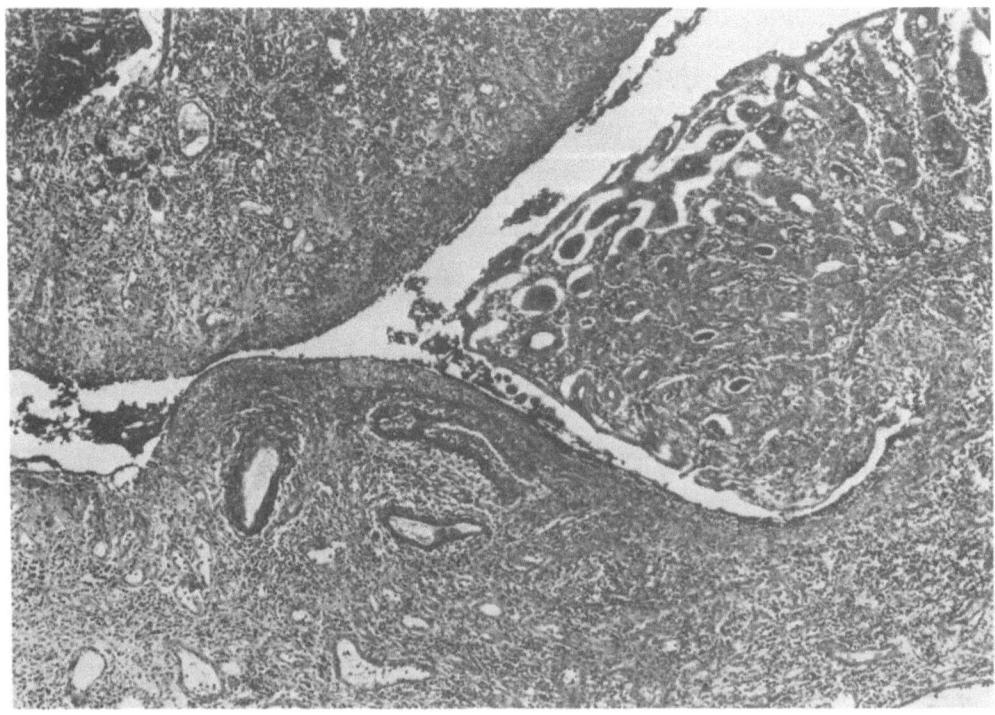

Fig. 26.22. Subchronic ulceration. Ulcer undermining remaining mucosa (HA × 30).

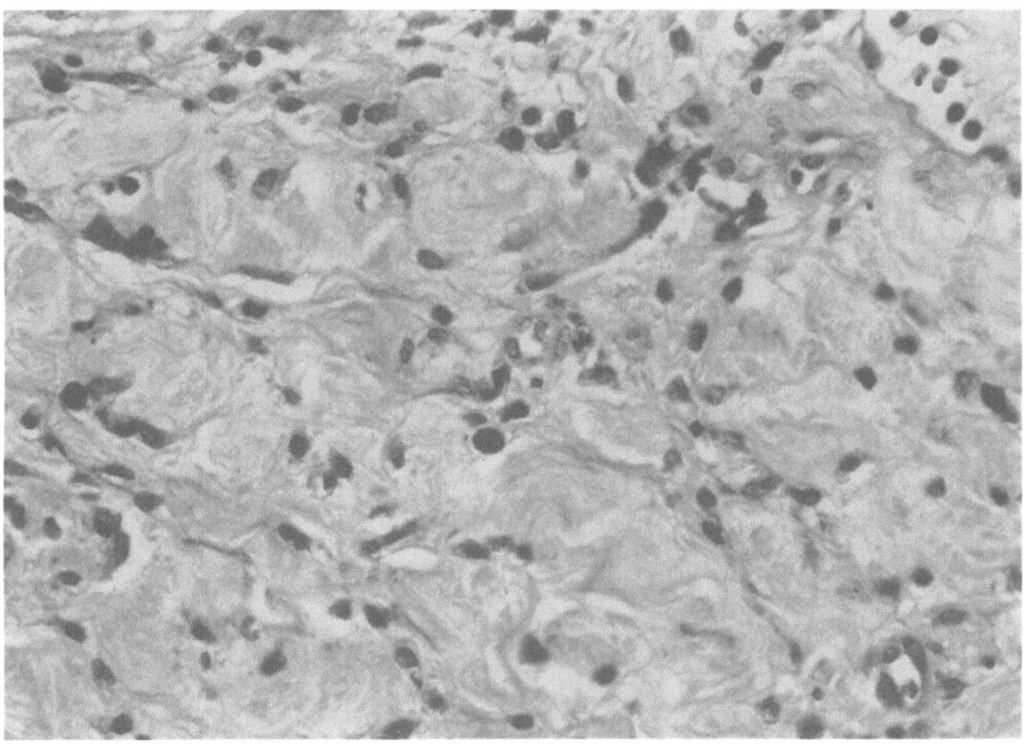

Fig. 26.23. Tubular stricture; fibrosis of submucosa; the dark staining cells are siderophages (= haemosiderin laden macrophages) containing iron (Prussian Blue × 300).

and the number of capillaries in the ulcer base will decrease. Fibroblasts increase in numbers and fibrotic changes will develop in which siderophages haemosiderin laden macrophages will at first be present (Fig. 26.23). A chronic persistent ulcerative process (Fig. 26.24) may also involve the inner muscularis propria: splaying of muscle fibres by granulation tissue which replaces necrotic muscle tissue may occur (Fig. 26.25). Obliterative vasculopathy (Fig. 26.26) may be seen in the ulcer base and occasionally the cause of bleeding may be evident (Fig. 26.27).

Lymphocytic or lymphoplasmacellular aggregates in a transmural distribution may mimick typical Crohn-like lesions (Fig. 26.28, 29), but granulomas have been absent in our material. Fragmentation of the outer layer of the muscularis propria may also occur (Fig. 26.30).

26.6.3.3 Regenerative phase. Superficial ischaemic lesions involving only the mucosal layer are capable of reconstitution to a normal appearance in 5–7 days (Whitehead, 1976).

After sloughing of necrotic tissue and removal of tissue debris by macrophages, reepithelialisation starts from crypt remnants and surface epithelium at the margin of the lesion. Newly formed crypts at first have a bizarre appearance due to crowding of nuclei and pleiomorphism of nuclei and glands (Fig. 26.31, 32). The hypercellularity of the lamina propria will gradually subside and a normal mucosa will eventually be reconstituted.

Deeper lesions will often result in residual abnormalities in the microscopical appearance. When muscle tissue either of the muscularis mucosae or of the muscularis propria is destroyed there will be no regeneration of these layers. Epithelial regeneration takes place from bordering preserved mucosa. A lining of the ulcer base by a flat layer of undifferentiated cells may result (Fig. 26.33, 34) as well as pseudopolyp formation with distorted regenerated glands (Fig. 26.35). Pseudopyloric or Panethcell metaplasia may also occur.

26.6.3.4 Obstructive ischaemic colitis. Depending on the rapidity of onset with which the intralume-

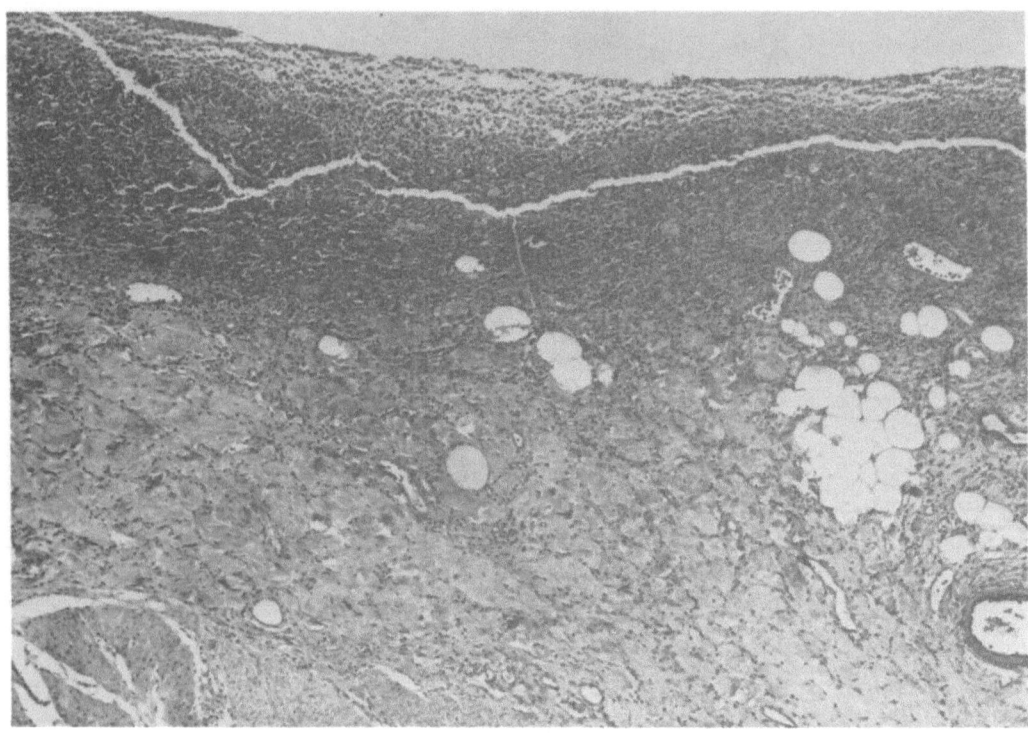

Fig. 26.24. Chronic persistent ulcerating ischaemic colitis. Chronic ulceration with fibrosis of submucosa. The ulcer base is covered by fibrinopurulent exudate (EG × 48).

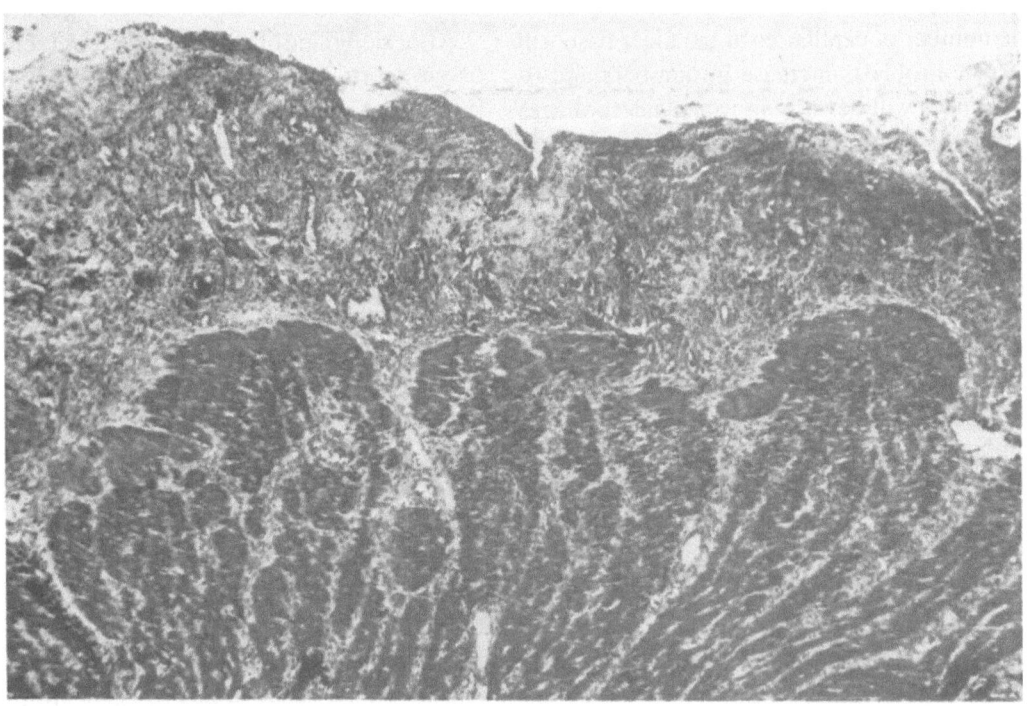

Fig. 26.25. Chronic 'non resolving' ischaemic colitis. Chronic ulceration; there is splaying of fibres of the muscularis propria by granulation tissue and fibrosis (HA × 30).

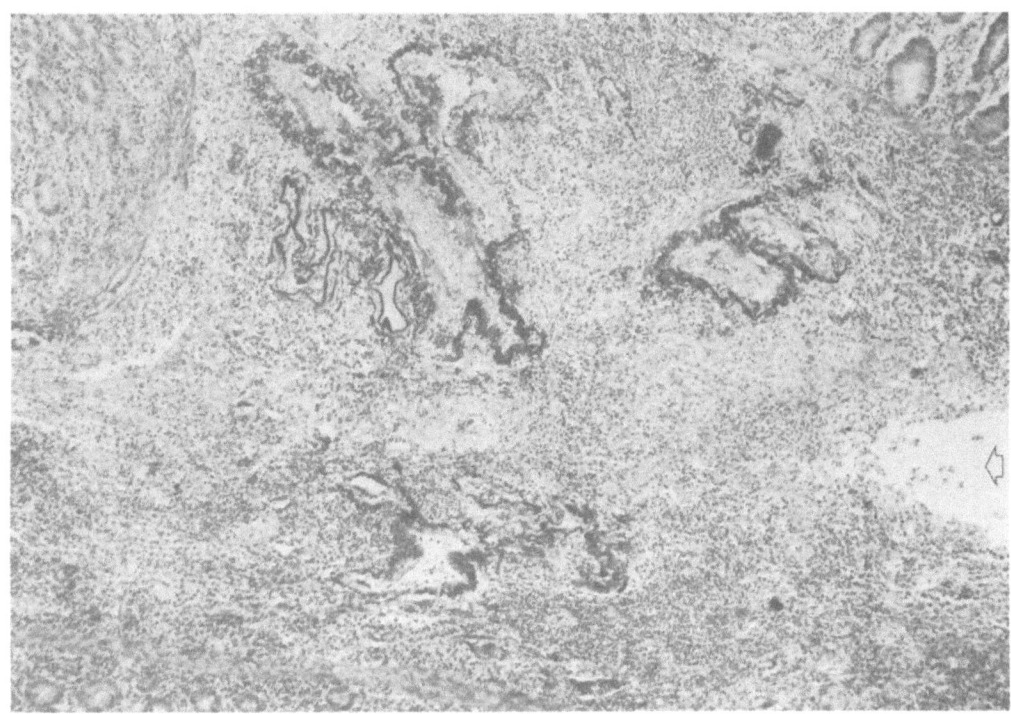

Fig. 26.26. Obliterative vasculopathy in submucosa bordering on the edge of an undermining ulcer (arrow) (EG × 120).

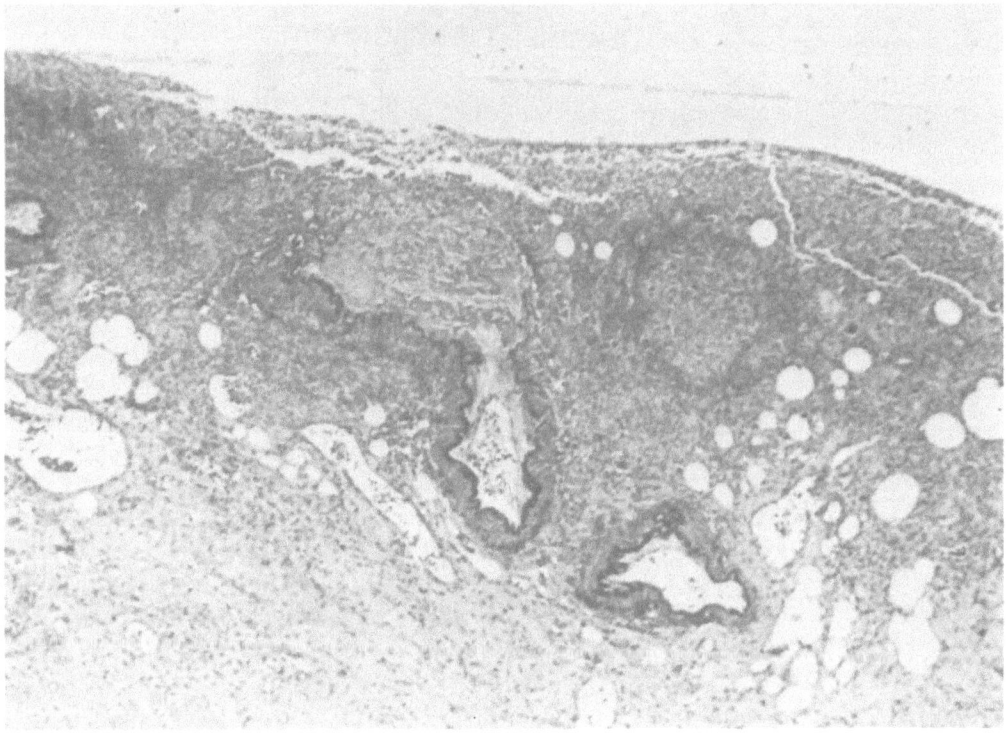

Fig. 26.27. Ulcer base with destruction and thrombosis of submucosal artery (HA × 48).

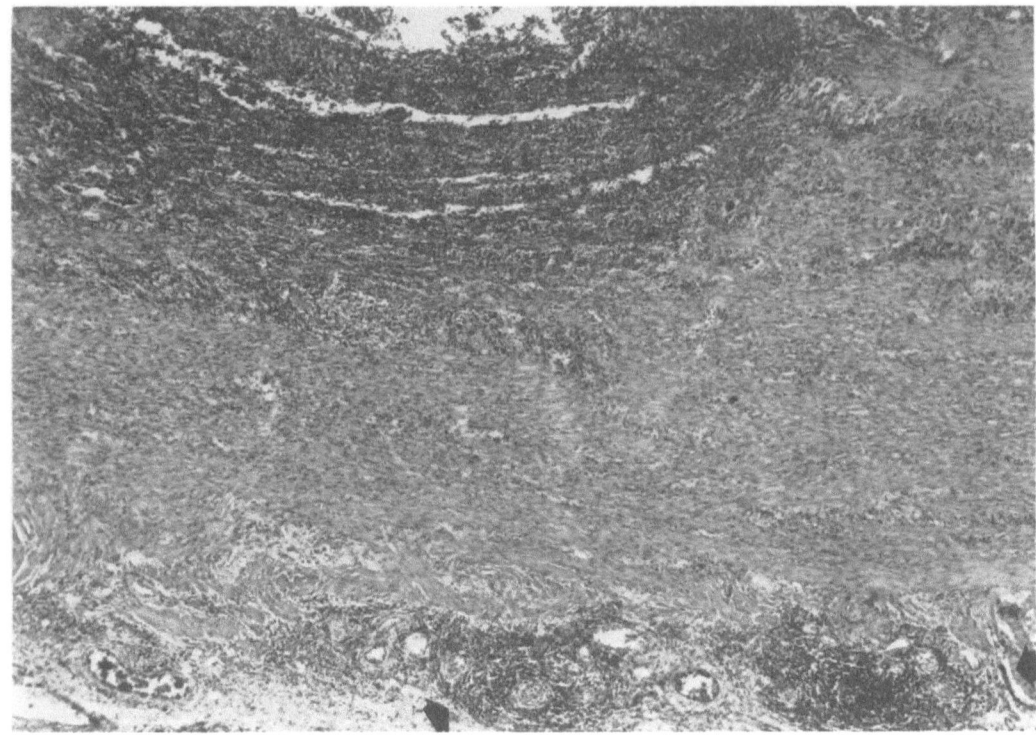

Fig. 26.28. Crohn-like aspect of ulceration with lymphoplasmacellular infiltrates (arrows) at outer border of muscularis (HA × 4).

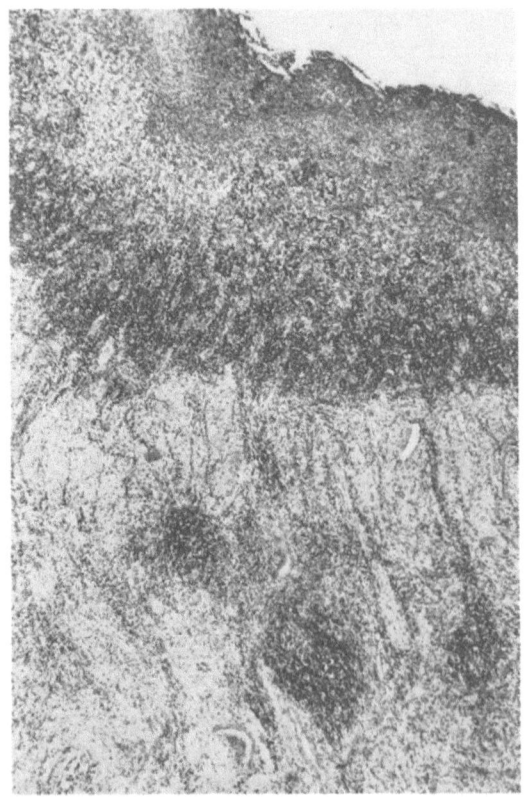

Fig. 26.29. Crohn-like pattern of transmural mononuclear infiltrate in subchronic ischaemic ulcerative colitis (HA × 48).

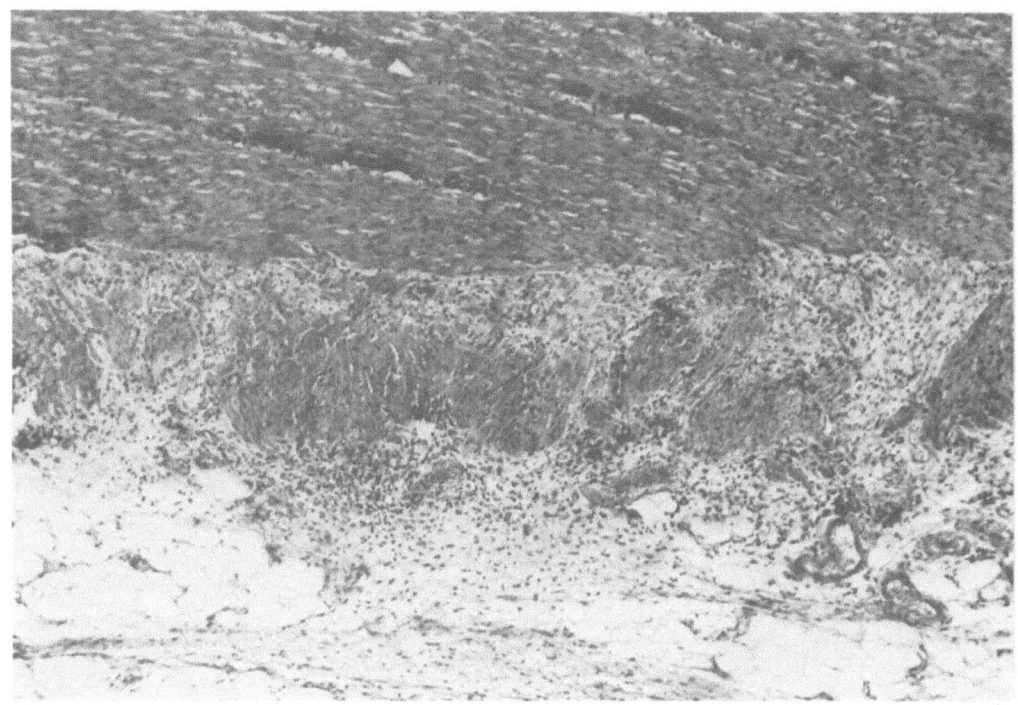

Fig. 26.30. Fragmentation of outer layer of muscularis propria in a case of chronic persisting ischaemic colitis (HA × 48).

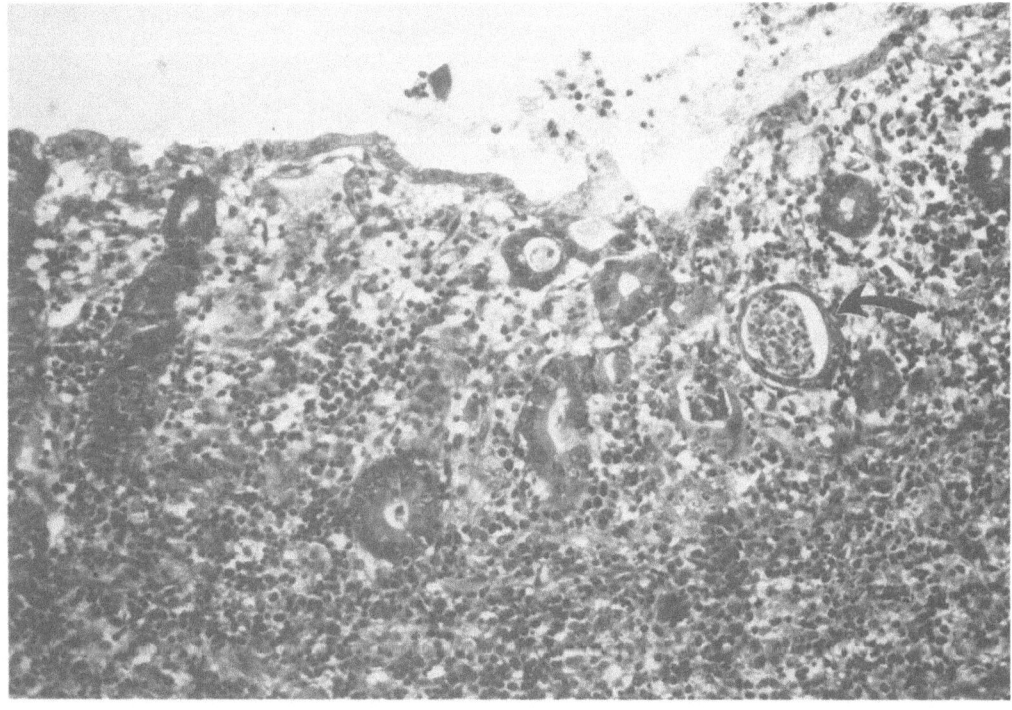

Fig. 26.31. Regenerating mucosa at the margin of an ischaemic ulcer. Abnormal surface epithelium and crypts: note crypt abscesses (arrow) (HA × 120).

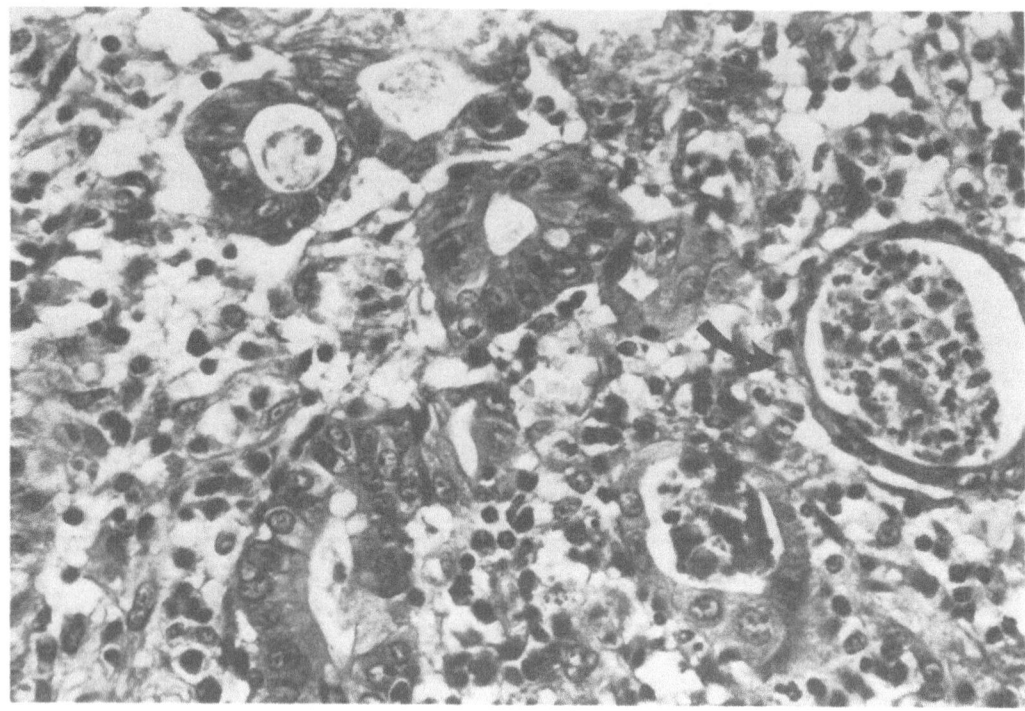

Fig. 26.32. Magnification of detail from previous figure. Crowding of nuclei; nuclear and gland pleiomorphy (HA × 300).

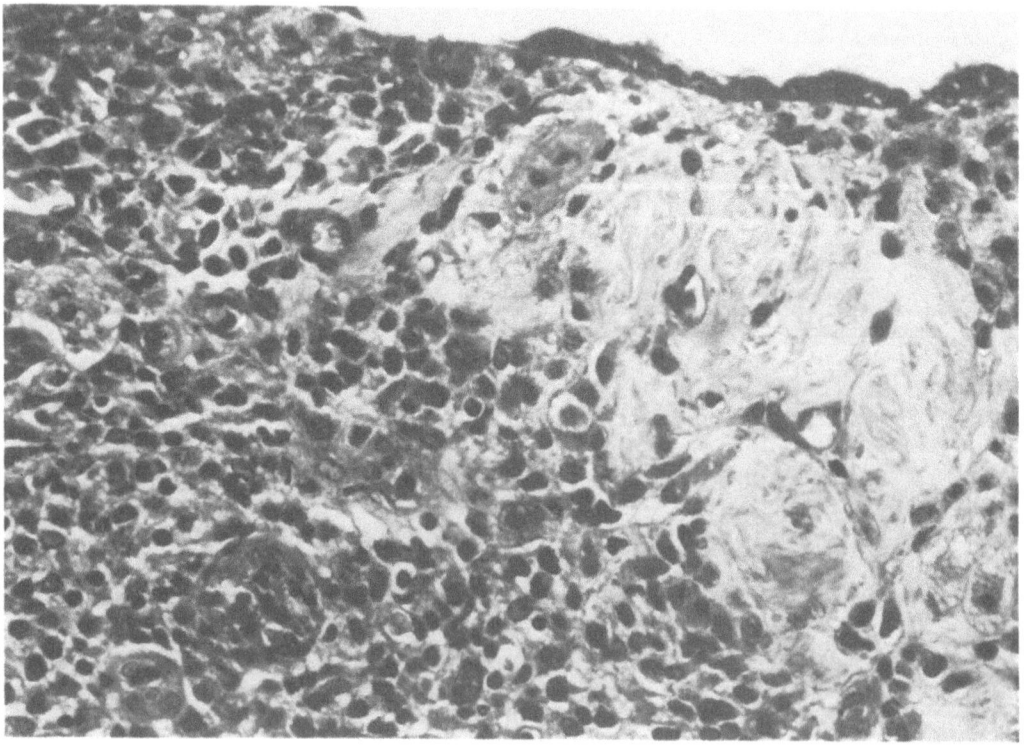

Fig. 26.33. Reepithelialisation of chronic ulceration; note area of fibrosis in dense lymphoplasmacellular infiltration (HA × 300).

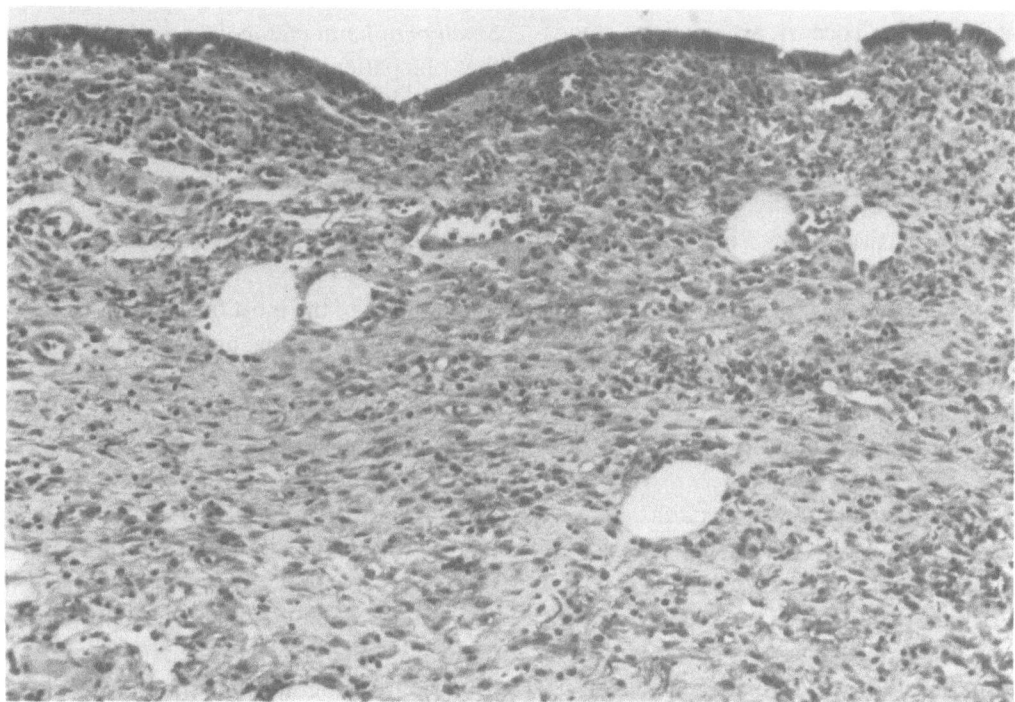

Fig. 26.34. Reepithelialisation of chronic ulceration. The cellular infiltration gradually decreases in density. The number of round cells declines; fibroblasts increase in number: early fibrosis (HA × 120).

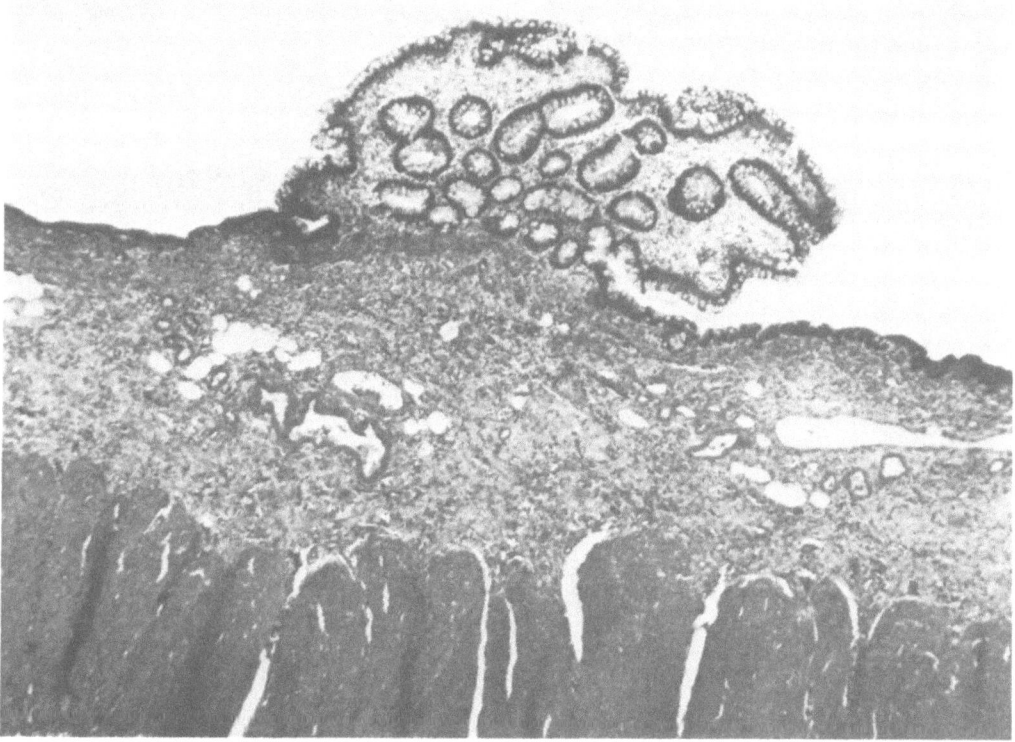

Fig. 26.35. Incomplete regeneration of mucosa following chronic ischaemic ulceration in a case of tubular stenosis. The submucosa shows fibrosis and contains but little inflammatory infiltrate; mucosal pseudopolyp with chaotically arranged plump crypts; the remainder of the previous ulcer base is covered by flat epithelium (HA × 48).

138

nal pressure elevation occurs, proximal to a stenosing process in the distal colon and on the virulence of the bacterial flora, various types of ischaemic lesions may ensue.

A (focal) transmural necrosis with or without perforation will preferentially occur in the most dilated part of the colon. Focal transmural phlegmonous inflammation resulting in peritonitis may also be observed (Fig. 26.36), in which the muscularis propria may have vanished almost completely. A subacute or chronic ulcerating colitis in which there is lysis of the inner layer of the muscularis propria is depicted in Fig. 26.37.

26.6.3.5 Stenosing lesions of mesenteric vessels

Large mesenteric vessels. Various types of lesions (thrombi, atherosclerosis, emboli) were encountered in the large mesenteric vessels in 67 cases as shown in table 26.4. The vessels were reported as being normal in 13 cases. In the remainder of our patient material the large vessels were not examined.

Small peripheral mesocolic vessels. Due to the fact that our patient material was collected from various hospitals in which often no special attention had been given to the state of the peripheral mesocolic arteries, the figures given in table 26.4 do not give a correct impression of the importance of small vessel disease in the pathogenesis of ischaemic colitis.

Examples of the most frequently occurring types of small vessel lesions are given in figures 26.38–26.45.

In 63 of those cases under consideration, various types of lesions were encountered in the small peripheral vessels. The vessels were reported as being normal in 30 patients. In the remaining patient material (72 patients) the peripheral vasculature of the mesocolon had not been studied specifically. Cholesterol embolism of the small mesocolic arteries was encountered in 3 patients, in 1 of them following angiography of the aorta (Fig. 26.38). Necrotizing arteritis (periarteritis nodosa type) was

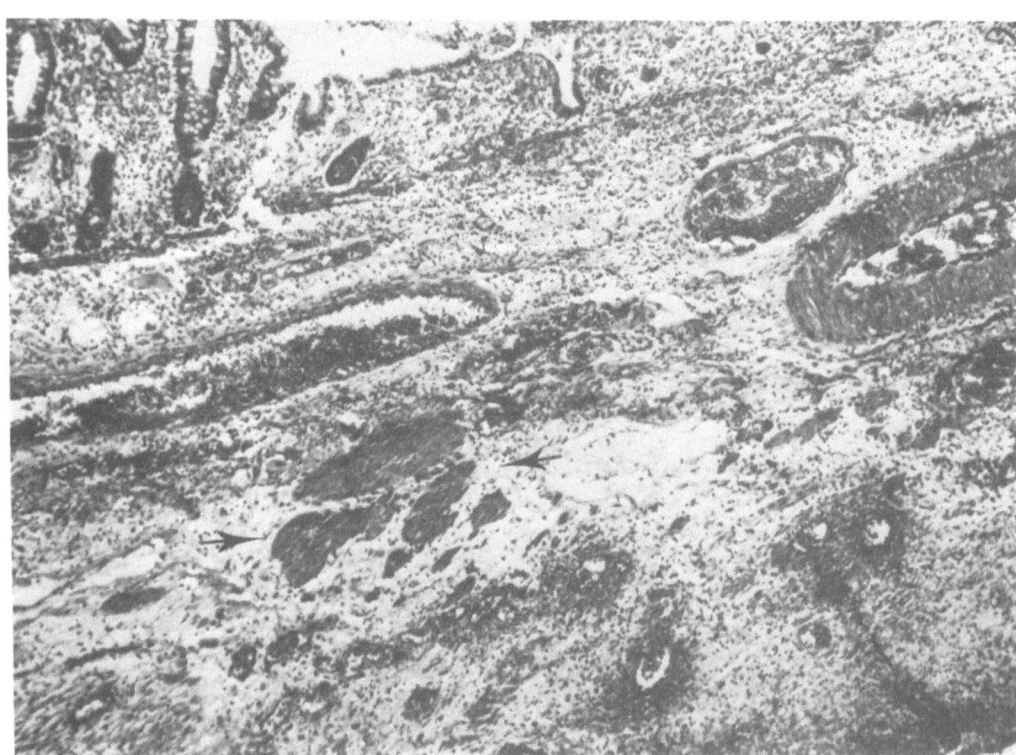

Fig. 26.36. Focal acute transmural phlegmonous inflammation and early ulceration in the ascending colon secondary to intralumenal pressure elevation, caused by stenosing adenocarcinoma of the sigmoid. The muscularis propria has vanished almost completely; small remnants are visible left of the centre (arrow) (HA × 48).

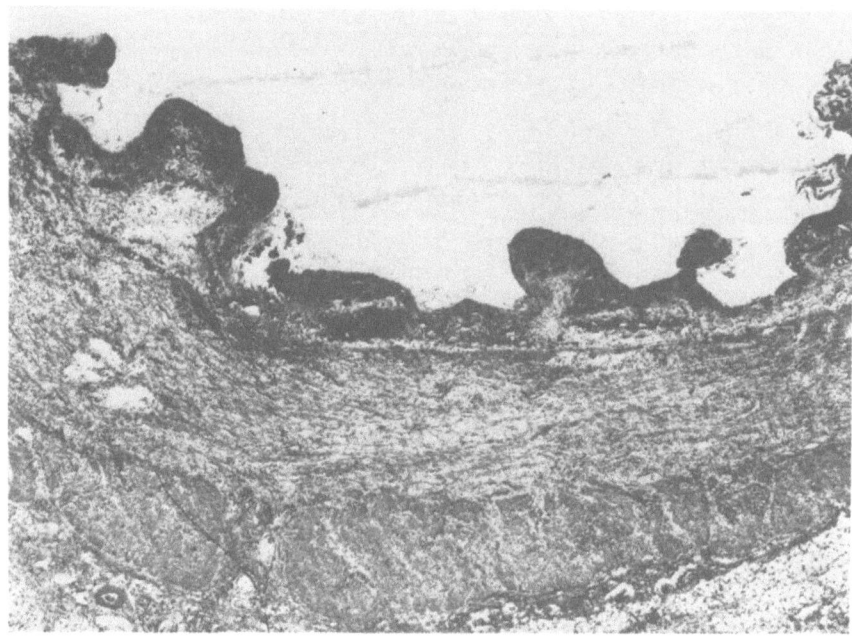

Fig. 26.37. Chronic ulcerating ischaemic colitis proximal to obstructive lesion in the sigmoid. Irregular ulcerations with intervening mucosal remnants. The inner part of the muscularis propria shows lysis of muscle fibres, oedema and neutrophil infiltration (HA × 4).

observed in only 1 patient (Fig. 26.39, 40). Vasculitis secondary to lupus erythematosus disseminatus and rheumatoid arthritis occurred in 4 cases.

Elastosis secondary to tumour invasion was present in 1 case (Fig. 26.41, 42).

Radiation vasculopathy, seen in 5 of our patients, is shown in Fig. 26.43.

Amyloid deposition in small mesenteric vessels was encountered in 3 patients (Fig. 26.44).

As was to be expected, diabetes mellitus was associated with more severe peripheral atherosclerosis than occurred in non diabetic patients. In 15 of the 34 patients with hypertension the mesocolic vessels were studied histologically.

In all these patients there was a tendency for lumenal narrowing caused by hyperplasia of delicate loose fibrous connective tissue and myocytes in the intima (Fig. 26.45). These changes were especially severe in patients in whom both diabetes and hypertension occurred.

26.6.3.6 Biopsies

Early stage of colonic ischaemia. In some biopsy specimens the characteristic appearance of the early stage of colonic ischaemia was present – i.e.-

Table 26.4. Pathology of the colonic vessels (165 observations)

Large mesenteric vessels		Small peripheral mesocolic vessels	
Not examined	85	Not examined	72
Stenosis SMA	–	Tumour induced	
Stenosis IMA	5	elastosis	1
Stenosis SMA + IMA	2	Thrombi (diffuse	
Occlusion SMA	24	intravascular	
Occlusion IMA	19	coagulation)	31
Occlusion			
SMA + IMA	17	Vasculitis	5
Normal	13	Amyloiddeposition	3
		Cholesterolemboli	3
		Irradiation-vasculopathy	5
		Proliferative intima-	
		hyperplasia with	
		lumenal narrowing	15
		Normal	30
Total	165	Total	165

superficial oedema, haemorrhage and necrosis of the surface and crypt epithelium, with thrombi in (sub)mucosal vessels and dilated mucosal vessels.

Late stage of colonic ischaemia. The appearance of the later stages of ischaemic colitis in biopsy specimens was that of a non specific chronic ulceration.

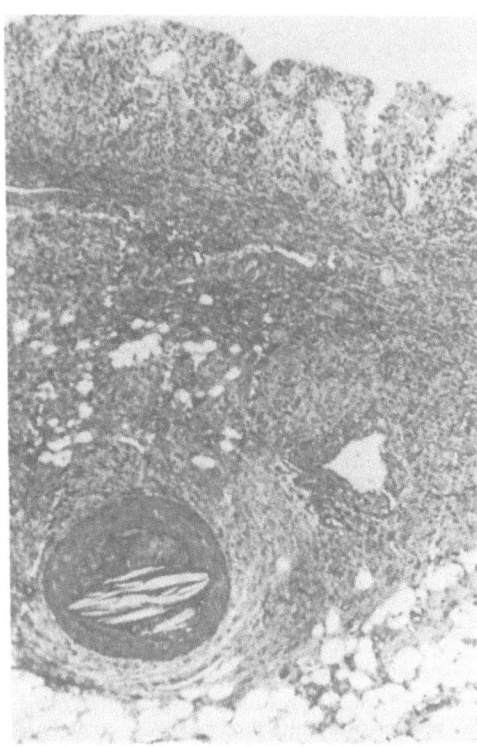

Fig. 26.38. Haemorrhagic necrosis of mucosa and submucosa; cholesterolemboli in su! mucosal artery, following angiography of aorta (HA × 48).

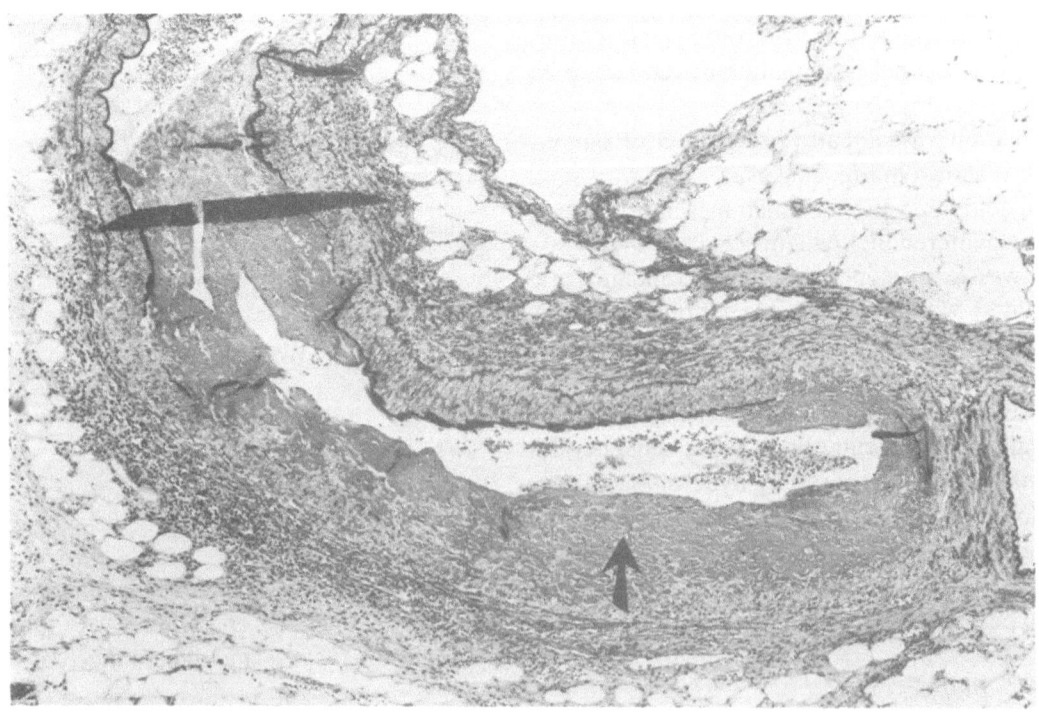

Fig. 26.39. Patient with focal ulcerative ischaemic colitis due to necrotizing arteritis. A branch of a colonic artery near the wall of the colon. Arrow points to necrosis of the arterial wall (EG × 20).

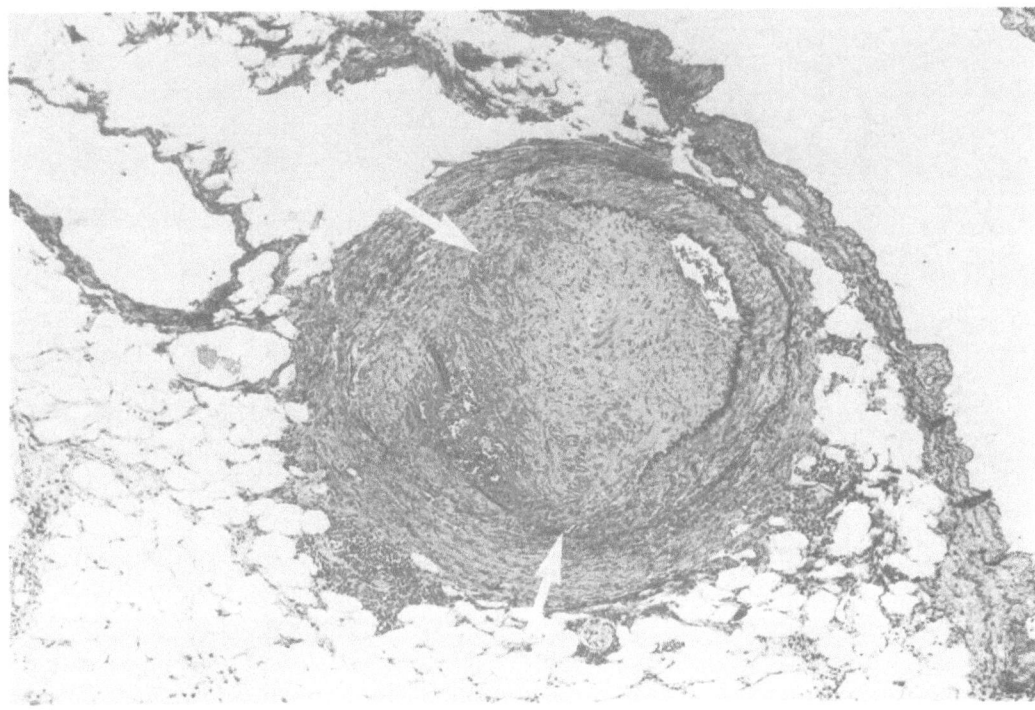

Fig. 26.40. Same patient as Fig. 26.39. Another branch is obstructed by fibrosing thrombus. Note destruction of the media and elastica interna by scar tissue, following acute necrotizing arteritis (HA × 48).

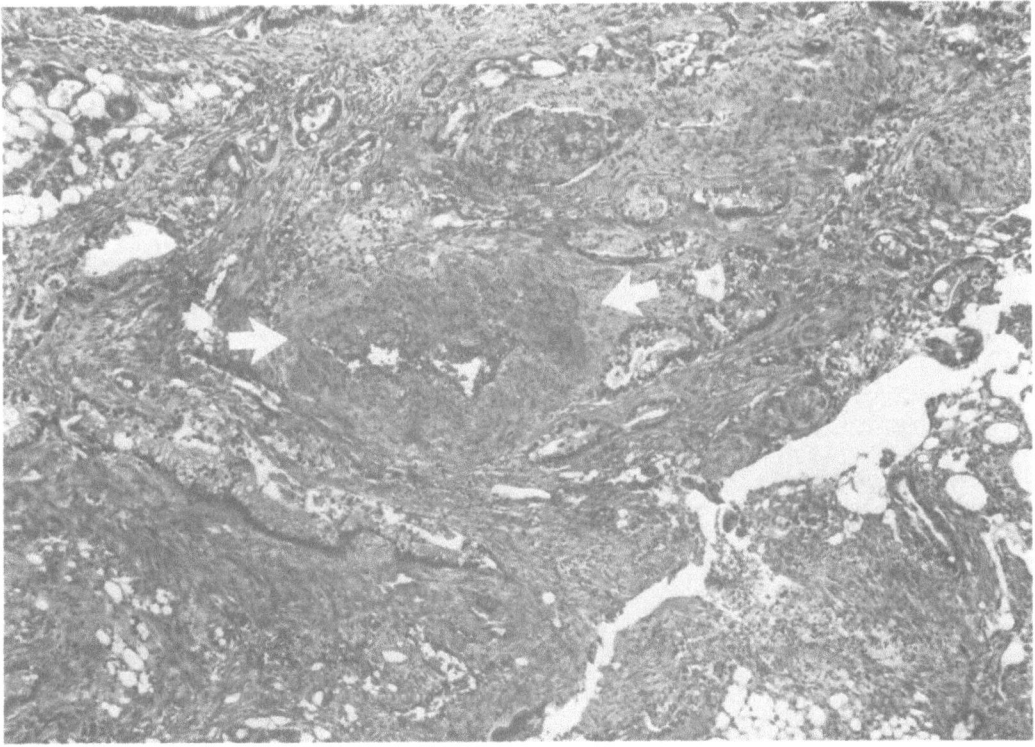

Fig. 26.41. Ischaemic colitis due to adenocarcinoma encroaching on mesocolon vessels near outer edge of colon transversum (HA × 48).

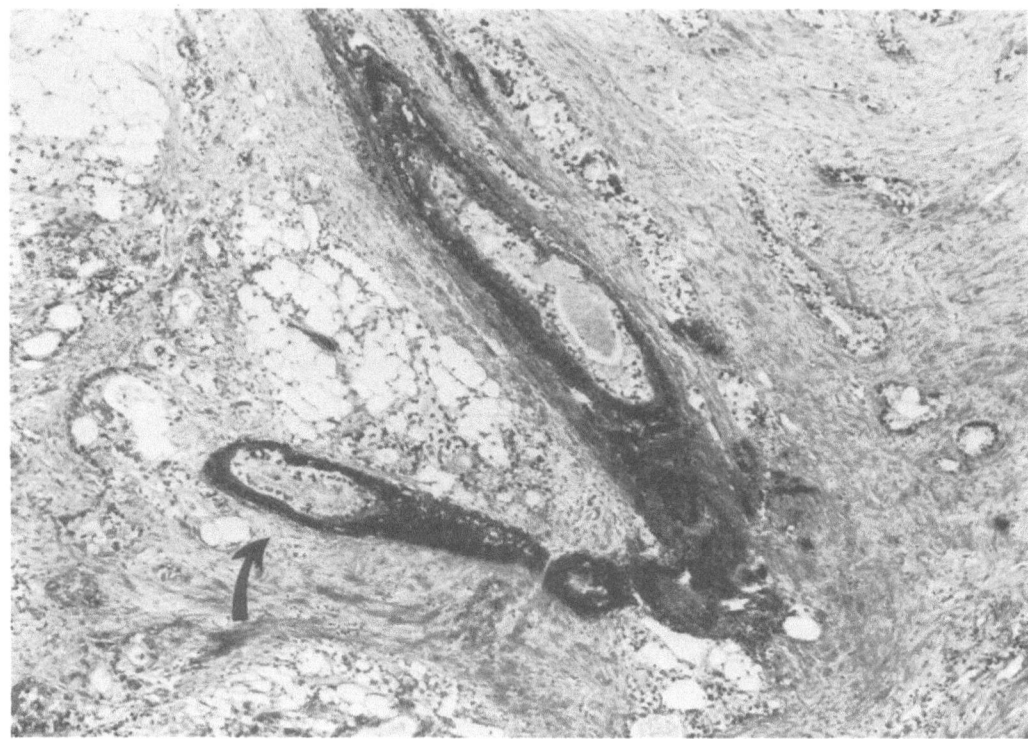

Fig. 26.42. Obliteration of arterial branches by tumor and tumor induced elastosis (HA × 48).

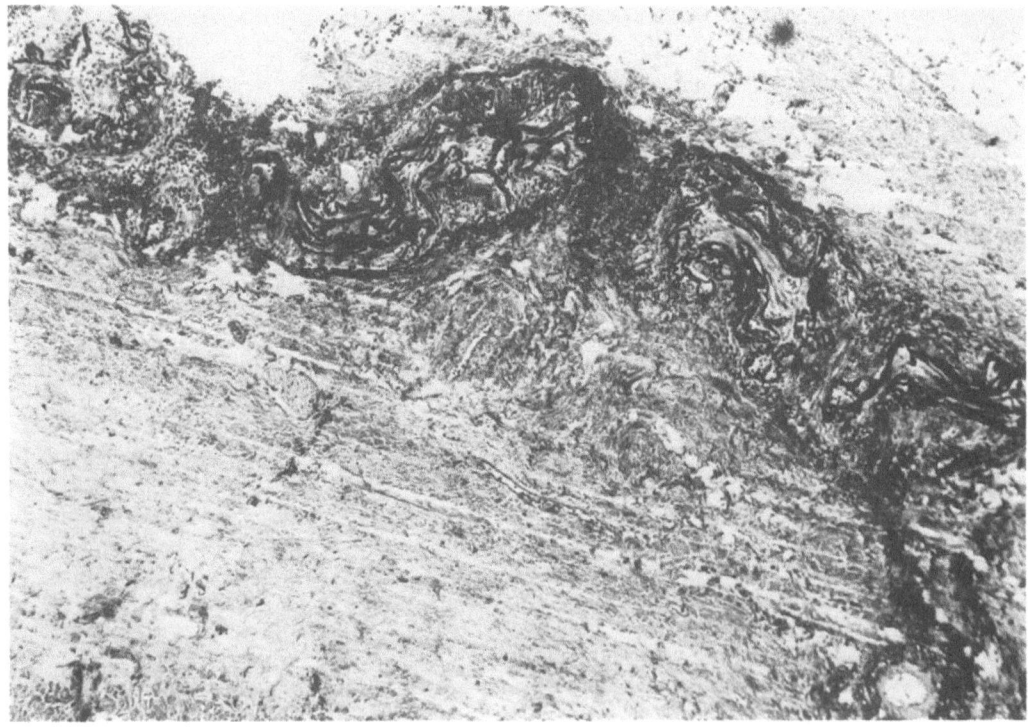

Fig. 26.43. Obliterative vasculopathy caused by radiation treatment. Elastotic obliteration of subserosal arterial branch (EG × 48).

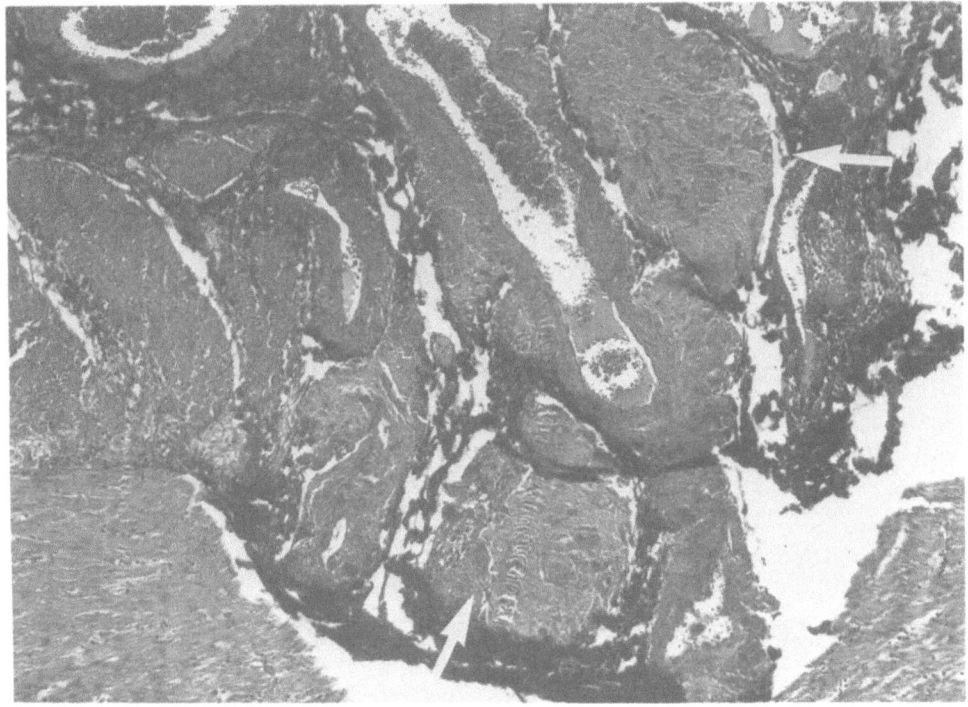

Fig. 26.44. Patient with ischaemic colitis secondary to small vessel disease. Intramural branches of artery and vein obliterated by amyloid deposition (HA × 48).

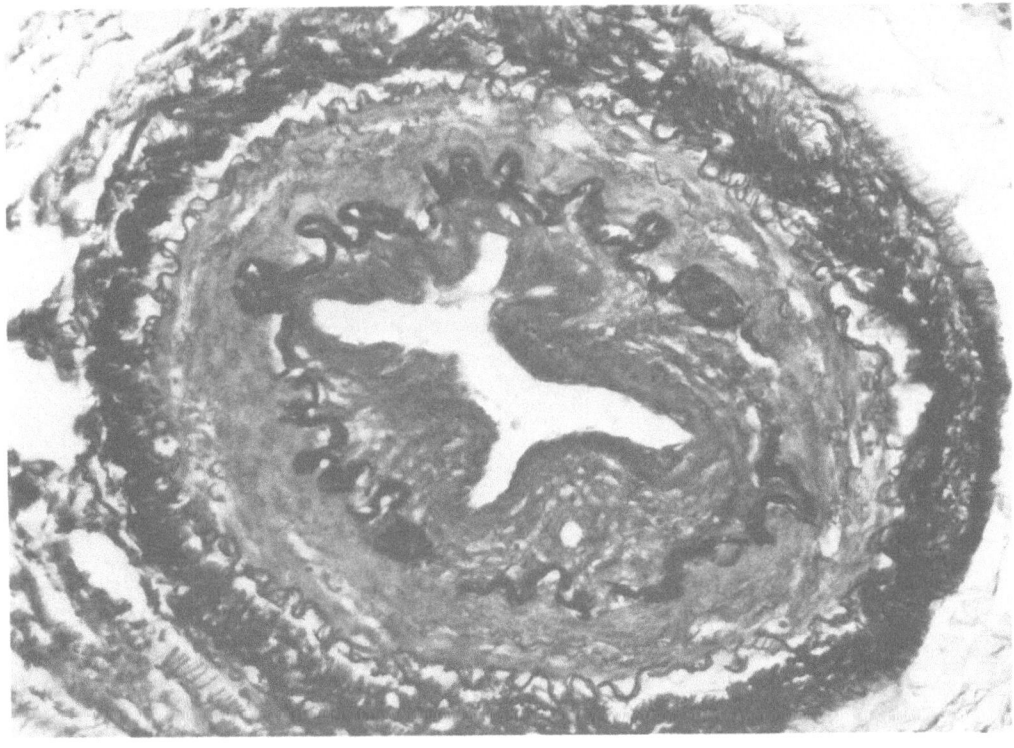

Fig. 26.45. Peripheral branch of mesenteric artery, folded lamina elastica interna. Fibrosis of proliferated intima with severely narrowed lumen (EG × 120).

27. THERAPEUTIC METHODS FOR ISCHAEMIC COLITIS

27.1 *Introduction*

27.2 *Conservative treatment*

27.3 *Surgical treatment*
    27.3.1 Non gangrenous forms of ischaemic
        colitis
        Mucosal form (synonymous with
        transient ischaemic colitis)
        Stricturing (mural) form
        Chronic 'non resolving' (mural) form
    27.3.2 Gangrenous form of ischaemic
        colitis
        Gangrenous (transmural) ischaemic
        colitis
    27.3.3 Arterial reconstruction

27.4 *Relationship between the depth of the isch-*
aemic lesion, the surgical resection technique
used and the circulatory state of the resection-
ends

27.5 *Complications and mortality following con-*
servative and/or surgical treatment

27.1 Introduction

In our series of 199 patients 98 patients (49%) were treated conservatively and 101 patients (51%) surgically (Fig. 27.1; Table 27.1).

27.2 Conservative treatment

Ninety-eight patients were treated with conservative measures alone throughout their hospital stay; 66 of 101 surgically treated patients were treated conservatively in the first stage. Due to progression of the clinical and physical signs and increasing peritoneal tenderness or due to stricture formation they underwent a colonic resection in a

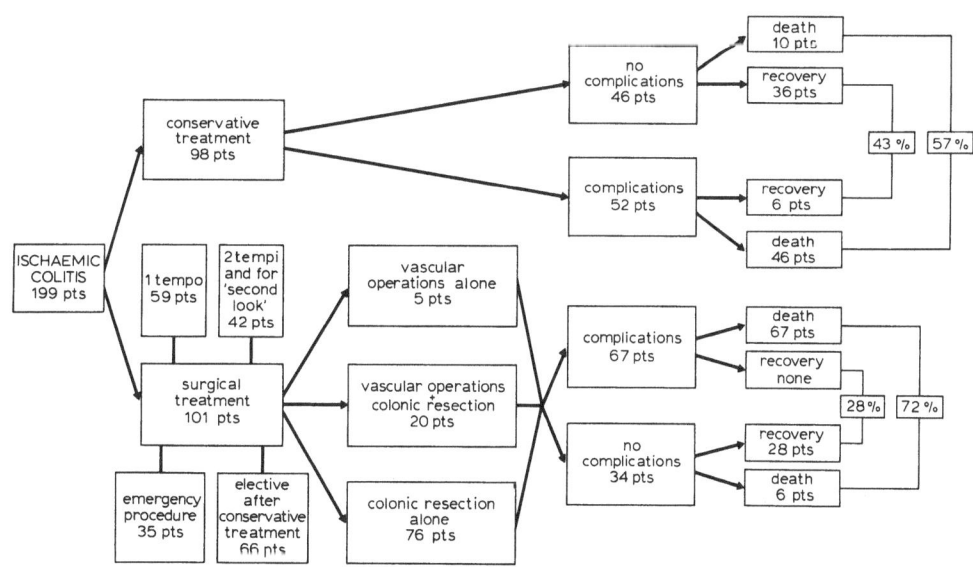

Fig. 27.1. Methods and results of therapy of our patients with ischaemic colitis. pts = patients.

Table 27.1. Treatment in the different forms of ischaemic colitis.

	Mucosal form of ischaemic colitis			Mural form						Transmural form		
				Stricturing ischaemic colitis			Chronic 'non resolving' ischaemic colitis			Gangrenous ischaemic colitis ± perforation		
Total number of patients	35			15			18			131		
Methods of treatment	S	C+S	C	S	C+S	C	S	C+S	C	S	C+S	C
Number of patients	1	1	33	4	3	8	5	11	2	25*	51	55
Result Death	1	–	1	2	1	1	1	3	–	20	43	54
Recovery	–	1	32	2	2	7	4	8	2	5	8	1

S = Surgical treatment alone.
C + S = Initially conservative treatment, followed by surgical treatment in a later stage.
C = Conservative treatment alone.
* = Vascular operations included.

later stage. Bedrest, oral restriction, parenteral nutrition, correction of acidosis and polyvalent antibiotic treatment were the most frequently presented forms of conservative treatment. In addition, cardiac glycosides (digitalis) were continued in some patients.

27.3 Surgical treatment

Hundred and one patients were treated surgically (tables 27.1, 27.2). In 35 of the 101 cases an emergency surgical procedure followed immediately after admission into the hospital. All these 35 patients had severe clinical symptoms and presented with signs of an acute abdomen.

In 66 of the 101 cases the clinical symptoms were mild initially without signs of peritoneal tenderness. In a later stage, inspite of conservative treatment, signs of peritonitis had developed. Surgical treatment followed. Mesenteric vascular operations alone were performed in 5 of the 101 cases; mesenteric vascular operations in combination with colonic resection were performed in 20 cases; colonic resection alone was performed in 76 cases.

Colonic resection (with/without partial small bowel resection) and an end-to-end anastomotic procedure were performed in 43 cases. Colonic resection with colostomy was performed in 46 cases.

Explorative laparotomy without colonic resection was carried out in 7 cases.

27.3.1 Non gangrenous forms of ischaemic colitis
Table 27.2 shows the correlation between the different types of surgical treatment and the different forms of ischaemic colitis.

Mucosal form (synonymous with 'transient form'). In the group of 35 patients with mucosal ischaemic colitis 33 patients were treated on a conservative basis and 2 patients had to be treated surgically for a distal obstructive colonic lesion. The colonic segment proximal to the colonic obstruction showed histological evidence of mucosal ischaemia.

Stricturing (mural) form. In this group of 15 patients, 8 patients were treated conservatively, because there were no signs of obstruction.

Seven patients were treated surgically, due to progression of stricture formation with signs of colonic obstruction.

Chronic 'non resolving' (mural) form. In this group of 18 patients, 2 patients were treated conservatively and 16 patients were treated surgically.

Six patients had a colonic resection with an end-to-end anastomosis; 9 patients had a colonic resection with a colostomy and in 1 patient explorative laparotomy was performed.

Table 27.2 Correlation between the different types of operations and the different types of ischaemic colitis, the presence of colonic ischaemia at the suture-line or colostomy-end(s) and the results of treatment in 96 patients with ischaemic colitis, who underwent surgery.

Different types of operation	Mucosal form of ischaemic colitis	Mural form: Stricturing ischaemic colitis	Mural form: Chronic 'non resolving' ischaemic colitis	Transmural form: Gangrenous ischaemic colitis ± perforation	Circulatory state of suture-line or colostomy-end(s) −	+	no histology	Result: Death	Recovery
End-to-end procedures									
Left hemicolectomy end-to-end	−	1	3	4	4	4	−	3	5
Right hemicolectomy end-to-end	−	−	1	3	2	1	1	3	1
Ileocoecal resection	−	−	1	2	2	1	−	2	1
43 cases Partial small bowel resection	−	−	−	5	1	3	1	5	−
Partial small bowel resection + right hemicolectomy	−	1	−	6	1	6	−	5	2
Partial small bowel resection + partial colonic resection	1	−	−	5	2	4	−	4	2
Partial small bowel resection + colonic resection	−	−	−	1	1	−	−	1	−
Partial colonic resection end-to-end	1	1	1	6	4	4	1	5	4
Total number of patients	2	3	6	32	17	23	3	28	15
Colostomy procedures									
Left hemicolectomy + Hartmann procedure	−	−	4	6	2	7	1	7	3
Left hemicolectomy + double colostomy	−	2	−	10	4	4	4	10	2
46 cases Right hemicolectomy + double colostomy	−	−	−	2	−	2	−	2	−
Partial colonic resection + colostomy	−	1	2	10	5	4	4	6	7
Total colectomy/colostomy; blind closure	−	1	3	5	4	3	2	6	3
Total number of patients	−	4	9	33	15	20	11	31	15
Explorative laparotomy	−	−	1	6	−	−	7	7	−

− = Free of (sub)mucosal ischaemic necrosis.
+ = Not free of (sub)mucosal ischaemic necrosis.

148

27.3.2 Gangrenous form of ischaemic colitis
Gangrenous (transmural) ischaemic colitis. In the group of 131 patients with gangrenous ischaemic colitis, surgical colonic procedures were performed in 71 cases. In 32 cases a colonic resection with an end-to-end anastomosis, and in 33 cases a colonic resection with colostomy was carried out (table 27.2). In 6 cases explorative laparotomy without colonic resection was performed. 4 Patients died due to progression of gangrene and 1 patient died due to sepsis.

In 2 patients a postmortem examination was refused, so the cause of death could not be verified. Five patients underwent a vascular operation. Fifty-five patients received conservative methods of therapy alone. In all these 55 cases gangrene of the bowel was either misdiagnosed initially, or the necrosis had progressed too far at the time of initial diagnosis.

27.3.3 Arterial reconstruction
In 25 cases an arterial reconstruction was performed; in 20 cases this was prior to resection of the colon. Vascular procedures consisting of an aortic bifurcation prosthesis in 15 cases, lower aortic vessel reconstruction in 1 case, ligation of the IMA in 1 case and embolectomy/thrombectomy of aorta/ mesenteric vessels in 8 cases, were carried out.

27.4 Relationship between the depth of the ischaemic lesion, the surgical resection technique used and the circulatory state of the resection-ends

Table 27.2 shows the relation between the depth of the ischaemic lesion, the circulatory state at the anastomosis and the various surgical resection procedures performed. In 75 patients the ends of the resected colonic segments were histologically examined.

Forty-three surgical procedures of end-to-end anastomosis had been performed of which 40 were checked histologically for signs of ischaemic damage. In 23 (58%) of these 40 cases the colonic suture line was *not* free from ischaemic damage. In 17 cases the colonic suture lines had a normal histological appearance. Forty-six surgical colostomy procedures had been performed of which 35 were checked histologically for ischaemic lesions. In 20 (57%) of these 35 cases the resection-end(s) were found to contain ischaemic lesions.

In 15 of these patients the end(s) were not ischaemic. Table 27.3 shows the relation between the different groups of ischaemic colitis and the ischaemic involvement of colonic resection-ends. In summary it can be concluded, that histological evidence for ischaemia of the colonic resection-ends was apparent in 57% (43/75) of the cases. Due to anastomotic leakage and progression of gangrene at the anastomosis or colostomy-end 35 of the 43 patients with ischaemia of the colonic resection-ends died (81%).

Table 27.3. Correlation between histology of colonic resection-ends (free- or not free of ischaemia) and the different forms of ischaemic colitis.

Different types of ischaemic colitis	Mucosal form	Mural form	Mural form	Transmural form	Total number of patients	Result	
Histology of colonic resection-ends	Transient ischaemic colitis	Stricturing ischaemic colitis	Chronic 'non resolving' ischaemic colitis	Gangrenous ischaemic colitis ± perforation		Death	Recovery
Colonic resection-ends free of ischaemia	–	5	8	19	32	12	20
Colonic resection-ends not free of ischaemia	–	4	6	33	43	35	8
Total number of patients	–	9	14	52	75	47	28

Table 27.4. Complications after surgical treatment (with or without conservative treatment initially): 96 laparotomies, in our patient material of 199 patients.

Type of operation	Total number of operations	(1) Shock	(2) Sepsis	(3) Necrosis of anastomosis or colostomy-end(s)	(4) Peritonitis	(5) Bleeding	(6) Cardiac arrhytmia	2+3+4	1+2+4	Progressive gangrene +1	None
End-to-end procedure 43 cases											
Left hemicolectomy end-to-end	8	1	–	–	–	–	–	1	–	1	5
Right hemicolectomy end-to-end	4	1	1	–	–	–	–	1	–	–	1
Ileococecal resection	3	2	1	–	–	–	–	–	–	3	–
Partial small bowel resection	5	1	–	–	–	–	–	1	–	3	–
Partial small bowel resection + right hemicolectomy	7	–	1	1	–	–	–	1	1	1	2
Partial small bowel resection + partial colonic resection	6	1	1	–	–	–	–	2	–	1	1
Partial small bowel resection + colonic resection	1	1	–	–	–	–	–	–	–	–	–
Partial colonic resection end-to-end	9	1	–	–	–	–	–	3	–	–	5
Total number of patients	43	8	4	1	–	–	–	9	1	6	14
Colostomy procedure 46 cases											
Left hemicolectomy + Hartmann procedure	10	1	1	–	–	1	1	1	–	3	2
Left hemicolectomy + double colostomy	12	3	–	4	–	1	–	–	1	1	2
Right hemicolectomy + double colostomy	2	–	–	2	–	1	–	–	–	1	–
Partial colonic resection + colostomy	13	1	–	1	–	–	–	3	3	2	6
Total colectomy/colostomy; blind closure.	9	2	2	–	–	–	–	–	1	1	3
Total number of patients	46	7	3	7	–	2	1	1	5	7	13
Explorative laparotomy	7	–	1	–	–	–	–	–	–	4	2

27.5 Complications and mortality following conservative and/or surgical treatment

In the group of 98 conservatively treated patients, 52 patients (53%) suffered from complications (table 27.5). Forty-six of the 52 patients died and 6 patients recovered. In 46 of the 98 patients no complications occurred. Ten of these 46 patients died for unknown reasons. In the group of 96* patients who underwent surgical treatment, (including all emergency-procedures) 67 patients (66%) suffered from complications (table 27.4). All 67 patients died. In 29 of these 96 patients (34%) no complications occurred. Following the 35 emergency procedures complications occurred in all patients (table 27.6). In the 5 patients with vascular operations alone no complications occurred. Sepsis, shock and progression of gangrenous infarction, with subsequent peritonitis and septic shock were the most frequently observed complications (tables 27.4, 27.5 and 27.6).

In 10 patients (10%) an anastomotical necrosis occurred after an end-to-end surgical procedure, due to (histologically proven) transmural ischaemic necrosis. In 8 patients necrosis of the colostomy end(s) occurred. In all of them it occurred after a colonic resection for a distal colonic obstruction (tables 18.6, 18.8). All the 18 patients with postoperative necrosis of the anastomosis or colostomy end(s) died.

Table 27.1 and Figure 27.1 show also the mortality rates in the groups of conservatively and surgically treated patients. In the group of patients with conservative treatment alone, 43% recovered and 57% died and in the group of patients which had undergone surgical treatment 28% recovered and 72% died.

Ninety-five % of the patients with complications (following conservative and/or surgical treatment) died. Table 27.7 shows the correlation between the treatment, the type of ischaemic colitis, and the mortality in our series of 199 patients.

In the group of patients with *non gangrenous* ischaemic colitis, 95% of the 43 patients recovered after conservative treatment and only 68% of the 25 patients who had undergone surgical treatment recovered.

* The 5 patients with vascular operations alone are not included.

Table 27.6. Complications following surgical treatment alone: 35 patients.

Complications	Result Death	Recovery	Total number of patients
Shock	15	–	15
Necrosis of the suture-line or colostomy-end(s)	8	–	8
Progression of gangrene + septic shock	12	–	12
Total number patients	35	–	35

Table 27.5. Complications following conservative treatment alone: 52 patients.

Complications	Result Death	Recovery	Total number of patients
Shock	30	5	35
Sepsis	6	1	7
Peritonitis	1	–	1
Progression of gangrene + septic shock	9	–	9
Total number of patients	46	6	52

Table 27.7. Correlation between result following conservative and surgical treatment and the main groups of ischaemic colitis in 199 patients.

Main groups of ischaemic colitis	Result following conservative and surgical treatment	Following conservative treatment	Following surgical treatment
Non-gangrenous ischaemic colitis	Recovery	95% (41)	68% (17)
	Death	5% (2)	32% (8)
Gangrenous ischaemic colitis	Recovery	2% (1)	18% (13)
	Death	98% (54)	82% (63)

The number of patients is indicated in brackets.

In those patients diagnosed as having a *gangrenous* form of ischaemic colitis, 98% of the 55 patients died after conservative treatment and 82% of the 76 patients who had undergone surgical treatment died.

In summary, in our study of 199 patients with ischaemic colitis 72 patients (36%) recovered and 127 patients (64%) died.

PART III

Reduction of the colonic arterial blood pressure after vessel occlusion, small vessel disease, low flow state and increased intralumenal pressure secondary to distal obstruction will lead to (sub) mucosal blood flow reduction, (sub)mucosal hypoxia, capillary wall damage, intestinal oedema and haemorrhage (Fig. 3.1).

The severity of the ischaemic involvement is dependent upon the rapidity of onset, the duration and the extent of the blood flow impairment.

Aetiology: In our studies ischaemic colitis developed spontaneously in 78% and secondary to a surgical procedure in 22% of the patients.

In this last group, left sided colonic ischaemia occurred in 5% of our patients after aortic bifurcation prosthesis, due to ligation of the IMA in the absence of a well developed collateral circulation. This incidence of 5% is higher than the findings of other authors who found an overall incidence of 1–2% (Johnson and Nabseth, 1974; Papadopoulos et al., 1974; Ernst et al., 1976).

Our results and the high incidence of 10% suggested by Smith and Szilagyi (1960) might be attributed to differences in operative technique, inappropriate ligation of the IMA, ligation of one or both hypogastric arteries and associated atheromatous lesions in other vessels.

In the other 17% of the patients we studied in this group postoperative shock and/or sepsis were probably the main cause of ischaemic colitis.

In 65% of our patients only one single demonstrable aetiopathogenic factor was present, whilst in 20% a combination of two or more of such factors were evident (Fig. 18.1). In 15% of our patients (all with a transient (mucosal) form of ischaemic colitis) no aetiopathogenic factor could be found.

Occlusive ischaemic colitis: Arterial occlusion: Obliterative atherosclerosis and thrombosis of the main stem or branches of the SMA and/or IMA were found in 16% of the cases we studied, which is a lower incidence than was suggested by Reiner et al., (1963). In our series the percentage incidence of embolism, found in one or both mesenteric arteries was also lower (13.5%) than previously reported, especially for the IMA.

The SMA seems to be a more frequent site for emboli (8%), compared to the IMA (2%) in our series, presumably due to the greater diameter and less acute angle of origin of the SMA (Demos et al., 1962; Dickson, 1968).

The IMA was frequently occluded as a result of aortic arteriosclerosis or abdominal aortic aneurysms. These patients were usually asymptomatic since the marginal vessel which extends from the middle colic to the left colic artery was capable of maintaining the viability of the left colon.

In the presence of an abdominal aneurysm, acute thrombosis of arterial branches appeared to be the main cause of colonic ischaemia. This frequently develops when, in addition to the anatomical factors, there is also hypovolaemia, hypotension and haemoconcentration, due to massive extravasation of blood in the retroperitoneal space and mesosigmoid. Our 5% incidence of this occurrence corresponds with that which has been reported in the literature (Young et al., 1963; Humphreys and Graham, 1977).

Compression of mesenteric arteries due to haemorrhage was encountered in 1.5%.

Venous occlusion: Venous occlusion was a not frequent causative factor in our cases (4%).

Hypercoagulable states (polycythaemia rubra vera, essential thrombocytosis) (2%), tumor infiltration into mesenteric veins and portal thrombosis (1%) were rare both in our series and in the literature (Dickson, 1968).

Necrotizing pancreatitis with compression of mesenteric veins by the necrotic infammatory mass and thrombophlebitis had caused ischaemic colitis in 0.5% of our cases.

In our retrospective studies no cases were present of venous thrombosis caused by the use of oral contraceptives (Reed and Coon, 1963; Barcewicz and Welch, 1980).

We found occlusive ischaemic colitis (arterial- and venous occlusion) in about 50% of the patients. The other 50% can be accounted for by non-occlusive ischaemia.

Non-occlusive ischaemic colitis: Low flow state: a diminution in circulating blood volume, due to cardiogenic haemorrhagic or septic shock or to dehydration, resulting in spasm of the splanchnic vessels appeared to be the second most frequent aetiopathogenic factor in ischaemic colitis in our study (35.5%).

Angiographically, surgically and even at post mortem examination the mesenteric arteries and veins appear to be patent, when traced from their origin to the bowel wall. Congestive heart failure, cardiac arrhythmia, and myocardial infarction, resulting in low left ventricular output was considered to have led to blood flow reduction to the colon and secondarily to ischaemic colitis in 16% of our patients. The difference between the relative infrequency (7%) with which we found cardiac arrhythmia as a cause of low flow state leading to ischaemic colitis, and the much higher incidence (50%) found by Renton (1972) is probably accounted for by patient selection. In most cases of cardiopathy, a combination with other factors, such as narrowing of large colic arteries and/or small vessel stenosis may have added to the risk of colonic ischaemia.

Digitalis (Pawlik and Jacobson, 1974) and antihypertensive medication (O'Connell, 1976) which have a vasoconstrictive action on the splanchnic circulation, may potentiate the decrease in circulatory volume in cardiac patients and lead to colonic ischaemia.

A massive circulatory volume deficit ('low flow') and haemoconcentration, as a result of dehydra-

tion, with or without a prolonged medication of diuretics (Sharefkin and Silen, 1974) may also lead to colonic ischaemia which happened in 4% of our patients.

Thus, a prolonged or too intensive treatment with diuretics may be dangerous and cause ischaemic colitis, especially in elderly patients with generalized arteriosclerotic vessel disease.

Small vessel disease: Small vessel disease may play an important role in the development of ischaemic colitis, when combined with a diminished circulating blood volume and an already compromised splanchnic circulation. It occurred in 7.5% of our patients. We can endorse the suggestion of Whitehead (1971) that diffuse intravascular coagulation may play a part in the pathogenesis of non-occlusive colonic ischaemia.

We have also regularly found capillary and venular thrombi in the bowel wall of our patients with ischaemic colitis. Microangiopathy (proliferative intima hyperplasia) due to diabetes and/or hypertension, in combination with low flow state was found in 8% of our patients with ischaemic colitis. This strong correlation has already been suggested earlier by various authors (Arosemena and Edwards, 1967; Detry et al., 1979; McGregor et al., 1980; Raghunatha et al., 1983). Vasculitis of the mesenteric arteries, due to immunological disorders such as systemic lupus erythematosus, rheumatoid arthritis and polyarteritis nodosa may have led to a critical reduction in mesenteric blood flow with resultant multifocal ischaemic lesions in 3% of our cases.

Qan (1968) suggested that enterocolitis secondary to irradiation vasculopathy could become manifest several months to many years after radiation treatment. In 5 of our patients such lesions were present.

The interval between radiation treatment and onset of ischaemic colitis varied between 2 weeks and 11 years. Narrowing of peripheral mesenteric vessels, due to amyloidosis as a additional aetiopathogenic factor of ischaemic colitis (Perarnau et al., 1982) was encountered in 2% of our patients.

Obstructive ischaemic colitis: The incidence of proximal colonic ischaemia in the presence of a more distally located stenosing malignancy is

1–4.7% according to various authors. Some authors, however, (Saegesser and Sandblom, 1975; Lewin and Hahn, 1979) noted an incidence below 1%. Schwartz and Boley (1972) on the other hand noted an incidence of 10%. We found this type of ischaemic colitis in 12 patients (6%). No data on the frequency of occurrence of ischaemic colitis proximal to benign stenosing lesions is available in the literature: this occurred in 2% of our patients and was due to benign diverticular disease (Thijn, 1973) and in 2% after faecal impaction (de Boer and van Unnink, 1968; Hay, 1978). In addition to dilatation and elevation of the intralumenal pressure, the virulence of bacterial overgrowth in stagnant material, hypermotility, repetitive straining and increased muscular spasm should also be considered as important factors in the aetiology of ischaemic colitis secondary to obstruction (Boley et al., 1978).

Obstructive colitis caused by either benign or malignant stenosing disease occurred in 10% of our cases, but was only rarely diagnosed before surgery. We consider that:

– The radiologist should be alert to the possibility of such proximal ischaemic damage in studying colorectal cancer. A barium enema during the initial phase of the illness is the most important method to make the diagnosis.
– For the surgeon it is necessary to examine the entire colonic segment that is removed for car cinoma to exclude the presence of ischaemia in the proximal resection end, since such involvement may lead to dehiscence or stricture formation.

Classifications: Various classifications of ischaemic colitis have been introduced by different authors; these have been based upon clinical (Marston et al., 1966; Brown, 1968; van Dongen et al., 1982), histological (Morson, 1971; Swerdlow et al., 1981) or endoscopical (Favier et al., 1976; Scowcroft et al., 1981) findings.

The clinical classification after Marston et al., (1966) – sometimes in a modified version (Brown, 1968; van Dongen et al., 1981) – has been most frequently used.

However, the heterogeneity of the different classifications may cause confusion. For a greater practical usefulness we employed a classification which combines the clinical classification (after Marston et al., 1966) with the histological classification (after Morson, 1971 and Swerdlow et al., 1981) (Fig. 19.1) as follows.

The non gangrenous type of ischaemic colitis may be subdivided into a (reversible) transient (mucosal) ischaemic colitis, and an (irreversible) (mural) ischaemic colitis, which may present as a persistent ulcerating form (chronic 'non resolving' ischaemic colitis) or may be complicated by fibrosis (stricturing form). A gangrenous (transmural) necrotizing form of ischaemic colitis may occur with or without perforation. An ischaemic process may heal after the acute phase has subsided, or, in unfavourable conditions (prolonged hypertension, small vessel disease, inadequate collateral circulation etc.), progress to deeper layers or extend in surface area.

In the collected literature (1950–1982) the non gangrenous form has been reported in 52% of the cases investigated and the gangrenous form in 48%. With 54% in our material, we found a higher incidence of gangrenous (transmural) ischaemic colitis than in the literature; this may probably be accounted for by patient selection.

Age/sex ratio: Most of the 199 patients studied with ischaemic colitis were between the 6th–9th decade. The mean age of patients in our studies (69.1 years) was higher than that which we found after reviewing the literature (60 years); again this was most probably due to the selection of our patient material predominantly from autopsy studies (51%).

A study of the sex-ratio of our patients with ischaemic colitis (1.14 men : 1 woman) and the sex-ratio of cases reported in the literature between 1950 and 1982 (1.5 men : 1 woman) indicates that men are slightly more prone to ischaemic colitis than are women.

Patients with a low flow state were relatively older than patients without demonstrable low flow state and patients in whom we could not find a clear aetiopathogenic factor were older than patients in whom one or more aetiopathogenic factors were found.

Associated diseases: According to Marcuson (1972) it should nearly always be possible to find a single predisposing factor in patients below 50 years of age. However, in our material in only 3 of the 11 patients below 50 years of age a single cause could be detected. Above 50 years of age Marcuson reported the diagnosis of pre-existing disease in 57% of the cases. He did not comment on particular combinations of predisposing factors. In our series of patients above 50 years of age 64% had associated diseases (53% single and 11% multiple). It is remarkable that hypertension was found in 17% of the patient group older than 50 years (either alone (7%) or in combination with other diseases e.g. diabetes (10%)). We conclude that hypertension and diabetes is an important combination of factors in the development of non-occlusive colonic ischaemia.

Clinical symptoms/signs: Comparing our clinical data with those reported in the literature, we can corroborate the nature and incidence of the different clinical signs. Acute onset of intermittent colicky pain, mostly localized in the left hypochondrium and paraumbilical region was the most frequently found clinical sign both in the literature and in our patients, followed by passage of dark or bright red blood, diarrhoea, nausea and vomiting.

In our material no correlation between histological depth of ischaemia and severity of clinical symptoms was apparent. Swerdlow et al., (1981) came to the same conclusion.

Physical symptoms/signs: Distension, peritoneal tenderness and pressure pain upon palpation occurred in all forms of ischaemic colitis, but most frequently within the group of gangrenous (transmural) ischaemic colitis. However, a complete lack of physical signs was apparent in 18–23% of the patients examined, whatever the form of ischaemic colitis including those with gangrenous ischaemic colitis (21%).

It seems from these studies therefore, that any form of ischaemic colitis can be associated with the full spectrum of physical and clinical symptoms and signs or, on the contrary, may go completely unnoticed.

Localisation of the ischaemic lesion: Both in the 1,024 case reports collected from the literature (Fig. 10.1) and in own patient material (Fig. 23.1) the left side of the colon (descending colon and sigmoid) showed the greatest predisposition to is-

chaemia, 73% and 62% respectively. On the left side of the colon, especially at the splenic flexure (Griffith's point) the marginal artery of Drummond, which is a major connection between the middle colic artery and the left colic artery may be poorly developed or even absent (Meyers, 1976).

The blood flow to the left side of the colon can therefore be precarious and may easily lead to blood flow impairment in the event of a low flow state.

Right sided colonic ischaemia is more usually the consequence of distal colonic obstruction (4% in our series) or a result of embolism of the main branch of the SMA (30%).

Because both these aetiopathogenic factors were included in our studies, we found a higher incidence of ischaemic damage at the right side (34%) than was reported in the literature (23%).

Right sided colonic ischaemia was also seen in two young adults with evanescent ischaemic colitis. While some authors initially considered rectal ischaemia as rare or non existent, (Egger and Kellock, 1970; O'Connell, 1976), other authors suggested (Alschibaja and Morson, 1977) that rectal involvement represented 4–16% of the cases. Both in the literature studied and in our series, rectal ischaemia was apparent in only 4% of the cases. This low incidence can be explained by the particularly rich vascularisation of the rectum (Fig. 2.4). Major obstruction of sacral arterial branches would be necessary before rectal ischaemia may develop.

No definite correlation between the colonic segment involved and particular aetiopathogenic factors could be found.

Laboratory investigation: Reports of laboratory investigations are scarce in the literature (Marston et al., 1966). Because the results are often non-specific, the investigations usually offer little help in making the diagnosis.

The WBC count and ESR were elevated and both independent of the depth of colonic ischaemia. Owing to haemoconcentration there may also be a rise in the haematocrit.

Serumenzyme levels (AF, SGOT, SGPT, LDH) may be elevated. Stool- and blood cultures were of little or no value in diagnosing ischaemic colitis in our own material. The Guajac test for occult blood was positive in most of our cases (84%).

Radiology: Barium enema: In the cases reviewed in the literature 92% of the 402 barium enemas, and in our series 77% of 75 (first) barium enemas showed one or more positive signs for ischaemic colitis. 'Thumbprinting', defined as a translucent oval or rounded filling defect due to submucosal haemorrhage and/or oedema was found in 67% of the cases recorded in the literature and in 57% in our series. They are circumferentially, but often asymmetrically distributed over the colonic wall. It may be temporary and was most frequently (74%) shown in the early stage (1–7 days) of colonic ischaemia. In 43% of our own cases it was still present in the second week and in 25% persisted into the third week. This supports the finding of Gore et al., (1979), who also reported that thumbprints may persist for a duration of several weeks. Usually, however, the thumbprints disappear after 48–72 hours by resorption of blood or oedema. This is frequently accompanied by spasm, which was indeed found in 29% of our cases and in a higher percentage (56%) of those cases reported in the literature. Loss of haustration, due to submucosal haemorrhage and/or oedema in the early stage and fibrosis in a later stage, was also detected in a lower percentage (19%) in our studies than in those reported in the literature (52%). The lower incidence of both signs in our series is probably due to the retrospective analysis of barium enemas, thus missing the spastic contractions which would occur during the 'dynamic phase' of the examination.

'Transverse ridging', deep transverse contractions running perpendicular to the colonic axis and symmetrically distributed over the colonic wall, were found in 19% of our cases. Most authors did not mention this feature (Table 11.1), although Wittenberg et al., (1975) reported an incidence of 32% of this phenomenon in the early stages of ischaemic colitis. Because we found transverse ridging only in the first 2 weeks, we consider it as an early sign for colonic ischaemia. We did not find it in later stages.

Ulceration, which appears as a ragged saw tooth irregularity or spiculation on a barium enema, seems in our studies to be independent of the time of performing the barium enema. Ulceration occurred in 42% of the cases reported in the literature and in 48% in our series.

Sacculation – wide mouthed outpouchings or pseudodiverticula of the colonic wall on the anti-mesenteric side – occurred in our material in a late stage of colonic ischaemia after 1–3 months. It is commonly found associated with tubular narrowing or stricturing. Sacculation was seen in 24% of our cases, whilst the literature gives an incidence of only 11%. Stricturing and/or tubular narrowing were described in 20% of the cases reported in the literature and in 17% of our cases. In all patients it occurred in the final stage of ischaemic colitis (between 3 weeks and 12 months after onset of clinical symptoms).

We consider tubular stenosis and/or stricturing and sacculation of the bowel as a radiological expression of the reparative scarring of the bowel wall and a final stage of ischaemic colitis (Marston et al., 1966; Marshak and Lindner, 1968; Williams, 1971; Alschibaja and Morson, 1971; Gore et al., 1979). To demonstrate evolutionary changes during ischaemic colitis and to document stricturing lesions or tubular narrowing secondary to chronic 'non resolving' ischaemic colitis, a follow-up barium enema is recommended.

Following study of both the cases reported in the literature and those included in our own series, we conclude that the single- our double contrast barium enema is a sensitive and accurate radiographic method for detection of the early signs of ischaemic colitis (thumbprinting, transverse ridging, spasm, loss of haustration, ulceration), especially if it has been performed in the early stage of the disease, preferably within the first week after the onset of symptoms. A follow-up barium enema (between 3 weeks and 3 months later) should be performed to establish whether or not there are chronic or late stage signs of ischaemic colitis (tubular narrowing, stricturing, sacculation, loss of haustration, ulceration).

The combination of an appropriate clinical history and a barium enema with characteristic findings permits an accurate differential diagnosis between ischaemic ulcerative inflammatory colonic disease and colon carcinoma to be made in the majority of cases.

Angiography: Angiography was performed in 195 of the 1,024 patients (19%), reported in the collected literature (1950–1982). Occlusion and stenosis of one or both mesenteric arteries were frequently found. However, in 26% of the cases (51 patients) the mesenteric arteries were patent. In 33 of our 199 patients (17%) angiography was performed. In 11 of these 33 patients (35%) the mesenteric arteries were patent.

It is evident from studying the literature as well as our own experience that it is often difficult to correlate clinical symptoms with mesenteric vessel occlusion as shown by arteriography. We agree with many authors that the occurrence of a stenosis or occlusion of one of the colic arteries on the angiography does not necessarily imply that such lesions were the primary cause of ischaemic colitis.

In the first place a rich collateral network can prevent ischaemia of a colonic segment despite occlusion of one or more main colic vessels. Secondly, the occurrence of colon gangrene without demonstrable vascular occlusion can be caused by a low flow state of elevation of intralumenal pressure due to distal colonic obstruction. (A combination of these two aetiopathogenic factors was even more frequently (45.5%) found in our series than was arterial occlusion (43%)). Furthermore it is difficult to detect a flow obstruction in peripheral vessels, because they are too small to be visualized by angiography. Therefore a 'negative' arteriography does not exclude ischaemic colitis.

'Early venous filling' and intense blushing of the bowel wall can also be found in other inflammatory ulcerative colonic lesions and are therefore non-specific.

The only advantage of angiography, in our opinion, is that aortography or selective angiographic studies of the IMA and SMA can give information about the presence and adequacy of collateral circulation and the condition of the main mesenteric vessels preoperatively. This additional information may allow the surgeon to anticipate the need for the reimplantation of the IMA or the revascularization of the SMA or coeliac artery.

Endoscopy: Colonoscopy, which was indicative for ischaemic colitis, was performed in 20% of our patients in different stages of the disease.

Oedema and haemorrhage (bulbous protrusions corresponding with the thumbprinting seen on a barium enema) were more frequently (88%) present in the early stage of the disease, but we also occasionally found late manifestations of thumb-printing corresponding with the observations of Gore et al., (1979) and Schmutz et al., (1980).

Ulceration was present at the end of the first week, with a peak frequency in the 4th–6th week; thereafter the frequency of occurrence decreases.

Reepithelialisation was most frequently found in the chronic stage of ischaemia, usually after 2 weeks. This observation corresponds with the time sequence of epithelial cell regeneration at the margins of the mucosal ulcers, such as described by Morson (1971).

Stricturing and/or tubular narrowing and sacculations were found in the late stages (4 weeks and later) of colonic ischaemia and they represent an end result of survival of the bowel wall; this is accompanied by progressive fibrosis and mucosal reorganisation.

Early and late findings as shown in fig. 28.1 correspond with our radiological and endoscopical findings and those of several authors (Marston et al., 1966; Schmutz et al., 1980). The different endoscopical classifications of ischaemic colitis, according to severity (Favier et al., 1976) and according to duration (Scowcroft et al., 1981) are not useful in our opinion, because there may be many gradations and overlaps in the different stages of ischaemic colitis (Alschibaja and Morson, 1977).

Histopathology: In studying the histopathology of ischaemic colonic disease a combination of two classifications was used in the microscopical analysis of 165 pathological specimen examined, – one based upon depth (Swerdlow et al., 1981) and one based upon stage (Morson, 1971) of the ischaemic lesion. In transient ischaemic colitis the damage was limited to the mucosa; in the stricturing or chronic 'non resolving' form the depth of damage was mural and in gangrenous ischaemic colitis the lesions were transmural.

The microscopical features of ischaemic colitis in our studies did not differ from earlier descriptions by Morson, (1971) and Whitehead, (1972).

The susceptability of the colon to ischaemia was evident in our autopsy material in which careful microscopical examination often revealed early mucosal lesions as a result of preterminal circulatory collapse.

Depending on the rapidity of onset, the type and extent of vascular occlusion and the quality of the

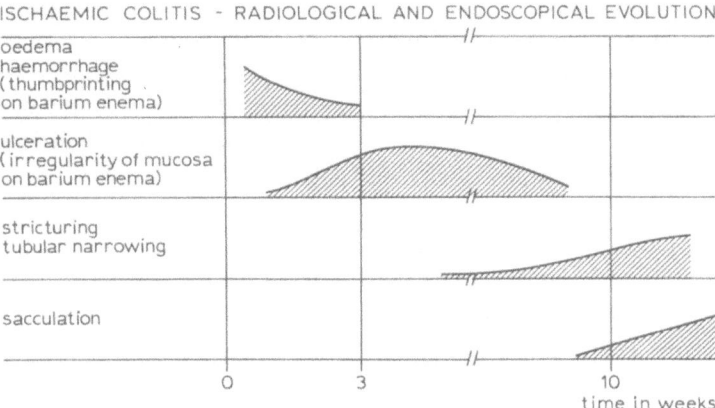

ISCHAEMIC COLITIS - RADIOLOGICAL AND ENDOSCOPICAL EVOLUTION

oedema
haemorrhage
(thumbprinting
on barium enema)

ulceration
(irregularity of mucosa
on barium enema)

stricturing
tubular narrowing

sacculation

0   3   10
time in weeks

Fig. 28.1.

collateral circulation colonic necrosis may have a pale ischaemia or a congestive red haemorrhagic appearance due to blood extravasation in the tissues.

The haemorrhagic type can be expected to occur in patients with venous occlusion or with slowly developing occlusive- and non-occlusive ischaemic lesions, but no clear correlation could be established with the various types of aetiopathogenic factors in our material. It was not difficult to diagnose the acute stages of gangrenous and non gangrenous ischaemic colitis. However, it was sometimes hard to differentiate the chronic ulcerating form from 'ulcerative colitis' or 'Crohn's disease of the colon'. This concerns most likely cases, which are described in the literature as 'ulcerative colitis of undetermined origin'. Such lesions represent 9% of our histological material. 'Wedge shaped' ulcerations, that may penetrate the muscularis propria or ulcers that undermine edges of adjacent unaffected mucosa may occur in this chronic 'non resolving' form. Also Crohn-like lesions with transmural lymphoplasmacellular infiltrations were encountered and these sometimes make differentiation from other inflammatory ulcerative colonic lesions more difficult. However, the combination with the clinical history and the results of radiological and endoscopical studies may lead to a correct diagnosis.

Since Marston et al., (1966) noted that 'haemosiderin-laden' macrophages are a prominent feature of the cellular infiltrate in ischaemic colitis, many authors have considered this finding as being pathognomonic for colonic ischaemia. Whilst there is evidence for this phenomenon in early lesions, it has been not so evident in the more persisting lesions in our experience.

In case of obstructive ischaemic colitis the ischaemic mucosa is particularly susceptible to penetration by a faecal flora which has become more pathogenic as a consequence of bacterial overgrowth of more virulent species as occurs in the blind loop syndrome. The histological appearance of this form of colitis is quite varied. One may encounter superficial mucosal ulceration, subchronic ulcerative colitis, focal phlegmonous inflammation with peritonitis or transmural necrosis and perforation. A segment of relatively normal mucosa may be found between the site of obstruction and the segment with ischaemic damage. This occurred in 13% of our cases and in 31% of those cases reported in literature.

With only a few exceptions (Aboumrad et al., 1963; Arosemena and Edwards, 1967; Williams, 1969; Pierce and Brokenbrough, 1970; McGregor et al., 1980; Raghunatha et al., 1983), most authors have not discussed the possible role of stenosing lesions of the small mesenteric arteries. This suggests that small mesenteric vessels are rarely examined histologically at autopsy or in resection material in patients with ischaemic vascular diseases. This unfortunately also applies to the case material of our own study. In 44% of our own histological material no mention was made of the condition of the small mesenteric vessels in the initial pathology report or there was no material available for histological examination.

Obstruction or disease at the level of distal meso-colic arteries in patients with ischaemic colitis may exist, without the presence of obstructing athe-romas in the larger mesenteric- or submucosal vessels.

As could be expected, diabetes was associated with more severe peripheral atherosclerosis than occured in non diabetic patients. A strong correla-tion between hypertension and stenosing lesions in terminal mesenteric arteries was suggested by Arosemena and Edwards (1967) and Pierce and Brokenbrough (1970): our observations support this association. In 24% of our patients with hyper-tension the distal mesenteric vessels were histo-logically examined. All showed lumenal narrow-ing, caused by intimal proliferation.

Especially the combination of diabetes and hy-pertension may lead to peripheral vessel narrow-ing. Without any examination of the peripheral vasculature, the importance of other small vessel diseases as vasculitis, amyloidosis, radiation damage, cholesterol emboli, as aetiopathogenic factors of ischaemic colitis will stay underes-timated.

It is our conclusion that, widespread intimal hy-perplasia of the small terminal mesocolic arteries, in association with diabetes and/or hypertension as well as other small vessel diseases, may play an important role in adding to the deleterious effects of large vessel disease and of poor circulation.

We agree with the conclusion of Whitehead (1973) and Hunt and Buchanan (1979) that the usefulness of colonic biopsies in the diagnosis of ischaemic colitis is limited, because of the superfi-cial nature of the specimen and the lack of specif-icity of the microscopical findings in chronic cases. The appearance of the early necrotic lesion in isch-aemic colitis may be characteristic, but in the ul-cerating phase the histological changes are those of non-specific chronic ulceration.

Other diagnostic procedures: Other diagnostic pro-cedures such as ultrasound (te Strake, 1983; Ike, 1983), Doppler ultrasound flow measurements (Hobson et al., 1976; Cooperman et al., 1979), computed tomography (Jones et al., 1982) and ra-dionuclide imaging (Bardfeld et al., 1977; Barth et al., 1978, 1979; Dutcher et al., 1981) might prove to be useful in the diagnosis of ischaemic colitis in the near future. To date the reports in the literature are very scarce.

Differential diagnosis: Ischaemic colitis must be distinguished from diverticular disease, tuber-culous colitis, bacillary dysentery, amoebiasis, campylobacter colitis, pseudomembranous colitis, carcinoma, irradiation colitis and particularly ul-cerative colitis and Crohn's disease of the colon (Price, 1977). We consider that the combination of clinical and physical signs with the results of radi-ological, endoscopical and histological examin-ation, are important in differentiating ischaemic colitis from other ulcerative inflammatory bowel diseases. Results of laboratory analysis are usually not specific. The distribution and character of the lesions are the two main diagnostic features by which the physician can distinguish ischaemic col-itis from ulcerative colitis and Crohn's disease of the colon (tables 15.1–15.5).

Therapeutic management: Non gangrenous form of ischaemic colitis: Recognition of the clinical entity of ischaemic colitis is the first vital step in deciding upon the appropriate treatment of patients with ischaemic colitis. Once the disease is diagnosed, therapy may be guided by the clinical picture.

In the non gangrenous forms of ischaemic colitis the symptoms were frequently mild and the disease self limiting. In the entire non gangrenous group of our patients with ischaemic colitis 95% recovered after regular monitoring and conservative treat-ment. A review of the collected literature (1950–1982), indicates that 90% of the patients in this group recovered after conservative treatment.

Oral food and fluid restriction, gastric aspiration if necessary, total parenteral nutrition, correction of acidosis, reequilibration of body water and elec-trolytes, polyvalent antibiotic treatment (ery-thromycine or neomycine) constitute the appropri-ate primary management of all patients with non gangrenous ischaemic colitis. If possible, cortico-steroids should be avoided, because these are use-less and may perhaps increase the chance of phlegmonous enteritis and colonic perforation and secondary infection.

Gangrenous form of ischaemic colitis: The gang-renous (transmural or necrotizing) form of ischaemic colitis is important because of the high mortality rate within this group (79% in the collected literature and 98% of patients in our series who had received conservative treatment only).

The decision as to whether or not to operate is determined by the clinical picture (Abel and Russell, 1983).

If, despite regular monitoring and the failure of initial conservative therapy, the condition of the patient deteriorates, and progressive peritoneal signs develop, then the need for operative intervention becomes urgent.

A review of the literature indicates that there is a considerable divergence of opinions concerning surgical treatment of patients with gangrenous ischaemic colitis (Kaminski et al., 1973; Heikkinen et al., 1974; Hunt, 1977; Rausis et al., 1977; Saegesser et al., 1981; Milleret, 1981; Guivarc'H et al., 1982). After studying the collected literature on 302 patients with gangrenous ischaemic colitis the mortality after colonic resection with end-to-end anastomosis was high (56%) with an anastomotic 'leakage' in 7% of the cases. In our material the mortality rate after this type of resection was even higher (65%). In 23% of the patients, necrosis of the suture line was found clinically and histologically.

An analysis of the literature reports on patients who had undergone a colostomy showed a mortality rate of 54%, whilst in our own material it was 67%. In 17% of our patients necrosis of the colostomy-end(s) was found clinically and histologically. Most problems, due to necrosis of the suture line or colostomy-end(s) occurred because of a too limited colonic resection, particularly when the extent of the disease was not carefully established at laparotomy or when perforation had already occurred.

Indeed, in 58% of the cases with histologically checked suture lines, the suture line was not free from (mucosal) ischaemia. In 57% of the histologically checked colostomy-end(s), the resection-end(s) were found to contain (mucosal) ischaemic lesions.

From these results it is evident that the extent of the ischaemic process may not be readily apparent from the normal looking serosa (Rosen et al., 1973; Williams and Wittenberg, 1975).

The mucosa may be severely damaged micro-scopically and even necrotic, while the vascular supply to the serosa remains intact, giving the bowel a healthy pink appearance at laparotomy. This is the reason why these superficially extended ischaemic lesions often remained unrecognized. Therefore we consider a wide colonic resection with colostomy at both ends followed by re-establishment of continuity after 4–6 weeks as the treatment of choice. Colonic resection with end-to-end anastomosis should only be considered if a wide resection is performed and furthermore, if the colonic resection-end(s) are histologically checked for early ischaemic necrosis. This is also the therapy of choice in cases of chronic 'non re-solving' (mural) ischaemic colitis.

If the postoperative physical signs deteriorate this procedure should be followed by a 'second look' procedure (Schennach and Flora, 1972; Lubbers, 1982).

Considering the high mortality rate (86%) in our group of patients who underwent explorative laparotomy without colonic resection, because the appearance of the colon was not suggestive of serious ischaemic disease, we suggest that, had a 'second look' procedure been done, the mortality rate might have been lower.

The decision as to the timing of a second operation must be made at the time of completion of the first laparotomy, since the symptoms and clinical signs during the next 24 hours are unreliable (16.3.1.2).

Complications: The occurrence of complications was frequently not mentioned in the literature. After conservative treatment, we found a high complication rate in our own cases (53%). Most frequent complications were shock (58%), progression of gangrene with subsequent peritonitis and septic shock (17%), and sepsis (12%).

After surgical treatment complications occurred in an even higher percentage (66%) of our cases.

Septic shock (34%), necrosis of the suture line or colostomy-end(s) (27%) and progressive gangrene (25%) were the most frequently observed postoperative complications in our series. In a retrospective review of 18 patients with ischaemic colitis by Abel and Russel (1983) the mortality rate after conservative treatment was 45%, in the collected literature reviewed 25% and in our material 57%.

The mortality rates after surgical treatment were respectively 55%, 43% and 72%.

The high complication- and mortality rates in our series are probably due to the following features:

– A frequent misdiagnosis of ischaemic colonic disease and subsequent inappropriate treatment: elderly patients were frequently treated for 'ulcerative colitis' or 'Crohn's colitis', while the disease had an ischaemic basis;

– Gangrenous (transmural) ischaemic colitis can frequently pass unrecognized despite the evidence of clinical symptoms, since there may be a complete absence of physical signs;

– Not recognizing ischaemia as a causative factor of colonic disease;

– A too limited colonic resection. All patients with progressive necrosis at the resection line or colostomy-end(s) died; This selection procedure skews the patient representation into the more severe end of the spectrum.

However, the 'in-depth study' of these more severe cases will hopefully improve our understanding of this disease and lead to a better patient management.

29 LITERATURE AND REFERENCES

The articles used for the study about 'increased intralumenal pressure secondary to colonic obstruction' are marked with an □.
The articles used for the review study of ischaemic colitis in general are marked with an ○.

Abel, M.E., Russell, T.R.: Ischemic colitis; comparison of surgical and non-operative management. Dis. Colon & Rectum 26, 2, 113–115, 1983.

Aboumrad, M.H., Fine, G., Horn, R.C. Jr.: Intimal hyperplasia of the small mesenteric arteries. Arch. Path. Lab. Med. 75, 98–102, 1963.

Addleman, W.: Obstructing carcinoma with acute proximal ulcerative colitis. Amer. J. Gastroenterology 40, 174–178, 1963. (□)

Agrawal, N.M., Gyrr, N., McDowell, W., Font, R.G.: Intestinal obstruction due to acute pancreatitis. Am. J. Dig. Dis. 19, 179, 1974.

Aldrete, J.S., Han, S.Y., Laws, H.L., Kirklin, J.W.: Intestinal infarction complicating low cardiac output states. Surg. Gynec. Obstet. 144, 371–375, 1977.

Alschibaja, T., Morson, B.C.: Ischaemic bowel disease. J. Clin. Pathol. 30, suppl. (Roy. Coll. Path.) 11, 68, 1977.

Ambruoso, V.N., Feraru, F.: Massive gangrene of the colon due to distal obstruction. Surgery 61, 228–230, 1967. (□)

Andersen, J.F., Eklöf, O.: Segmental vascular occlusion of the colon. Pediatr. Radiol. 11, 5–7, 1981.

Anderson, R.E., Witkowski, C.J., Pontius, G.V.: Radiation stricture of the small intestine. Surgery 38, 605–609, 1955.

Anderson, P.E.: Ischaemic colitis caused by angiography. Clin. Radiol. 20, 414–417, 1969.

Anthony, P.P.: Gangrene of the small intestine: a complication of argentaffin carcinoma. Brit. J. Surg. 57, 118–122, 1970.

Archibald, R.B., Burnstein, A.V., Knackstedt, V.E., Tolman, K.G., Holbrook, J.H.: Ischaemic colitis in a young adult due to inferior mesenteric vein thrombosis. Endoscopy 12, 140–143, 1980. (○)

Arkin, A.: A clinical and pathological study of periarteritis nodosa. A report of 5 cases, one histologically healed. Am. J. Path. 6, 401, 1930.

Arosemena, E., Edwards, J.E.: Lesions of the small mesenteric arteries underlying intestinal infarction. Geriatrics 22, 122–138, 1967.

Aubia, J., Lloveras, J., Munne, A., et al.: Ischaemic colitis in chronic uremia. Nephron 29, 146–150, 1981.

Avnet, N.L., Elkin, M.: Unusual appearance of the colon following sigmoid volvulus. Radiology, 77, 836–838, 1961. (□)

Baas, E.U.: Die ischämische Kolitis. Dtsch. med. Wschr. 100, 1247–1248, 1975.

Baghwat, A.G., Hawk, W.A.: Terminal haemorrhagic necrotizing enteropathy. Amer. J. Gastroenterology 45, 163, 1966.

Balslev, I., Jensen, H.E., Nørgaard, F., Poll, P.: Ischemic colitis. Acta Chir. Scand. 136, 235–242, 1970. (○)

Balz, J., Minton, J.P.: Mesenteric thrombosis following splenectomy. Ann. Surg. 179, 126–128, 1975.

Bane, A.E., Austen, W.G.: Superior mesenteric artery embolism. Surg. Gynec. Obstet. 116, 474, 1963.

Barcewicz, P.A., Welch, J.P.: Ischaemic colitis in young adult patients. Dis. Colon & Rectum 123, 109–114, 1980. (○)

Bardfeld, P.A.A., Boley, S.J., Sammartano, R., Bowtemps, R.: Scintigraphic diagnosis of ischaemic intestine with technetium 99m sulphur colloid labelled leucocytes. Radiology 124, 439–443, 1977.

Barth, K.H., Alderson, P.D., Strandberg, J.D., Strauss, H.W., White, R.I.: ^{99m}Tc pyrophosphate imaging in experimental mesenteric infarction relationship of tracer uptake to the degree of ischaemic injury. Radiology 129, 491–495, 1978.

Barth, K.H., Alderson, P.O., Strandberg, J.D., Fara, J.W.: Early imaging of experimental intestinal infarction with ^{99m}Tc pyrophosphate. Radiology 133, 459–462, 1979.

Bartram, C.J.: Obliteration of thumbprinting with double contrast enemas in acute ischemic colitis. Gastrointest. Radiol. 4, 85–88, 1979. (○)

Bar-Ziv, J., Ayoub, J.I.G., Fletcher, B.D.: Hemolytic uremic syndrome: a case presenting with acute colitis. Pediatr. Radiol. 2, 203–205, 1974.

Bekheit, F.: Ischaemic colitis, study of 17 cases. Egypt. Med. Ass. 58, 20–26, 1975.

Benacerraf, R., Delage, Y., Bléry, M., Bismuth, V.: Les aspects radiologiques des colites ischémiques: Etude de huit observations. Ann. Radiol. 19, 5, 495–504, 1976. (○)

Berenquer, J., Cabades, F., Gras, M.D., Pertejo, V., Rayon, M., Sala, T.: Ischemic colitis attributable to a cleansing enema; case report. Hepato-gastroenterol. 28, 173–175, 1981. (○)

Bergan, J.J., Dry, L., Conn J. Jr., Trippel, O.H.: Intestinal ischemic syndromes. Ann. Surg. 169, 120, 1969.

Berger, R.L., Lium, R.: Abdominal post-ganglionic sympathectomy. A method for the production of an ulcerative-colitis-like-state in dogs. Ann. Surg. 152, 266, 1960.

Berger, R.L., Byrne, J.J.: Intestinal gangrene associated with heart disease. Surg. Gynec. Obstet. 112, 529–533, 1961.

Bernatz, P.E.: Necrosis of colon following resection for abdominal aortic aneurysm. Arch. Surg. 81, 373, 1960.

Bernstein, W.C., Bernstein, E.F.: Ischaemic ulcerative colitis following inferior mesenteric arterial ligation. Dis. Colon & Rectum 6, 54–61, 1963.

Berry, C.L.: Persistant changes in the large bowel following the enterocolitis associated with Hirschsprung's disease. J. Path. 97, 731–736, 1969. (□)

Bertelsen, S., Egeblad, K.: Necrosis of the colon and the rectum complicating abdominal aortic resection. Acta Chir. Scand. 134, 151–156, 1968.

Bicks, R.O., Bale, G.F., Howard, H., McBurney, R.F.: Acute and delayed colon ischaemia after aortic aneurysm surgery. Arch. Intern. Med. 122, 249–253, 1968. (○)

Bienenstock, H., Minick, C.R., Rogoff, B.: Mesenteric arteritis and intestinal infarction in rheumatoid disease. Arch. Intern. Med. 119, 359–364, 1967.

Bill, A.H., Chapman, N.D.: The enterocolitis of Hirschsprung's disease. Am. J. Surg. 103, 70–74, 1962. (□)

Binns, J.C., Isaacson, P.: Age-related changes in the colonic blood supply: their relevance to ischaemic colitis. Gut 19, 384–390, 1978.

Bircher, J., Bartholomew, L.G., Cain, J.C., Adson, M.A.: Syndrome of intestinal arterial insufficiency. Arch. Intern. Med. 117, 632, 1966.

Birnbaum, W., Rudie, L., Wylie, E.J.: Colonic and rectal ischaemia following aortic aneurysmectomy. Dis. Colon & Rectum 7, 293, 1964.

van Blankenstein, M., Gratama, S.: Een acute buik bij een patient met migraine. Ned. T. Geneesk. 123, 4, 124–129, 1979.

Blom, J.M.H.: Ischemische colitis. Ned. T. Geneesk. 118, 1974.

Bluestone, R., MacMahon, M., Dawson, J.M.: Systemic sclerosis and small bowel involvement. Gut 10, 185, 1969.

de Boer, H.H.M., van Unnink, J.A.: Necrotizing colitis in patients undergoing long term treatment with phenothiazine derivates. Arch. Chir. Neerl. 20, 163, 1968. (○)

Boley, S.J., Schwartz, S., Lash, J., Sternhill, V.: Reversible vascular occlusion of the colon. Surg. Gynec. Obstet. 116, 53, 1963. (○)

Boley, S.J., Krieger, H., Schultz, L., Robinson, K., Siew, F.P., Allen, A.C., Schwartz, S.: Experimental aspects of peripheral vascular occlusion of the intestine. Surg. Gynec. Obstet. 121, 789–794, 1965.

Boley, S.J., Agrawal, G.P., Warren, A.R., Veith, F.J., Levowitz, B.S., Treiber, W., Dougherty, J., Schwartz, S.S., Gliedman, M.L.: Pathophysiologic effects of bowel distention on intestinal blood flow. Am. J. Surg. 117, 228–234, 1969.

Boley, S.J., Schwartz, S.S.: Colitis complicating carcinoma of the colon. Vascular disorders of the intestines. Butterworths, London 40, 631–642, 1971.

Boley, S.J., Brandt, L.J., Veith, F.J.: Current problems in surgery. Ischaemic disorders of the intestines. Year book Med. Publishers Chicago, London, vol. 15, 4, 1978.

Bookstein, J.J.: Non-occlusive ischemic colitis; angiographic aspects in a canine model. Invest. Radiol. 13, 506–513, 1978.

Boreham, P.: Benign strictures of the colon. Proc. R. Soc. Med. 50, 601–604, 1957.

Bounous, G., McArdle, A.H., Hodges, D.M.: Biosynthesis of intestinal mucin in shock: relationship to tryptic haemorrhagic enteritis and permeability to curare. Ann. Surg. 164, 13–22, 1966.

Bounous, G.: Role of the intestinal contents in the pathophysiology of acute intestinal ischaemia. Am. J. Surg. 114, 368, 1967.

Bounous, G., McArdle, A.H.: Release of intestinal enzymes in acute mesenteric ischaemia. J. Surg. Res. 9, 339, 1969.

Bounous, G.: Ischemic bowel disease; Mucosal injury in low flow state. Canad. J. of Surg. 17, 434–437, 1974.

Boylan, R.C., Sokoloff, L.: Vascular lesions in dermatomyositis. Arthr. Rheum. 3, 379, 1960.

Boysen, E.: Mesenteric angiography. In Abrams H.L. Angiography: Little, Brown, Boston, 1971.

Brandt, L.J., Gomery, P., Mitsudo, S.M., Chandler, P., Boley, S.J.: Disseminated intravascular coagulation in non occlusive mesenteric ischaemia: the lack of specificity of fibrin thrombi in intestinal infarction. Gastroenterology 71, 954, 1976.

Brandt, L.J., Boley, S.J., Goldberg, L.: Colitis in the elderly: A reappraisal. Amer. J. Gastroenterology 76, 239–245, 1981.

Braunwald, E., Childsey, C.A.: The adrenergic nervous system in the control of the normal and failing heart. Proc. R. Soc. Med. 58, 1063–1066, 1965.

Brennan, M.F., Clarke, A.M., Macbeth, W.A.A.G.: Infarction of the midgut associated with oral contraceptives. New Engl. J. Med. 279, 1213–1214, 1968.

Briggs, R.S.J., Barrand, K.G., Levene, M.: Ischemic colitis and drug abuse. Brit. Med. J. 1478, 1977. (○)

Brindle, M.J., Henderson, I.N.: Vascular occlusion of the colon associated with oral contraception. Canad. Med. Assoc. J. 100, 681–682, 1969.

Britt, L.G., Cheek, R.C.: Non-occlusive mesenteric vascular disease. Ann. Surg. 169, 704–711, 1969.

Brody, I.A., Wertlake, P.T., Laster, L.: Causes of intestinal symptoms in primary amyloidosis. Arch. Intern. Med. 113, 512, 1964.

Brom, B., Bank, S., Marks, I.N. Milner, Ch.B.G., Baker, P.: Ischemic colitis, gastric ulceration and malabsorption in a case of primary amyloidosis. Gastroenterology 57, 319, 1969.

Brown, P., Dey, M.M.: Gangrene due to embolus of the inferior mesenteric artery. Brit. Med. J. 1, 186–187, 1932.

Brown, Ch., Shirey, E.K., Hasenick, J.R.: Gastrointestinal manifestations of splenic lupus erythematosus. Gastroenterology 31, 649, 1956.

Brown, A.R., Szakes, J.E.: Intestinal bleeding and perforation complicating treatment with vasoconstrictors. Ann. Surg. 150, 790–798, 1959.

Brown, R.B., Borowsky, M.: Further observations in intestinal lesions associated with phaeochromocytoma. Ann. Surg. 151, 683–692, 1960.

Brown, A.R.: Diagnosis and management of non gangrenous ischemic colitis. Gut 9, 737, 1968.

Brown, A.R.: Non gangrenous ischemic colitis. A review of 17 cases. Brit. J. Surg. 59, 6, 463–472, 1972. (○)

Brownlee, T.J.: Regional colitis as an acute abdominal emergency. Brit. J. Surg. 38, 507–513, 1972.

Bryk, D.: Ulcerative colitis proximal to an obstructing surgical colonic stricture. Radiology 91, 786–787, 1968. (□)

Buchhardt Hansen, H.J., Qigaard, A.: Embolization to the superior mesenteric artery: arteriography and embolectomy in four cases. Acta Chir. Scand. 142, 451, 1976.

Byrd, B.F., Sawyers, J.L., Bomar, R.L., Klatte, E.G.: Reversible vascular occlusion of the colon: Recognition and management. Ann. of Surg. 167, 6, 901–908, 1968.

Calem, W.S., Gandino-Ruiz, M., Pochaczevsky, R., Papadakis, L.: Ischemic lesion of the transverse colon. Arch. Surg. 96, 939, 1968.

Cannon, J.A.: Discussion. Am. J. Surg. 315, 1955.

le Capon, J., Galian, A., Potet, Fr.: Colites ischémiques (type Marston); Etude anatomopathologique, à propos de six cas. Sem. Hôp. Paris, 15, 1039–1047, 1972. (○)

Carasquilla, C., Arbulu, A.: Cecal perforation due to adynamic ileus. Dis. Colon & Rectum 13, 252, 1970. (□)

Carlin, M.S., Manashil, G.B.: Ischaemic colitis proximal to incarcerated left inguinal hernia. Amer. J. Gastroenterology 59, 547–550, 1973. (□)

Carter, R., Vannix, R., Hinshaw, D.B., Stafford, C.E.: Inferior mesenteric vascular occlusion: sigmoidoscopic diagnosis. Surgery 46, 845–846, 1959.

Carvajal, J.A., Anderson, R., Weiss, L., Grissmer, J., Berman, R.: Atheroembolism, an etiologic factor in renal insufficiency, gastrointestinal haemorrhages and peripheral vascular diseases. Arch. Intern. Med. 119, 593, 1967.

Carvalho, A.C.A., Vaillancourt, R.A., Carbral, R.B. et al.: Coagulation abnormalities in women taking oral contraceptives Jama, 237, 3: 875–878, 1977.

Castagnoli, E.N.: Verblutung aus vaskulären Dickdarm-Geschwüren bei hypertensiver Arteriolonekrose. Schweiz. med. Wschr. 95, 400, 1965.

Castelli, M.F., Qizilbash, A.H., Salem, S., Fyshe, I.G.: Ischemic bowel disease. Canad. Med. Assoc. J. 111, 935–941, 1974. (○)

Chandrasekhara, R., Levitan, R.: Ischemic colitis. Ill Med. J. 139, 266–269, 1971.

Chino, S., Johnson, J.C., Keith, L.M.: New clinical and radiographic signs in ischemic colitis. Am. J. Surg. 128, 640–643, 1974. (○)

Civetta, J.M., Kolodny, M.: Mesenteric venous thrombosis association with oral contraceptives. Gastroenterology 58, 713, 1970.

Claiborn, T.S.: Fibromuscular hyperplasia, report of a case with involvement of multiple arteries. Am. J. Med.49, 103, 1970.

Clark, A.W., Lloyd-Mostyn, R.H., de C. Sadler, M.R.: Ischaemic colitis in young adults. Brit. Med. J. 4, 70–72, 1972. (○)

McClennan, B.L.: Ischaemic colitis secondary to Premarin: report of a case. Dis. Colon & Rectum 19, 618–620, 1976. (○)

Cogbill, C.L., Makhar, J., Campana, H.D., Park, Y.S.: Ischemic colitis. Am. Surgeon 43, 3, 137–143, 1977. (○)

Coligado, E.Y., Fleshler, B.: Reversible vascular occlusion of the colon. Radiology 89, 432–434, 1967. (○)

Colin, R., Balmes, J.L., Favier, C.: L'endoscopie dans le diagnostic des colites ischémiques régressives. Chirurgie 100, 49–51, 1974. (○)

O'Connell, Th.X., Kadell, B., Tompkins, R.K.: Ischemia of the colon. Surg. Gynec. Obstet. 142, 337, 1976. (○)

Cooling, C.I., Protheroe, R.H.B.: Infarction of the colon. Postgrad. Med. J. 34, 494–498, 1958.

Cooperman, M., Pace, W.G., Martin, E.W. Jr., Pflug, B.,

168

Keith, L.M., Evans, W.E. et al.: Determination of viability of ischaemic intestine by Doppler ultrasound. Surgery 83, 705, 1978.

Cooperman, M., Martin E.W. Jr., Evans, W.E., Carey, L.C.: Assessment of anastomotic blood supply in operations upon the colon by Doppler ultrasound. Surg. Gynecol. Obstet. 149, 15, 1979[1].

Cooperman, M., Martin E.W. Jr., Keith, L.M., Carey, L.C.: Use of Doppler ultrasound in intestinal surgery. Am. J. Surg. 138, 856–859, 1979[2].

Cooperman, M.: Intestinal ischaemia. Futura Publishing Co, Mount Kisco, 1983.

Corbett, R.: Stenosed segment of descending colon associated with trauma. Proc. R. Soc. Med. 50, 271, 1957.

Corday, E., Irving, D.W., Gold, H., Bernstein, H., Skelton, R.B.T.: Mesenteric vascular insufficiency. Intestinal ischemia induced by remote circulatory disturbances. Am. J. Med. 33, 365–376, 1962.

Cormier, J.M.: Desoutter, P.: Ischémie aiguë du côlon. 23 Observations. J. Chir. (Paris) 117, 6–7, 355–360, 1980. (○)

McCort, J.J.: Infarction of the descending colon due to vascular occlusion. New Engl. J. Med. 262, 168–172, 1960. (○)

Cotton, P.B., Thomas, M.L.: Ischemic colitis and the contraceptive pill. Brit. Med. J. 3, 27–28, 1971. (○)

Courbier, R., Jausseran, J.M., Reggi, M.: L'arcade de Riolan: signification hémodynamique – déductions thérapeutiques. Schwelz. med. Wschr. 106, 363–367, 1976.

Couris, G.D., Block, M.A., Rupe, C.E.: Gastrointestinal complications of collagen diseases. Arch. Surg. 89, 695, 1964.

Courty, A., Carli, G.: Invagination intestinale aiguë après aortographie essai d'interprétation: déductions pratiques. Gaz. Méd. France 57, 719, 1950.

Curr, J.F.: Rectal stricture due to ischemia following ruptured ectopic gastation. Gut 8, 178–179, 1967.

Cynn, W.S., Richert, R.R.: Ischemic proctosigmoiditis. Dis. Colon & Rectum 16, 537, 1973.

Dallemand, S., Farman, J., Stein, D., Waxman, M., Mitchell, W.: Colonic necrosis complicating pancreatitis. Gastroint. Radiol. 2, 27–30, 1977.

Davis, J.E.:Reversible vascular occlusion of the colon. Ann. Surg. 171, 789, 1970.

Dawson, M.A., Schaeffer, J.W.: The clinical course of reversible ischaemic colitis. Observations on the progression of sigmoidoscopic and histological changes. Gastroenterology 60, 4, 577–580, 1971. (○)

Degos, R.: Malignant atropic papulosis: a fatal cutaneo-intestinal syndrome. Brit. J. Dermatol. 66, 304–307, 1954.

Delavierre, Ph., Vayre, P., Gueraud, J.P., Laffite, Ph., Jost, J.L., Parrot, A.M.: Les colites ischémiques. Sem. Hôp. Paris 49, 28, 2062–2064, 1973. (○)

Deleu, H.W.O.: Necrotic colitis in the presence of normal vascularization of the colon. Arch. Chir. Neerl. 55–62, 1976. (○)

Deloyers, L.: Colite ischémique chez un jeune homme – forme sténosante rectosigmoidienne. Acta Gastroent. Belg. 33, 800–803, 1970.

Demos, N.J., Bahuth, J.J., Urnes, P.D.: Comparative study of arteriosclerosis in the inferior and superior mesenteric arteries with a case of gangrene of the colon. Ann. Surg. 155, 599, 1962.

Demuth, W.E., Fitts, W.T., Patterson, L.T.: Mesenteric vascular occlusion; Collective review. Int. Abstr. Surg. 3, vol. 108, 209–223, 1959.

Dencker, H., Lindgarth, C., Muth, T., Olin, T.: Massive gangrene of the colon secondary to carcinoma of the rectum. Acta Chir. Scand. 135, 357–361, 1969. (□)

Descotes, J., Bonchet, A., Sisteron, A., George, P.: La reimplantation de l'artérie mésentérique supérieure dans le traitement de l'insuffisance artérielle intestinale. Lyon Chir. 59, 5–8, 1963.

Detry, R., De Vroede, G., Madarnas, P., Haddad, H., Gysling, E.: Ischemic colitis associated with hypertension. Canad. J. of Surg. 22, 3, 256–257, 1979. (○)

Dewbury, K.C.: Ischaemic and evanescent colitis. Radiology 69, 617, 1976.

Dharia, K.M., Ngo, N.L., Marino, A.W.M., Mancini, H.W.N., Shali, I.C.: Reversible ischemic colitis, report of four cases. Dis. Colon & Rectum 16, 211–215, 1973. (○)

Dickson, G.H.: Three cases of ischaemic colitis. Gut 9, 376–380, 1968.

Diemel, H., Rau, G., Schmitz-Dräger, H.G.: Die Riolansche Kollaterale. Ihre diagnostische Bedeutung für die Angiographie bei Verschlusskrankheiten der Mesenterial Arterien. Fortschr. Röntgenstr. 101, 253–264, 1964.

Dietz, M.W.: Unique vascular colon stenoses. Radiology 93, 385–386, 1969. (□)

Dilenge, D.: Angiography in ischemic bowel disease. Canad. J. of Surg. 17, 438–443, 1974.

de Dombal, F.T., Fletcher, D.M., Harris, R.S.: Early diagnosis of ischemic colitis. Gut 10, 131, 1969.

McDonald, H., Hourihane D.O'B.: Ischaemic lesions of the alimentary tract. J. Clin. Pathol. 25, 99–105, 1972.

van Dongen, R.J.A.M., Tytgat, G.N., Schwilden, E.D.: Gefässbedingten Erkrankungen des Kolons und Rektums. Handbuch der inneren Medizin, K. Müller-Wieland, (Ed.) Verdauungsorgane. Springer Verlag, Berlin, Heidelberg, N.Y. 1021–1058, 1982.

O'Donnell, J.A., Hobson, R.W.: Operative confirmation of Doppler ultrasound in evaluation of intestinal ischaemia. Surgery 87, 1, 109–112, 1980.

Dosik, G.M., Luna, M., Valdivieso, M., McCredie, K.B., Gelran, E.A., Gil-Extremero, B., Smith, T.L., Bodey, G.P.: Necrotizing colitis in patients with cancer. Am. J. of Med. 67, 646–656, 1979.

Drucker, W.R., Davis, J.H., Holden, W.D., Reagan, J.R.: Hemorrhagic necrosis of the intestine. A clinical syndrome presence without organic vascular occlusion. Arch. Surg. (Chicago) 89, 42–52, 1964.

Drummond, H.: The arterial supply of the rectum and pelvic colon. Brit. J. Surg. 1, 677–685, 1913–1914.

Dudley, H.A.F.: Ischaemic colitis without predisposing cause. Brit. Med. J. 3, 637–638, 1971. (○)

Duffy, T.J.: Reversible ischaemic colitis in young adults. Brit. J. Surg. 68, 34–37, 1981. (○)

Dunbar, J.D.: Reversible cecal infarction: A case report with angiographic follow up study. Am. J. Surg. 112, 447, 1966.

Dutcher, J.P., Schiffer, C.A., Johnson, G.S.: Rapid migration of ^{111}Indium labelled granulocytes to sites of infection. New Engl. J. Med. 304, 586–589, 1981.

Eastcott, H.H.G.: Ischaemic colitis. Proc. R. Soc. Med. 59, 890, 1966.

Edwards, A.J.: Intestinal ischaemia. A.H. Marcus and L. Adamson 'Arteries and veins'. Churchill Livingstone, London, N.Y., 1975.

Egger, G., Kellock, T.D.: Akute regionäre Kolitis – ischämische Kolitis. Schweiz. med. Wschr. 100, 1264–1272, 1970. (○)

Egger, G., Härtel, M., Halter, F., Laissue, J.: Die nicht gangränöse ischämische Kolitis Klinik und radiologische Diagnostik. Fortschr. Röntgenstr. 115, 4, 432–439, 1971.

Eisenberg, R.L., Montgomery, C.K., Margulis, A.R.: Colitis in the elderly: Ischemic colitis mimicking ulcerative and granulomatous colitis. AJR 133, 1113–1118, 1979. (○)

Ellis, K., Heifetz, C.J.: Mesenteric venous thrombosis in two women taking oral contraceptives. Am. J. Surg. 125, 641, 1973.

Ende, N.: Infarction of the bowel in cardiac failure. New Engl. J. Med. 258, 879–881, 1958.

Engelhardt, J.E., Jacobson, G.: Infarction of the colon, demonstrated by barium enema. Radiology 67, 573–575, 1956.

Ernst, C.B., Hagihara, P.F., Daugherty, M.E., Sachatello, C.R., Griffen, W.O.: Ischaemic colitis incidence following abdominal aortic reconstruction. A prospective study. Surgery, 80, 417–421, 1976.

Fagin, R.R., Kirsner, J.B.: Ischemic diseases of the colon. Adv. internal Med. 17, 343–362, 1973.

Fagniez, P.L., Julien, M., Germain, A.: Colite ischémique et pancreatite nécrosante. Med. Chir. Dig. 5, 283–285, 1976. (○)

Farinon, A.M., Battistini, C., Zanella, E.: Aspetti endoscopici delle coliti ischemiche. G. Clin. Med. 58, 339–358, Fasc. 9–10, 1977. (○)

Farinon, A.M.: Coloscopy: A necessary aid in the diagnosis of transient ischaemic colitis. Endoscopy 10, 112–114, 1978.

Farman, J.: Vascular lesions of the colon. Brit. J. Radiol. 39, 575–582, 1966.

Farman, J., Betancourt, E., Kilpatrick, Z.M.: The radiology of ischemic proctitis. Radiology 91, 302, 1968.

Faust, H., Hartweg, H.: Ischämische Darmerkrankungen. Fortschr. Röntgenstr. 119, 3, 273–285, 1973. (○)

Favier, C., Bonneau, H.P., Tran Minh, V., Devic, J.: Diagnostic endoscopique des colites ischémiques régressives. La Nouvelle Presse Médicale 5, nr. 2, 77–79, 1976. (○)

Favriel, J.M., Couturier, D., Gouerou, H., Cassaigne, J.Y., Rosen, J., Debray, C.: Colite ischémique régressive de l'angle gauche. Gastroenterol. Clin. Biol. 1, 1035–1041, 1977. (○)

Felsen, J.: The sigmoidoscopic diagnosis of periarteritis nodosa. Ann. intern. Med. 15, 251, 1941.

Ferguson, C.D.: Gangrene and perforation due to embolus of the inferior mesenteric artery. Brit. Med. J. 1, 840–841, 1932.

Ferrara, J.J., Spontaneous ischaemic colitis. In: Intestinal ischaemia; Edited by M. Cooperman. Futura Publishing Co (Mount Kisco), 245–261, 1983.

Ferrer, M.I., Bradley, S.E., Wheeler, H.O., Enson, Y., Preisig, R., Harvey, R.M.: The effect of digoxin in the splanchnic circulation in ventricular failure. Circulation 32, 524–537, 1965.

Fineberg, C., Schechter, D.C., Barrick, C.W.: Gangrene of the large intestine and ovaries after translumbar aortography. JAMA 167, 1232, 1958.

Finkbiner, R.B., Decker, J.P.: Ulceration and perforation of the intestine due to necrotizing arteriolitis. New Engl. J. Med. 268, 14, 1963.

Fitts, W.T. Jr., Erde, A., Peskin, G.W., Frost, J.W.: Surgical implication of polycythaemia vera. Ann. Surg. 152, 548, 1960.

Fogarty, T.J., Fletcher, W.S.: Non occlusive mesenteric ischaemia. Am. J. Surg. 11, 130, 1965.

Forde, K.A., Lebwohl, O., Wolff, M., Voorhees, A.B.: Reversible ischemic colitis – correlation of colonoscopic and pathologic changes. Amer. J. Gastroenterology, 72, 182–185, 1979.

Foster, F.P., Dadey, J.L.: Management of postoperative diarrheas and infections. Am. J. Surg. 92, 770–780, 1956.

Frenkel, M.: Ischemische colitis na ernstige hartritme stoornissen. Ned. T. Geneesk. 113, 509, 1969. (○)

170

Friedland, G.W., Filly, R.: Case reports. Evanescent colitis in a child. Pediatr. Radiol. 2, 73–74, 1974.

Frodl, F.K.O.: Roentgenologisch beeld van een locaal colon-infarct in het ulcereuze stadium. Tijdschrift voor Gastro-enterologie 7, 1, 90–95, 1964.

Furnemont, E.: Colite ischémique réversible (Un cas). J. Radiol. Electrol. 59, 1, 65–67, 1978. (O)

Gaal, C.S., Nemeth, L.: Mit Signatumor vergesellschaftete Nekrose des Colon descendens. Chirurg 44, 478–479, 1973. (□)

Gage, T.P., Gagnier, J.M.: Ischaemic colitis in a patient with sickle cell anaemia. Gastroenterology 84, 171–174, 1983. (O)

Le Gall., J.R., Germain, A., Rapin, M., Pinandeau, Y., Regnier, B., Lange, F., Simonian, S.: Les enterites aiguës nécrosantes post operatives. Nouv. Presse méd. 2, 2787–2790, 1973.

Ganchrow, M.I., Clark, J.F., Ferguson, J.A.: Ischemic proctitis with obliterative vascular change. Dis. Colon & Rectum 13, 470–471, 1970.

Ganchrow, M.I., Clark, J.F., Benjamin, H.G.: Ischaemic colitis proximal to obstructing carcinoma of the colon; case report. Dis. Colon & Rectum 34, 38–42, 1971. (□)

Gatch, W.D., Gulbertson, C.G.: Circulatory disturbances caused by intestinal obstruction. Ann. Surg. 102, 619, 1935. (□)

Gazes, P.C., Holmes, C.R., Mosely, V., Pratt-Thomas, H.R.: Acute haemorrhage and necrosis of the intestines associated with digitalization. Circulation 23, 358–364, 1961.

Gelfland, M.D.: Ischemic colitis associated with a depot synthetic progestagen. Am. J. Dig. Dis. 17, 275–277, 1972.

Gharemani, G.G., Meyers, M.A., Farman, J., Port, R.B.: Ischaemic disease of the small bowel and colon associated with oral contraceptives. Gastrointest. Radiol. 2, 221–228, 1977.

Giessler, R., Hoffman, K., Heberer, G.: Akute und chronische Verschlüsse der Viszeralarterien. Dtsch. med. Wschr. 98, 1112, 1973.

Gilat, T., Spiro, H.M.: Amyloidosis and the gut. Am. J. Dig. Dis. 13, 619, 1968.

Gimmon, Z., Berlatzky, Y., Freund, U.: Tension pneumoperitoneum complicating non-gangrenous non-occlusive ischemic colitis. Am. J. of Proctol., Gastroent., Colo-rectal Surg. 8, 13, 24, 1980.

Glotzer, D.J., Roth, S.I., Welch, C.E.: Colonic ulceration proximal to obstructing carcinoma. Surgery 56, 950–956, 1963. (□)

Glotzer, D.J., Phil, B.G.: Experimental obstructive colitis. Arch. Surg. 92, 8, 1966.

Goldgraber, M.B., Kirsner, J.B.: The Schwartzman phenomenon in the colon of rabbits. Arch. Path. 64, 225, 1957.

Gore, M., Calenoff, L., Rogers, L.F.: Roentgenographic man-ifestations of ischemic colitis. J. Am. med. Ass. 241, 1171–1173, 1979.

Goulston, S.J.M., McGovern, V.J.: Pseudomembranous colitis. Gut 6, 207–212, 1965.

Goulston, St.: Ischemic colitis. Med. J. Austr. 1, 1194, 1973.

McGovern, V.J., Goulston, S.J.M.: Ischaemic enterocolitis. Gut 6, 213–220, 1965. (O)

McGowan, J.R.: Collateral circulation in sigmoid colon. Arch. Surg. 71, 531–537, 1955.

Granata, L., Huvos, A., Gregg, D.E.: Hemodynamic changes in coronary and mesenteric arterial beds following sympathetic nerve stimulation. Physiologist 4, 142, 1961.

Gratama, S.: Personal communications, Rotterdam, The Netherlands, 1982.

McGregor, D., Pierce, G.E., Thomas, J.H., Tilzer, L.L.: Obstructive lesions of distal mesenteric arteries. Arch. Path. Lab. Med. 104, 79–83, 1980.

Grendell, J.H., Ockner, R.K.: Mesenteric venous thrombosis. Gastroenterology 82, 358–372, 1982.

Greves, J.H., Bohlman, T.W., Frische, L.H., Katon, R.M.: Intramural barium in ischemic colitis. Am. J. Dig. Dis. 21, 257–263, 1976. (O)

Griffen, T.S., Hagihara, P.F.: Ischemic colitis in rats. Dis. Colon & Rectum 25, 7, 638–640, 1982.

Griffiths, J.D.: Surgical anatomy of the blood supply of the distal colon. Ann. Coll. Surg. 19, 241–256, 1956.

Griffiths, J.D.: Extramural and intramural blood supply of the colon. Brit. Med. J. 1, 323, 1961.

Griffiths, J.D., Marston, A., Mavor, G.E., Robertson, G.S., Thomas, M.L., Morson, B.C., Eastcott, H.H., Pheils, M.T.: Ischemic diseases of the colon. Proc. R. Soc. Med. 59, 881, 1966.

Guay, A., Janower, M.L., Bain, R.W., McCready, F.J.: A case of Buerger's disease causing ischemic colitis with perforation in a young male. Am. J. of Med. Sciences 271, 2, 239–240, 1976. (O)

Guilfoil, P.H.: Inferior mesenteric artery syndrome after trans-lumbar aortography. New Engl. J. of Med. 269, 12, 1963.

Guivarch, M., Roullet-Audy, J.C., De Margerie, V., Backet, J.: 22 Colitis ischémiques dont 18 gangréneuses. Chirurgie 8, 108, 633–645, 1982.

Guly, H.R., Stewart, I.P.: Ischaemic colitis with perforation in a patient with multiple injuries. Injury 14, 100–102, 1982.

Habboushe, F., Wallace, H.W., Nusbaum, M., Baum, S., Dratch, P., Blakemore, W.S.: Non occlusive mesenteric vascular insufficiency. Ann. Surg. 180, 819–823, 1974.

Hagihara, P.F., Parker, J.C., Griffen, W.O.: Spontaneous ischemic colitis. Dis. Colon & Rectum 20, 236–251, 1977. (O)

Hagihara, P.F., Ernst, C.B., Griffen, W.O.: Incidence of ischaemic colitis following abdominal aortic reconstruction. Surg. Gynec. Obstet. 149, 571–573, 1979. (O)

Hahnloser, P.: Maladie ischémique colo-rectale. New Chir. Acta 48, 813–822, 1981.

Hamilton, M.D., Barnett, A.J., Lowe, T.E.: Ischemic episodes in cardiac failure: Acute arterial insufficiency with and without structural blockage. Med. J. Austr. 2, 93, 1955.

Handel, J., Schwartz, S.: Gastrointestinal manifestation of the Schönlein-Henoch syndrome. Roentgenologic findings. AJR 78, 643, 1957.

Hannan, J.R., Jackson, B.F., Pipik, P.: Fibrosis and stenosis of the descending colon and sigmoid following occlusion of the IMA. AJR 91, 4, 826–832, 1964. (O)

Hansen, H.J.B., Jorgenson, S.J., Engell, H.D.: Acute mesenteric infarction caused by small vessel disease. Acta Chir. Scand. 472, 109–111, 1976.

Hardie, I.R.: Intestinal ischaemia: clinical review. Med. J. Austr. 2, 164–167, 1974.

Hardy, J.D., Alican, K.: Ischemic gangrene without major organic vascular occlusion: an enlarging concept. Surgery 50, 107–114, 1961.

Hardy, R., Scullin, D.R.: Thumbprinting in a case of amoebiasis. Radiology 98, 147, 1971.

Harrison, A.W., Croal, A.E.: Left colon ischaemia following occlusion or ligation of the inferior mesenteric artery. Can. J. of Surg. 5, 293–298, 1962.

Hay, A.M.: Association between chlorpromazine therapy and necrotizing colitis. Report of a case. Dis. Colon & Rectum 21, 5, 380–382, 1978. (O)

Hayward, R.H., Calhoun, T.R., Korompai, F.L.: Gastrointestinal complications of vascular surgery. Surg. Clinies of N.A. 59, 5, 885–903, 1979.

Heer, F.W., Silen, W., French, S.W.: Intestinal gangrene without apparent vascular occlusion. Am. J. Surg. 110, 231–238, 1965.

Heikkinen, E., Larmi, T.K.I., Huttunen, R.: Necrotizing colitis. Am. J. Surg. 128, 362–367, 1974. (O)

Heller, F.R., Gilbeau, J.D., Schmitz, A.: Ischemic colitis with involvement of the rectum. Case report. J. Belge Radiol. 60, 109–112, 1977. (O)

Hemet, J., Ducastelle, T., Teniere, D., Jouanneau, P., Metayer, J., Chleq, C.I.: Les colites en amont des cancers à propos de 7 observations. Sem. Hôp. Paris 38, 2139–2145, 1976. (□)

Herlinger, H.: Angiography of the visceral arteries. Clinics in Gastroent. 1, 547, 1972.

Hermanek, P., Mühe, E.: Ischämische Kolitis durch experimentellen Volvulus. Z. exper. Chirurgie, 4, 115–120, 1971.

Heron, H.C., Khubchandani, I.T., Trimpi, H.D., Sheets, J.A., Starik, J.J.: Evanescent colitis. Dis. Colon & Rectum 24, 7, 555–561, 1981.

Herrington, J.L., Grossmann, L.A.: Surgical lesions of the small and large intestine resulting from Buerger's disease. Ann. Surg. 168, 1079, 1968.

Herrmann, J.W., Paine, J.R., Stubbe, N.J.: Acute obstruction with gangrene of the colon secondary to carcinoma of the sigmoid. Surgery 57, 647–650, 1965. (□)

Hill, J.D., Mittal, A.K., Kerth, W.J., Gerbode, F.: Syndrome of acute hemorrhagic intestinal infarction and renal insufficiency following aortic valve replacement for aortic insufficiency. J. thorac, cardiovasc. Surg. 61, 430–437, 1971.

Hillemand, B.: Les colites ischémiques. Sem. Hôp. Paris, 48, 1607–1610, 1972.

Hingorani, K., Graham, G.S.: Small bowel necrosis due to arteritis in rheumatoid disease. Ann. phys. Med. 7, 68–71, 1963.

Hobson, R.W., Wright, C.B., Rich, N.M., Collins, G.J.: Assessment of colonic ischemia during aortic surgery by Doppler ultrasound. J. Surg. Res. 20, 231–235, 1976.

Hoffman, F.G., Zimmerman, S.L., Cardwell, E.S.: Massive intestinal infarction without vascular occlusion associated with aortic insufficiency. New Engl. J. Med. 263, 436, 1960.

Hope, J.W., Borus, P.F., Berg, P.K.: Roentgenologic manifestation of Hirschsprung's disease in infancy. AJR 95, 217–229, 1965. (□)

Horie, Y., Tsuchiya, S., Mishima, Y., Kagami, H., Hara, K., Ishikawa, K.: Ulcerogenic lesions of the intestine (colon) due to ischemia. Folia Angiologica 24, 116–118, 1976.

Horton, E.H., Murthy, S.K., Seal, R.M.E.: Haemorrhagic necrosis of small intestine and acute pancreatitis following open heart surgery. Thorax 23, 438–445, 1968.

Hubens, A., Dochez, Ch., Van Vooren, W.: Reversibele vasculaire segmentaire colitis. T. Gastroent. 11, 551, 1968.

Huber, F.B., Akovbiantz, A.: Zur Klinik und Therapie der segmentären ischämischen Enterokolitis. Helvetica Chirurgica Acta 1–2, 173–176, 1970. (O)

Huber, F.B.: Darminfarkt nach stumpfem Abdominal Trauma. Schweiz. med. Wschr. 102, 339, 1972.

Huber, F.B.: Darminfarkt als Folge einer spontanen mesenterialen und intramuralen Anticoagulantienblutung. Schweiz. med. Wschr. 107, 88, 1977.

Huber, F.B.: Ischämische Entero-Kolopatien 11–13. Verlag Hans Huber, Bern, Stuttgart, Wien, 1981. (O)

Huibregtse, K., Bartelsman, J.F.W.M., Tytgat, G.N.: Unusual presentation of ischemic colitis. Acta Gastroent. Belg. 43, 353–355, 1980. (O)

172

Humphreys, W.G., Graham, W.J.H.: Ischaemic colitis: a sequel to femoral artery laceration. Injury 10, 217–219, 1977.

Hunt, D.R., Mildenhall, P.: Etiology of strictures of the colon associated with pancreatitis. Digestive Diseases 20, 10, 941–946, 1975.

Hunt, D.R.: Surgical management of gangrenous ischaemic colitis: Report of five cases. Dis. Colon & Rectum 20, 1, 36–39, 1976.

Hunt, R.H.: Ischaemic colitis: Endoscopy. Clinics in Gastroenterology, W.B. Saunders Co. Ltd., 734, 1978.

Hunt, R.H., Buchanan, J.D.: Transient ischaemic colitis – colonoscopy and biopsy in diagnosis. J. of the Royal Naval Med. Service 65, 15–19, 1979.

Hurwitz, A., Khafif, R.A.: Acute necrotizing colitis proximal to obstructing neoplasms of the colon. Surg. Gynec. Obstet. 749–752, 1960. (○)

Hurwitz, R.L., Martin, A.J., Grossman, B.E., Waddell, W.R.: Oral contraceptives and gastrointestinal disorders. Ann. Surg. 172, 5, 892–896, 1970. (○)

Ike, B.: Personal communications, Amersfoort, The Netherlands, 1983.

Inman, W.H., Vessey, M.P., Westerholm, B., Engelund, A.: Thromboembolic disease and the steroidal content of oral contraceptives: A report to the committee on safety of drugs. Brit. Med. J. 2, 203–209, 1970.

Irving, D.W., Corday, E.: Effect of the cardiac arhytmias on the renal and mesenteric circulation. Am. J. Cardiol. 8, 32, 1961.

Irwin, A.: Partial infarction of the colon due to reversible vascular occlusion. Clin. Radiol. 16, 261–263, 1965.

Jackish, G.E.: Ischemic colitis: A common clinical entity? Geriatrics 81–87, 1972.

Jacobson, E.D., Lanciault, G.: The gastrointestinal vasculature. In: Scientific Basis of Gastroenterology (Ed.) Duthie H.L. & Wormsley K.G. pp. 26–48, Edinburgh, London, N.Y. Churchill Livingstone, 1979.

Jernstrom, P., Stasney, J.: Acute ulcerative enteritis due to polyarteritis; diagnostic dilemma. J. Am. med. Ass. 148, 544, 1952.

Johnson, W.C., Nabseth, D.C.: Visceral infarction following aortic surgery. Ann. Surg. 180, 312–318, 1974.

Jones, B., Fishman, E.K., Siegelman, S.S.: Ischaemic colitis demonstrated by computed tomography. J. Comp. Ass. Tom. 6, 6, 1120–1123, 1982.

Joyeux, R., Courty, A., Biscaye, A., Carli, G., Lisbonne, M.: Une complication abdominale grave et inédite de l'aortographie. Sem. Hôp. Paris 26, 152, 1950.

Joyeux, R., Sellanin, A.: Nècrose segmentaire du côlon gauche. Med. Chir. Dig. 2, 103, 1973.

Julien, M.: Nécrose totale du côlon. Mém. Acad. Chir. 91, 995, 1965. (□)

Kaminski, D.L., Keltner, R.M., Willman, V.L.: Ischaemic colitis. Arch. Surg. 106, 558–563, 1973. (○)

Karmody, A.M., Jordan, F.R., Zaman, S.N.: Left colon gangrene after acute IMA occlusion. Arch. Surg. 111, 972–975, 1976. (○)

Katz, P., Dorman, M.T., Aufses, A.H.: Colonic necrosis complicating post-operative pancreatitis. Ann. Surg. 179, 403–405, 1974.

Katz, S., Wahab, A., Murray, W., Williams, L.: New parameters of viability in ischaemic bowel disease. Am. J. Surg. 127, 136, 1974.

Kawarada, Y., Satinsky, S., Matsumoto, T.: Ischemic colitis following rectal prolapse. Surgery 76, 2, 340–343, 1974. (○)

Kellock, T.D.: Acute segmental ulcerative colitis. Lancet, 660–663, 1957.

McKeown, K.C., Ganguli, A.K.: Gastro-intestinal symptoms in polyarteritis nodosa; report of a case. Brit. J. Surg. 44, 308–312, 1956.

Kieny, R., Cinqualbre, J., Wenger, J.J., Tongio, J.: Les ischémies intestinales aiguës. Paris, Expansion scientifique française, 13–42, 1979.

Killen, D.A., Sewell, R., Foster, J.H.: Colonic injury resulting from angiographic contrast media. Am. J. Surg. 114, 904–909, 1967.

Killingback, M.J., Williams, K.L.: Necrotizing colitis. Brit. J. Surg. 49, 175–185, 1961. (□)

Kilpatrick, Z.M., Farman, J., Yesner, R., Spiro, H.M.: Ischemic proctitis. JAMA 205, 74–80, 1968.

Kilpatrick, Z.M., Silverman, J.F., Betancourt, E., Farman, J., Lawson, J.P.: Vascular occlusion of the colon and oral contraceptives. Possible relation. New Engl. J. Med. 278, 438–440, 1968.

Kim, M.W., Hundahl, S.A., Dary, C.R., McNamara, J.J., Straehley, C.J., Whelan, T.J.: Ischemic colitis after aortic aneurysmectomy. Am. J. Surg. 145, 392–393, 1983.

Kinkhabwala, M., Rabinowitz, J.G., Dallemand, S., Iyer, S.: 'Intersplanchnic steal syndrome': another cause for reversible distal colon ischaemia. Brit. J. Radiol. 47, 729–732, 1974.

McKinnell, J.S., Kearney, M.S.: Haemorrhagic necrosis of the intestine. Brit. Med. J. 460–463, 1967.

Kirks, D.R.: The radiology of enteritis due to haemolytic-uremic syndrome (abstract). Gastrointest. Radiol. 91, febr. 1982.

Kistin, M.G., Kaplan, M.M., Harrington, J.T.: Diffuse ischemic colitis associated with systemic lupus erythematosus; response to subtotal colectomy. Gastroenterology 75, 6, 1147–1151, 1978. (○)

Klein, E.: Embolism and thrombosis of the superior mesenteric artery. Surg. Gynec. Obstet. 33, 385–405, 1921.

Kleinman, P., Meyers, M.A., Abbott, G.: Necrotizing enterocolitis with pneumatosis intestinalis in systemic lupus erythematosus and polyarthritis. Radiology 121, 595–598, 1976.

Knox, W.G., West, J.D.: Abdominal aortography and femoral arteriography. Arch. Surg. 82, 656, 1961.

Kremen, A.J.: Acute colonic obstruction secondary to carcinoma of the sigmoid colon with gangrene of an extensive segment of the large bowel; case report. Surgery 18, 335–338, 1945. (□)

Kühner, W., Höchler, W., Seibb, H.J.: Nicht infektiöse Sonderformen der Colitis – Endoskopische-histologische Befunde. From: Entzündliche Erkrankungen des Dickdarms. Ed. Ottenjahn R., Fahrländer, H. Springer Verlag Berlin Ch. 13, 188–190, 1983.

Lambana, S., Yamamoto, K., Miyashita, T., Tsuchiya, K.: Irreversible ischemic colitis caused by stenosis of sigmoid branches; a case report. Surgery 74, 4, 587, 1973. (O)

Lambert, M., de Peyer, R., Muller, A.F.: Reversible ischemic colitis after intravenous vasopression therapy. Jama, 247, 5, 666–667, 1982.

Langeron, P., Thery, D.: Les stenoses ischémiques du côlon par lésions de l'artère mésentérique inférieure. J. des sciences med. de Lille, 8–9, 259–266, 1976. (O)

Larmi, T.K.J., Heikkinen, E., Huttunen, R.: Ischemic and necrotizing colitis. Ann. Chir. Gynaec. Fenn 64, 1, 1975.

Laufman, H., Nora, P.F., Mittelpunkt, A.I.: Mesenteric blood vessels. Advances in surgery and physiology. Arch. Surg. 88, 1021–1044, 1964.

Lazarovitch, I., Englender, M., Baratz, M., Solowiejczyk, M.: Necrotizing proctitis with perforation of the rectal wall due to barium enema. A case report and review of literature. Am. J. of Proctol., Gastroent., Colo-rectal Surg. 22–24, 1980. (O)

Lenz, H., Rohr, H.: Die Darmgegenschaltung und ihre Folgen für die Bewegungsmechanik. Fortschr. Röntgenstr. 97, 321, 1962.

Lescher, T.J., Bombeck, C.T.: Mesenteric vascular occlusion associated with oral contraceptive use. Arch. Surg. 112, 1231–1232, 1977.

Levesque, M., Fanck, C., Mornet, P., Barsamian, L., Lecronier, M., Vital, C.: Manifestations digestives de la dermatomyosite. J. Radiol. 62, 13–18, 1981.

Levrat, M., Pasquier, J., Leonard, J.P.: Les colites sévères réactionelles en amont des néoplasms coliques. Arch. Fr. Mal. App. Digest. 58, 201–214, 1969. (□)

Lewin, J.R., Hwei-Shien, L., Hahn, A.: Ischemic colitis associated with colonic carcinoma. Report of a case. Dis. Colon & Rectum 328–329, 1979. (□)

Lewis, M.I.: Reversible ischemic colitis. Dis. Colon & Rectum 16, 121, 1973.

Lindahl, K., Vejlsted, H., Backer, O.G.: Lesions of the colon following acute pancreatitis. Scand. J. Gastroenterol. 7, 375, 1972.

Lister, F., Jungmann, H.: Gangrene of the colon. Brit. J. Radiol. 29, 341–343, 1956.

Litten, M.: Über die Folgen des Verschlusses des Arteria Mesenterica Superior. Virchows Arch. Pathol. Anat. Physiol. Klin. Med. 63, 289, 1875.

Littman, L., Boley, S.J., Schwartz, S.: Sigmoidoscopic diagnosis of the colon. Dis. Colon & Rectum 6, 142–146, 1963. (O)

Long, B.W., Kees, C.J.: Ischemic colitis. J. of Mississipi State Med. Assoc. 16, 2, 31–34, 1975. (O)

Loose, K.E., van Dongen, R.J.A.M.: Atlas of angiography. Georg Thieme Verlag, Stuttgart, 1976.

Lozman, H., Rao, V.: Surgical treatment of ischemic colitis. Report of a case. Dis. Colon & Rectum 21, 7, 520–521, 1978. (O)

Lubbers, E.: Personal communications. Nijmegen, The Netherlands, 1983.

Lupi Herrera, E., Sanchez Tones, G., Marcushamer, J., Mispireta, J., Horwitz, S., Espino Vela, J.: Takayasu's arteritis, clinical study of 107 cases. Amer. Heart J. 93, 94, 1977.

Maas, D., Hamann, W., Noetzel, H., Kimpel, G., Schubothe, H.: Wegenersche Granulomatose. Schweiz. med. Wschr. 101, 141, 1971.

MacVaugh, H., Roberts, B.: Results of resection of abdominal aortic aneurysm. Surg. Gynec. Obstet. 113, 17–23, 1961.

Marcuson, R.W., Arthur, J.F., Chapman, M., Marston, A.: Experimental aspects of ischaemic colitis. Proc. R. Soc. Med. 62, 711, 1969.

Marcuson, R.W., Farman, J.: Ischaemic disease of the colon. Proc. R. Soc. Med. 64, 1080–1083, 1971.

Marcuson, R.W.: Ischaemic colitis. Clinics in Gastroent. 1, 3, 745–763, 1972. (O)

Marcuson, R.W., Stewart, J.O., Marston, A.: Experimental venous lesions of the colon. Gut 13, 1–7, 1972.

Marcuson, R.W.: Ischaemia of the colon. Brit. J. Hosp. Med. 11, 203–209, 1974.

Margaretten, W., Mackay, D.G.: Thrombotic ulcerations of the gastrointestinal tract. Arch. Int. Med. 127, 250–253, 1971.

Marosi, L., Ferenci, P., Pötzi, R., Pamperi, H., Lochs, H., Tscholakoff, D., Ulrich, W.: Ischaemische Kolitis. Wien. klin. Wchschr. 93, 23, 720–724, 1981.

Maroy, B., Ali, Y., Tubiana, J.M., Monnier, J.P.: Colite ischémique et volvulus du côlon pelvien. Ann. Radiol. 25, 3, 161–165, 1982.

174

Marrash, H.E., Gibson, J.B., Simeon, F.A.: A clinicopathologic study of intestinal infarction. Surg. Gynec. Obstet. 114, 323–328, 1962.

Marshak, R.H., Maklansky, D., Calem, S.H.: Segmental infarction of the colon. Am. J. Dig. Dis. 10, 86–92, 1965.

Marshak, R.H., Lindner, A.E.: Ischaemia of the colon. Semin. Roentgenol. 3, 81–93, 1968. (○)

Marshak, R.H., Lindner, A.E., Ruoff, M.: The radiology corner. Amer. J. Gastroenterology 61, 484, 1974.

Marston, A.: Massive infarction of the colon demonstrated radiologically. Brit. J. Surg. 49, 609, 1962. (○)

Marston, A.: Causes of death in mesenteric arterial occlusion: I: local and general effects of devascularization of the bowel. Ann. Surg. 158, 952–959, 1963.

Marston, A.: Patterns of intestinal ischaemia. Ann. Roy. Coll. Surg. (Engl.) 35, 151–181, 1964.

Marston, A.: Patterns of intestinal ischaemia. Lancet, 1, 491, 1965.

Marston, A., Pheils, M.T., Lea Thomas, M., Morson, B.C.: Ischaemic colitis. Gut 7, 1–15, 1966. (○)

Marston, A., Marcuson, R.W., Chapman, M., Arthur, J.F.: Experimental study of devascularization of the colon. Gut 10, 121–130, 1969.

Marston, A.: Reversible vascular lesions of the colon. Vascular disorders of the intestine. In: Boley, S.J., Schwartz, S.S., Williams, L.F. Jr. (Eds.) Butterworths, London 1971.

Marston, A.: Intestinal arterial disease. Proc. R. Soc. Med. 64, 1080, 1971.

Marston, A.: Diagnosis and management of intestinal ischemia. Ann Roy. Coll. Surg. (Engl.) 50, 29–44, 1972.

Marston, A.: Intestinal ischaemia, pp. 143–175 Edward Arnold, London, 1977.

Martin, D.W., Watts, H.., Smith, L.H.: Ischemic disease of the colon and oral contraceptives. Western J. of Med. 126, 378–385, 1977. (○)

Matolo, N.M., Albo, D.: Gastrointestinal complication of collagen vascular diseases – surgical implications. Am. J. Surg. 122, 678–682, 1971.

Matthews, J.G.W., Parks, T.G.: Ischemic colitis in the experimental animal. I. Comparison of the effects of acute and subacute vascular occlusion. Gut 17, 671–676, 1976. II. Role of hypovolaemia in the production of the disease. Gut 17, 677–684, 1976.

Mavor, G.E., Lyall, A.D., Chrystal, K.M.R., Tsapogas, M.: Mesenteric infarction as a vascular emergency. The clinical problems. Brit. J. Surg. 50, 219, 1962.

Mays, E.T., Noer, R.J.: Colonic stenosis after trauma. J. Trauma 6, 316–331, 1966.

Mazingarbe, A.: Nécroses coliques distales après colectomie. Chirurgie 99, 911–916, 1973.

McDowell, R.F.C., Thompson, I.D.: Inferior mesenteric artery occlusion following lumbar aortography. Brit. J. of Rad. 32, 378, 1959.

McIlrath, D.C.: Surgical treatment of ischemic bowel disease. Canad. J. of Surg. 17, 444–445, 1974.

McIlroy, M., Doyle, C., Whelton, M.J.: Ischaemic enterocolitis after femoral arthroplasty: with diagnosis by fibreoptic colonoscopy. J. Irish Med. Ass. 68, 10, 260–263, 1975. (○)

McKain, J., Schumacher, H.B.: Ischemia of the left colon associated with abdominal aortic aneurysms and their treatment. Arch. Surg. 76, 355–357, 1958. (○)

Menge, H.: Ischämische Colitis. From: Entzündliche Erkrankungen des Dickdarms. Ed. Ottenjahn, R., Fahrländer, H. Springer Verlag Berlin, Ch. 11, 168–175, 1983.

Mercadier, J., Clot, P., Vidal, B., Bartier, J.: Nécroses coliques sans oblitération vasculaire. Mém. Acad. Chir. 43, 310, 1967.

Meyers, M.A.: Griffiths' point: critical anastomosis at the splenic flexure. Significance in ischaemia of the colon. Radiology 126, 1, 77–94, 1976.

Meyers, M.A., Ghahremani, G.G.: Ischemic colitis associated with sigmoid volvulus: New observations. AJR 128, 591–595, 1977. (○)

Michels, N., Siddharth, P., Kornblith, P., Parke, W.: The variant blood supply to the descending colon, rectosigmoid and rectum based on 400 dissections. Dis. Colon & Rectum 8, 251–278, 1965.

Millar, D.M.: Colitis and antecedent carcinoma. Dis. Colon & Rectum 8, 243–247, 1965. (□)

Miller, R.E., Knox, W.E.: Colon ischemia following infrarenal aortic surgery. Ann. Surg. 163, 4, 639–642, 1966.

Miller, J.H., Bennett, R.C.: Ischemic strictures of the rectosigmoid complicating resection of abdominal aortic aneurysms. Austr. N.Z. J. Surg. 37, 345, 1968.

Miller, W.T., Scott, J., Rosato, E.F., Rosato, F.E., Crow, H.: Ischaemic colitis with gangrene. Radiology 94, 291–297, 1970.

Miller, W.T., De Poto, D.W., Scholl, H.W., Rattensperger, E.C.: Evanescent colitis in the young adult: A new entity? Radiology 100, 71–78, 1971. (○)

Miller, D.R.: Unusual focal mesenteric venous thrombosis associated with contraceptive medication. Ann. Surg. 173, 135–138, 1971. (○)

Ming, S.C., Levitan, R.: Acute haemorrhagic necrosis of the gastro-intestinal tract. New Engl. J. med. 263, 59–65, 1960.

Ming, S.C.: Haemorrhagic necrosis of the gastro-intestinal tract and its relation to cardiovascular status. Circulation 32, 332–340, 1965.

Mirkovitch, V., Winistörfer, B., Robinson, J.W.L.: Functional alterations in the dog colon mucosa following temporary ischaemia. Digestion 25, 138–144, 1982.

Mitchell, H.G., Coppola, F.S., Desmery, R., Iotti, R.: Colitis isquemicas. Acta Gastroenter. Latinoamer. 3, 61–70, 1971. (○)

Mogadan, M.: Necrotizing colitis associated with rheumatoid arthritis. Gastroenterology 57, 168, 1972.

Möller, C., Stjernvall, L.: Ischemic colitis. Acta Chir. Scand. 137, 75, 1971. (○)

Montessori, G., Liepa, E.V.: Ischemic colitis. Canad. Med. Assoc. J. 102, 377–380, 1970.

Moore, S.W.: Resection of the abdominal aorta with defect replaced by homologous graft. Surg. Gynec. Obstet. 99, 745, 1954.

Morgan, C.N., Griffiths, J.D.: High ligation of the inferior mesenteric artery during operations for carcinoma of the distal colon and rectum. Surg. Cynec. Obstet. 108, 641–650, 1959.

Morin, J.: La nécrose hémorrhagique du tractus digestif; ses relations avec l'état cardiocirculatoire. Thèse, Med. Paris, 485, 1967.

Moritz, A.R., Oldt, M.R.: Malignant nephrosclerosis. Am. J. Path. 13, 679–728, 1937.

Morson, B.C.: Histopathology of ischaemic colitis. Proc. R. Soc. Med. 59, 889, 1966.

Morson, B.C.: Histopathology of intestinal ischaemia. Ch. 6, 103–123 Vascular disorders of the intestine. Butterworths, London, 1971.

Moskowitz, M., Zimmerman, H., Felsen, B.: The meandering mesenteric artery of the colon. AJR 92, 1088, 1964.

Moss, A.A., Margulis, A.R.: Ischemic colitis with perforation. AJR 113, 338, 1971.

Movius, H.J.: Resection of abdominal arterio-sclerotic aneurysm. Am. J. Surg 90, 298, 1955.

Muggia, F.M.: Haemorrhagic necrosis of the intestine: its occurence with digitalis intoxication. Am. J. of Med. Sciences 253, 263–271, 1967.

Occhsner, J.L., Cooley, D.A., De Bakey, M.E.: Associated intra-abdominal lesions encountered during resection of aortic aneurysms; Surgical considerations. Dis. Colon & Rectum 3, 485–490, 1960.

Olivier, C., Robert, P., Di Maria, G., Favre, M., Baur, O.: Ischemic colopathy. Mém. Acad. Chir. 94, 628, 1968.

Oppenheimer, M.J., Mann, F.C.: Intestinal capillary circulation during distension. Surgery 13, 548, 1943.

Orr, G., Jones, P.F.: Ischaemic proctitis followed by stricture. Br. J. Surg. 69, 433–434, 1982.

Ostermiller, W., Carter, R.: Mesenteric venous thrombosis secondary to polycythaemia vera. Am. J. Surg. 35, 407–409, 1969.

Ottinger, L.W., Austen, W.G.: A study of 136 patients with mesenteric infarction. Surg. Gynec. Obstet. 124, 251–261, 1967.

Ottinger, L.W., Darling, R.C., Nathan, M.J., Linton, R.R.: Left colon ischemia complicating aorto-iliac reconstruction. Arch. Surg. 105, 841–846, 1972.

Ottinger, L.W.: Non occlusive mesenteric infarction. Surg. Clincs of North America 54, 3, 689–698, 1974. (○)

Ottinger, L.W.: Current concepts; Mesenteric ischemia. New Engl. J. Med. 307, 9, 535–537, 1982.

Padhi, R.K.: Fatal infarction of the descending colon after lumbar aortography. Canad. Med. Assoc. J. 82, 199, 1960.

Papadopoulos, C.D., Mancini, H.W., Marino, A.W.M.: Ischemic necrosis of the colon following aortic aneurysmectomy: collective review and case reports. J. Cardiovasc. Surg. (Torino) 15, 494–500, 1974.

Parks, T.G.: Ischemic colitis. Proc. R. Soc. Med. 65, 784, 1972.

Parks, T.G., Johnson, G.W., Kennedy, T.L., Gough, A.D.: Spontaneous ischemic proctocolitis. Scand. J. Gastroenterol. 7, 241–246, 1972.

Parks, T.G.: Experimental non-gangrenous mesenteric ischemia. Acta Gastroent. Belg. 37, 529–538, 1974.

Pawlik, W., Jacobson, E.D.: Effects of digoxin on the mesenteric circulation. Cardiovasc. Res. Cent. Bulletin 12, 80–84, 1974.

Payan, H., Levine, S., Bronstein, L., King, E.: Subtotal ischaemic infarction of the colon simulating ulcerative colitis. Arch. Path. 80, 530, 1965. (○)

Penn, I., Brettschneider, L., Simpson, K., Martin, A., Starzl, L.F.: Major colonic problems in human homotransplant recipients. Arch. Surg. 100, 61, 1970.

Penner, A., Bernheim, A.I.: Acute postoperative enterocolitis. A study on the pathologic nature of shock. Arch. Path. 27, 966–983, 1939.

Penner, A., Druckerman, L.J.: Enterocolitis as postoperative complication and its significance. Gastroenterology 11, 478–487, 1948.

Perarnau, J.M., Raabe, J.J., Courrier, A., Peiffer, G., Hennequin, J.P., Bene, M.C., Arbogast, J.: A rare etiology of ischemic colitis – amyloid colitis. Endoscopy 14, 107–109, 1982. (○)

Perdue, G.D., Lowry, K.: Arterial insufficiency to the colon following resection of abdominal aortic aneurysms. Surg. Gynec. Obstet. 115, 39, 1962.

Perloff, L.J., Chon, H., Petrella, E.J., Grossman, R.A., Barker, C.F.: Acute colitis in the renal allograft recipient. Ann. Surg. 77–83, 1976. (○)

176

Peterson, R.B., Meseroll, W.P., Shrago, G.G., Gooding, C.A.: Radiographic features of colitis associated with the hemolytic uremic syndrome. Radiology 118, 667–671, 1976.

Pheils, M.T.: Ischaemic colitis. Med. J. Austr. 2, 715–716, 1969.

Phillips, J.C., Howland, W.J.: Mesenteric arteritis in systemic lupus erythematosus. J. Am. med. Ass. 206, 1569, 1968.

Pierce, G.E., Brokenbrough, E.C.: The spectrum of mesenteric infarction. Am. J. Surg. 119, 233–239, 1970.

Polansky, B.J., Berger, R.L., Byrne, J.J.: Massive non-occlusive intestinal infarction associated with digitalis toxicity. Circulation 30, suppl. 3, 141, 1964.

Pollak, V.E., Grove, W.J., Kark, R.M., Muehrcke, R.C., Pirani, C.L., Steck, I.E.: Systemic lupus erythematosus simulating acute surgical condition of the abdomen. New Engl. J. Med. 259, 258, 1958.

Poupon, R., Bonnefond, A.: Les colites ischémiques. Nouv. Presse méd. 2, 2473–2476, 1973.

Poupon, R., Girodet, J., Sonsino, E., Vilotte, J.: Rectite ischémique nécrosante spontanée sans obliteration vasculaire. J. Chir. 108, 241, 1974.

Powis, S.J.A., Barnes, A.D., Dawson-Edwards, P., Thompson, H.: Ileocolonic problems after cadaveric renal transplantation. Brit. Med. J. 1, 99–101, 1972.

Pradhan, D.J., Ikins, P.M.: Ischemic colitis in esophageal substitution: an unusual and lethal complication of colon interposition. Am. Surgeon 427–428, 1975.

Prandi, D., Degott, C., Molas, G., Lortat-Jacob, J.L.: Entérites et colites ischémiques aiguës post-opératoires caractéristiques cliniques, anatomopathologiques et pathogéniques. Arch. Fr. Mal. App. Dig. 64, 209–214, 1975.

Price, A.B.: Difficulties in the differential diagnosis of ulcerative colitis and Crohn's disease. In: The Gastrointestinal tract; Chapter 1, 1–13; B.C. Morson (ed.) Williams and Wilkins Co., Baltimore, 1977.

De Prophetis, N., Khubchandani, I.T.: Colic angina and gangrene of the transverse colon in polycythaemia vera. Case report and review of literature. Dis. Colon & Rectum 12, 142, 1969.

Puylaert, C.B.A.J.: Fatal and nearly-fatal mesenterial infarction caused by intramural injection in translumbar biphasic aortography. Journ. Belge de Radiologie 48, 6, 671–695, 1965.

Qan, S.H.A.: Factitional proctitis due to irradiation for cancer of the cervix uteri. Surg. Gynec. Obstet. 126, 70, 1968.

Quesada, C., Dupré, A., Carpentier, E., Guidicelli, H., Meaulle, P.Y., Grautier, R.: Le risque colique en chirurgie aorto-iliaque. Chirurgie, 106, 362–368, 1980. (O)

Raghunatha, N.R., Hilliard, K., Wray, C.H.: Widespread intimal hyperplasia of small arteries and arterioles. Arch. Path. Lab. Med. 107, 254–257, 1983.

Ranninger, K., Scheiner, D.L.: Experimental bowel ischaemia. Arch. Surg. 95, 768, 1967.

Rasmussen, P.C., Thordsen, C.: Iskaemisk proktit. Ugeskr laeger 144, 3743–3744, 1982.

Rausis, C., Robinson, J.W.L., Mirkovitch, V., Saegesser, F.: Ischémic colique nécrosante et gangreneuse: faits cliniques et recherche expérimentale. Helvetica Chirurgica Acta 39, 251, 1972.

Rausis, C., Robinson, J.W.L.: Sensibilité de la muqueuse intestinale à l'insuffisance circulatoire. Schweiz. Rundschau Med. (Praxis) 61, 217–219, 1973.

Rausis, C., Robinson, J.W.L., Mirkovitch, V., Saegesser, F.: Désordres vasculaires du gros intestin; données expérimentalles et corrélations cliniques. Helevetica Chirurgica Acta 40, 295–305, 1973.

Rausis, C., Mirkovitch, V., Robinson, J.W.L., Roenspiess, U., Saegesser, F.: Die Ischämie der Dickdarmwand nach angioplastischen aortoiliacalen Eingriffen und andere Ischämieformen (experimentelle und klinische Beobachtungen). Schweiz. Rundschau Med. (Praxis) 63, 545, 1974.

Reed, D.L., Coon, W.W.: Thromboembolism in patients receiving progestational drugs. New Engl. J. Med. 269, 622–624, 1963.

Reeders, J.W.A.J., Rosenbusch, G., Tytgat, G.N.J.: Radiological aspects of ischaemic colitis. Diagnostic Imaging 50, 4–16, 1981.

Reeders, J.W.A.J., Rosenbusch, G., Tytgat, G.N.J.: Ischaemic colitis associated with carcinoma of the colon. Europ. J. Radiol. 2, 41–47, 1982.

Reiner, L., Jimenez, F.A., Rodriquez, F.L.: Atherosclerosis in the mesenteric circulation. Observations and correlations with aortic and coronary atherosclerosis. Am. Heart J. 66, 200, 1963.

Renton, C.J.C.: Massive intestinal infarction following multiple injury. Brit. J. Surg. 54, 399, 1967.

Renton, C.J.C.: Non occlusive intestinal infarction. Clinics in Gastroent. 1, 3, 655–673, 1972.

Reuter, S.R., Fry, W.J., Bookstein, J.J.: Mesenteric artery branch aneurysms. Arch. Surg. 97, 497, 1968.

Reuter, S.R., Kanter, I.E., Redman, H.C.: Angiography in reversible colonic ischaemia. Radiology 97, 371, 1970.

Reuter, S.R., Redman, H.C.: Gastrointestinal angiography. Saunders, Philadelphia, 1972.

Rickert, R., Johnson, R., Wignarajan, K.: Ischaemic colitis in a young adult patient. Dis. Colon & Rectum 17, 112–116, 1974. (O)

Roach, P.J.: Gastrointestinal bleeding in phaeochromocytoma and following the administration of norepinephrine (arterenol). Arch. Intern. Med. (Chicago) 104, 175–177, 1959.

Rob, Ch., Snyder, M.: Chronic intestinal ischemia: A complication of surgery of the abdominal aorta. Surgery 60, 1141, 1966.

Roberts, W.M.: Ischaemic lesions of the colon and rectum. Suid Afrikaanse Tijdschrift vor Chirurgie 3, 4, 141–161, 1965. (○)

Robinson, J.W.L., Rausis, C., Basset, P., Mirkovitch, V.: Functional and morphological response of the dog colon to ischaemia. Gut 13, 775–783, 1972.

Robinson, J.W.L., Menge, H., Mirkovitch, V.: The response of the dog colon to one hour's ischaemia. Res. Exp. Med. 165, 127–134, 1975.

Robinson, J.W.L., Mirkovitch, V., Winistörfer, B., Saegesser, F.: Progress report: Response of the intestinal mucosa to ischaemia. Gut 22, 512–527, 1981.

Rodriquez, M.A.: Ischaemic colitis and malignant atrophic papulosis. Amer. J. Gastroenterology 67, 2, 163–166, 1977. (○)

Roenigk, H.H., Farmer, R.G.: Degos' disease (malignant papulosis). J. Am. med. Ass. 206, 1508, 1968.

Rosati, L.A., Augur, W.A.: Ischemic enterocolitis in phaeochromocytoma. Gastroenterology 60, 581–585, 1971. (○)

Rosato, E.F., Rosato, F.E., Scott, J., Crow. H., Miller, W.T.: Ischemic dilatation of the colon. Am. J. Dig. Dis. 14, 922, 1969.

Rose, M.B.: Superior mesenteric vein thrombosis and oral contraceptives. Postgrad. Med. J. 48, 430, 1972.

Rosen, I.B., Cooter, N.B., Ruderman, R.L.: Necrotizing colitis. Surg. Gynec. Obstet. 137, 645, 1973.

Rosenkrantz, H., Bookstein, J.J., Rosen, R.J., Goff, W.B., Healy, J.F.: Postembolic colonic infarction. Radiology 142, 47–51, 1982. (○)

Ross, S.T.: Ischaemic colitis. Postgrad. Med. J. 51, 71–74, 1972. (○)

Rötzscher, V.M., Kremen, K., Zehle, A., Imig, H., Sandmann, W.: Ischämische Necrose des Colon und Rectum nach alloplastischem Gefäszersatz der Aorta abdominalis. Chirurg 47, 193–197, 1976.

Rowe-Jones, D.C.: Ischemic colitis. Brit. Med. J. 1, 361. 1969.

Roy, B., Jobard, P.: Un case de nécrose du côlon gauche sans obliteration vasculaire. Mém. Acad. Chir. 92, 49–50, 1966. (□)

Ruckert, R.F., Buchmann, P.: Ischämische Colon- und Rektumnekrosen, nach Resektion der Aorta abdominalis. Chirurg 53, 556–562, 1982.

Russell, J.Y.W.: Inferior mesenteric artery occlusion. Brit. J. Surg. 37, 321, 1950.

Rutledge, R.H.: Pseudoulcerative colitis proximal to obstructing colon carcinoma. Am. Surgeon 35, 384–388, 1969. (□)

Rijke, R.P.C., Gart, R.: Epithelial cell kinetics in the descending colon of the rat. I: The effect of ischaemia induced epithelial cell loss. Virchows Arch. (Cell Pathol.) 31, 15–22, 1979.

Rijsbosch, J.K.C.: Haemorrhagic infarction of the sigmoid colon as a result of thrombangitis obliterans. Arch. Chir. Neerl. 10, 124, 1958.

Saegesser, F., Gardiol, D., Hessler, C., Rausis, C.: Transitory ischemic colitis and obstructive colitis. Syndrome of inferior mesenteric arterial insufficiency. Chir. Gastroent. 5, 154, 1971.

Saegesser, F., Gardiol, D., Hessler, C., Rausis, C.: Colite ischémique transitoire. Schweiz. Rundschau Med. (Praxis) 61, 220, 1972.

Saegesser, F., Gardiol, D., Rausis, C.: Colites ischémiques occlusives non gangreneuses. Schweiz. med. Wschr. 102, 1669, 1972.

Saegesser, F., Chapuis, G., Rausis, C., Tabrizian, M., Sandblom, Ph.: Distention intestinale et ischémie colique. Les complications occlusives et perforations des cancer colo-rectaux. Chirurgie 100, 502–516, 1974. (□)

Saegesser, F., Sandblom, Ph.: Ischaemic lesions of the distended colon; a complication of obstructive colo-rectal cancer. Am. J. Surg. 129, 309–315, 1975. (□)

Saegesser, F., Roenspies, U., Garcia Gil A., Boomghar, M.: Rectites nécrosantes d'origine ischémique spontanées et après chirurgie angioplastique aorto-ilio-fémorale et sympathectomie lombaire. Chirurgie 103, 907–921, 1977.

Saegesser, F., Roenspies, U., Robinson, J.W.L.: Les maladies d'origine ischémique des parois du gros intestin: colites et rectites ischémiques. Chirurgie 105, 297–314, 1979.

Saegesser, F.: Acute abdomen arising from vascular disorders in the elderly, part II. Clinics in Gastroent. 10, 1, 1981.

Saegesser, F., Loosli, H., Robinson, J.W.L., Roenspies, U.: Ischaemic diseases of the large intestine. Int. Surg. 66, 103–117, 1981.

Sakai, L., Keltner, R.M., Willman, V.L.: Spontaneous and shock associated ischemic colitis. Am. J. Surg. 140, 755–760, 1980.

Sakurai, Y., Tsuchiya, H., Ikegami, F., Funatomi, T., Takasu, S., Uchikoshi, T: Acute right sided hemorrhagic colitis associated with oral administration of Ampicillin. Dig. Dis. and Sciences 24, 12, 910–915, 1979.

Salaman, J.R., Mahmood, K.: Recurrent mesenteric venous thrombosis complicating renal transplantation. Brit. J. Urol. 46, 257, 1974.

Samuel, E., Sinclair, D.J.: Plain film diagnosis of ischaemic lesions of the colon. Clin. Radiol. 19, 303–308, 1968.

Sawaf, H., Sharp, M.J., Youn, K.J., Jewell, P.A., Rabbani, A.: Ischaemic colitis and stricture after hemolytic uremic syndrome. Pediatrics 61, 2, 1978. (○)

Schennach, W., Flora, G.: Die Bedeutung der Second-look Operation beim akuten Mesenterial arterienverschluss. From

178

Intestinale Durchblutungsstorungen. V. Jahrestagung der österreichischen Gesellschaft für Gefässchirurgie und Angiologie, 13.–14. Oktober 1972. Facta Publication, Verlag H. Egerman, Wien, 1973.

Schmutz, G., Schutz, J.F., Kempf, F., Baumann, G., Weill, J.P.: Aspect radiologiques de l'ischémie colique non gangreneuse. J. Radiol. (Masson, Paris) 61, 10, 603–609, 1980. (○)

Schwartz, S.S., Sternhill, V., Lash, J., Boley, S.J.: Roentgenologic aspects of reversible vascular occlusion of the colon and in relationship to ulcerative colitis. Radiology 80, 625–635, 1963. (□)

Schwartz, S., Boley, S.J., Robinson, K., Krieger, H., Schultz, L., Allen, A.C.: Roentgenologic features of vascular disorders of the intestines. Radiol. Clin. North America 2, 71–87, 1964.

Schwartz, S.S., Boley, S.J.: Ischaemic origin of ulcerative colitis associated with potentially obstructing lesions of the colon. Radiology 102, 249–252, 1972.

Schwartz, S.S., Farman, J.: Ischemic colitis. Warren Teed, G.I tract 4–9, 1974.

Scowcroft, C.W., Sanowski, R.A., Kozarek, R.A.: Colonoscopy in ischemic colitis. Gastrointest. Endoscopy 156–161, 1981.

Selby, D.K., Bergan, J.J.: Colonic infarction due to inferior mesenteric artery occlusion. Q. Bull. Northw. Univ. Med. School 34, 244, 1960.

Senturia, H.R., Wald, S.M.: Ulcerative disease of the intestinal tract proximal to partially obstructive lesions. AJR 99, 45–51, 1967. (○)

Shanbour, L.L., Jacobson, E.D.: Digitalis and the mesenteric circulation. Am. J. Dig. Dis. 17, 9, 826–828, 1972.

Sharefkin, J.B., Silen, W.: Diuretic agents. Inciting factors in non occlusive mesenteric infarction? J. Am. med. Ass. 229, 1451–1453, 1974.

Shaw, R.A., Green, T.H.: Massive mesenteric artery ligation in resection of the colon for carcinoma. New Engl. J. Med. 248, 890, 1953. (○)

Shearburn, E.W., Connell, J., Hopkins, J.E.: Rectal ulceration due to ischaemic necrosis. Ann. Surg. 141, 563–566, 1955.

Shenoy, S.S., Satchidanand, S., Wesp, E.H.: Colonic ischemic necrosis following therapeutic embolization. Gastrointest. Radiol. 6, 235–237, 1981. (○)

Sherbon, K.J.: Radiology of ischaemic colitis. Austral. Radiol. 14, 46–55, 1970. (○)

Shinahan, M.X., Steedman, P.K.: Inferior mesenteric artery occlusion. Brit. J. Surg. 50, 533, 1962/1963.

Shinya, H., Avern, M., Wolf, G.: Colonoscopic diagnosis and management of rectal bleeding. Surg. Clinics of N.A. 62, 5, 897–903, 1982.

Sidi, E., Reinberg, A., Spinasse, J.B., Hincky, M.: Lethal cutaneous and gastrointestinal, arteriolar thrombosis (malignant atrophying papulosis of Degos). J. Am. med. Ass. 174, 1170–1173, 1960.

Singh, G., Hellstrom, H.R.: Lymphomatoid granulomatosis: report of a case without pulmonary lesions and with ischaemic colitis: probably a sequel to granulomatosis. Human Pathol. 9, 3, 364–366, 1978. (○)

Smith, R.R., Szilagyi, D.E.: Ischemia of the colon as complication of surgery of abdominal aorta. Arch. Surg. 80, 806, 1960. (○)

Smith, R.B., Perdue, G.D., Walker, L.G.: Posttraumatic aneurysm of the abdominal aorta with recurrent emboli to superior mesenteric artery. A case report. Surgery 64, 736–742, 1968.

Sonneland, J., Anson, B., Beaton, L.: Surgical anatomy of the arterial supply of the colon from the superior mesenteric artery based upon a study of 600 specimens. Surg. Gynec. Obstet. 106, 385–398, 1958.

Sørensen, F.H., Vetnet, M.: Haemorrhagic mucosal necrosis of the gastrointestinal tract without vascular occlusion. Acta Chir. Scand. 135, 439–448, 1969.

Spiro, H.M., Kilpatrick, Z., Yesner, R., Farman, J.: Spontaneous ischemic proctitis, a new entity. Ann. Int. Med. 68, 1150, 1968.

Standard, J.E.: Perforation of the colon in the newborn infant. Recovery following operation. Am. J. Surg. 83, 107–111, 1952.

Stellamor, K., Redtenbacher, M., Kosak, D., Karobath, M.: Über die sogenannte ischämisch-ulzeröse Darminnenwandläsion proximal stenosierender Darmprozesse. Fortschr. Roentgenstr. 126, 556–559, 1977. (□)

Stellamor, K.: Typische Wandveränderungen des Darmes oralwärts stenosierender Prozesse. Röntgenbl. 32, 375–378, 1979. (□)

Steward, J.A., Rankin, F.W.: Blood supply of the large intestine; its surgical considerations. Arch. Surg. 843–892, 1933.

Stillman, A.E., Weinberg, M., Mast, W.C., Palpant, S.: Ischemic bowel disease attributable to ergot. Gastroenterology 72, 1336–1337, 1977. (○)

Stillwell, G.K.: The law of Laplace. Some clinical applications. Mayo Chir. Proc. 48, 863, 1973.

te Strake, L.: Personal communications, Groningen, The Netherlands, 1983.

Strole, W.E., Clark, W.H., Isselbacher, K.J.: Progressive arterial occlusive disease. (Köhlmeier-Degos). New Engl. J. Med. 276, 195, 1967.

Sturdy, D.E.: Non specific (ischaemic) segmental colitis. Brit. J. Surg. 55, 2, 99–101, 1968.

Südeck, P.: Über die Gefässversorgung des Mastdarmes in Hinsicht auf die operative Gangrän. Münsch. med. Wschr. 54, 1314–1317, 1907.

Sutherland, N.G., Bounous, G., Gurd, F.N.: Role of intestinal mucosal lysosomal enzymes in the pathogenesis of shock. J. Trauma 8, 350–380, 1968.

Swenson, O.: Hirschsprung's disease. (Aganglionic megacolon). New Engl. J. Med 260, 972, 1959.

Swerdlow, S.H., Antonioli, D.A., Goldman, H.: Intestinal infarction: A new classification (letter to the editor). Arch. Path. Lab. Med. 105, 218, 1981.

Symmers, W.S.C.: Primary amyloidosis: A review. J. Clin. Path. 9, 187, 1956.

Tate, G.T., Thompson, H., Willis, A.T.: Clostridium Welchii colitis. Brit. J. Surg. 52, 194–197, 1965.

Tchang, S.: Amebiasis in Northern Saskatchewan; radiological aspects. Canad. Med. Assoc. J. 99, 688, 1968.

Terry, D., Dodds, W.J.: Association of ulcerating colitis with colon-carcinoma. Amer. J. Gastroenterology 59, 551–557, 1973. (□)

Thayer, W.R., Spiro, H.M.: Ileitis after ileostomy: prestomal ileitis. Gastroenterology 42, 547, 1962.

Theodore, C., Coste, Th.: Colite ischémique et cancer du sigmoide. Méd. Chir. Dig. 5, 39–41, 1976. (□)

Theuvenet, W.J., van Elk, P.J., Slot, B.: Non occlusive ischaemic colitis. Neth. J. Surg. 34, 4, 177–180, 1982.

Thomas, M.L.: Further observations on ischaemic colitis (summary). Proc. R. Soc. Med. 61, 341–342, 1968. (○)

Thomas, M.L.: Radiology: plain films and barium studies of the ischaemic bowel. Clin. Gastroenterol. 1, 581–595, 1972. (○)

Thomas, M.L., Wellwood, J.M.: Ischaemic colitis and abdomino-perineal excision of the rectum. Gut 14, 64–67, 1973. (○)

Thompson, H.: Vascular pathology of the splanchnic circulation. Clinics in Gastroent. 1, 597–612, 1972.

Thompson, W.M., Kelvin, F.M., Rice, R.P.: Inflammation and necrosis of the transverse colon secondary to pancreatitis. AJR 128, 943–948, 1977.

Thomson, F.R.: Ischemic infarction of the left colon. Canad. Med. Assoc. J. 58, 183, 1948.

Thijn, C.J.P.: Irritable colon. A preliminary stage of colonic diverticulosis. Radiol. Clin. Biol. 42, 468, 1973.

Tingaud, R., Serise, J.M., le Heron, D., Cerquetta, P., Janvier, G., Couzigou, P.: L'ischémie colique aiguë dans le cadre de la chirurgie de restauration aorto-iliacue. Lyon Chir. 379–386, 1981. (○)

Todd, I.A.D., Pearson, F.G.: Mesenteric vascular occlusion: analysis of a series of cases and report of a successful embolec-tomy. Canad. J. Surg. 6, 33, 1963.

Tomchik, F.S., Wittenberg, J., Ottinger, L.W.: The roentgenographic spectrum of bowel infarction. Radiology 96, 688–695, 1970.

Tonitza, P., Ionescu, M.: Nécrose totale du côlon sans obliteration vasculaire au cours de l'évolution d'un neoplasme sigmoidien. Mém. Acad. Chir. 92, 648–649, 1966. (□)

Trotter, L.B.C.: Embolism and thrombosis of mesenteric vessels. London, Cambridge University Press, 1913.

Tsuchiya, M., Okazahi, I., Asakura, H., Ohkubo, T.: Radiographic and endoscopic features of colonic ulcers in systemic lupus erythematosus. Amer. J. Gastroenterology 64, 277–285, 1975.

Turnbul, A.R., Isaacson, P.: Ischaemic colitis and drug abuse. Brit. Med. J. 1000, 1977. (○)

Tytgat, G.N.J.: Symposium Abdominale vasculaire pathologie. Ned. Ver. voor Gastroenterologie, Noordwijkerhout, 2 okt. 1982.

Tytgat, G.N.J., Reeders, J.W.A.J.: Die ischämische Kolitis unter besonderer Berücksichtigung der Endoskopie. Internist 24, 75–80, 1983.

Ulano, H.B., Treat, E., Chang, A.C.K.: Splanchnic circulatory responses to maintain in shock. Surgery 70, 678–684, 1971.

Vandamme, J.P., Vandamme, J., Maenhoudt, R., Bonte, J., van der Schueren, G.: The importance of venous thrombosis in acute intestinal infarction. Arch. Chir. Neerl. 24, 4, 341–351, 1972. (○)

Vandamme, J.P.J., van der Schueren, G.: Re-evaluation of the colic irrigation from the superior mesenteric artery. Acta anat. 95, 578–588, 1976.

Vandamme, J.P.J., Bonte, J., van der Schueren, G.: Re-evaluation of the colic irrigation from the inferior mesenteric artery. Acta anat. 112, 18–30, 1982.

Varga, A.T., Currie, D.T.: Inferior mesenteric vascular occlusion. Canad. J. Surg. 8, 87–92, 1965.

De Villiers, D.R.: Ischaemia of the colon: an experimental study. Brit. J. Surg. 53, 497, 1966.

Voegeli, E.: Die Angiographie bei Dünndarm und Dickdarmerkrankungen. Thieme Stuttgart 1974.

De Vroede, G.J.: Differential diagnosis of colitis. Canad. J. of Surg. 17, 369–374, 1974.

Wald, M.: Gangrene of the distal two thirds of transverse colon, left colon, rectum and anal canal due to superior mesenteric vascular insufficiency. Dis. Colon & Rectum 7, 303–305, 1964.

Wang, C.C., Reeves, J.D.: Mesenteric vascular disease. AJR 83, 895–908, 1960. (○)

Wangensteen, O.H.: Intestinal obstruction, physiological,

180

pathological, clinical considerations with emphasis on therapy, including description of operative procedures. Ed. 3., Springfield, Charles C. Thomas 1955. (○)

Ward, G.W., Stevenson, J.R.: Colonic disorder and oral contraceptives. New Engl. J. Med. 278, 910, 1968.

Watanabe, H., Horimukai, F.: Personal communications with H. Shirakabe. Juntendo University, Tokyo, Japan, 1983.

Waye, J.D., Hunt, R.H.: Colonoscopic diagnosis of inflammatory bowel disease. Surg. Clinics of N.A. 62, 5, 905–913, 1982.

Wessler, S., Gitel, S.N., Wan, L.S., Pasternack, B.S.: Estrogen-containing oral contraceptive agents: a basis for their thrombogenicity. Jama, 236: 2179–2182, 1976.

West, B.R., Ray, J.E., Gathright, J.B.: Comparison of transient ischemic colitis with that requiring surgical treatment. Surg. Gynec. Obstet. 1, 366–368, 1980.

Westcott, J.L.: Angiographic demonstration of arterial occlusion in ischemic colitis. Gastroenterology 63, 3, 486–489, 1972. (○)

Whitehead, R.: Ischaemic enterocolitis; an expression of the intravascular coagulation syndrome. Gut, 12, 912–917, 1971. (○)

Whitehead, R.: The pathology of intestinal ischaemia. Clin. Gastroenterol. 1, 613–637, 1972.

Whitehead, R.: Mucosal biopsy of the gastrointestinal tract. Vol. 3, Major problems in pathology. W.B. Saunders Co., Ltd. 155–166, 1973.

Whitehead, R.: Reversible ischemic colitis. Practitioner 213, 54, 1974. (□)

Whitehouse, G.H., Watt, J.: Ischaemic colitis associated with carcinoma of the colon. Gastrointest. Radiol. 2, 31–35, 1977. (□)

Wielinga, W.J., Kuipers, F.C.: Een patiente met buikklachten. Ned. T. Geneesk. 113, 12, 527–531, 1969. (○)

Wilk, P.J.: Ischemic colitis with perforation of the gallbladder. J. Mt. Sinai Hosp. 42, 119–126, 1975.

Williams, L.F., Anastasia, L.F., Hasiotis, C., Bosniak, M.A., Byrne, J.J.: Non occlusive mesenteric infarction. Am. J. Surg. 114, 376–381, 1967.

Williams, L.F., Anastasia, J.F., Hasiotis, C.A., Bosniak, M.A., Byrne, J.J.: Experimental non occlusive mesenteric isch-

aemia. Am. J. Surg. 115, 82–88, 1968.

Williams, L.F., Bosniak, M.A., Wittenberg, J., Manuel, B., Grimes, H., Byrnes, J.J.: Ischaemic colitis. Am. J. Surg. 117, 254–264, 1969.

Williams, L.F.: Vascular insufficiency of the intestines. Gastroenterology 61, 5, 757–777, 1971.

Williams, L.F., Wittenberg, J.: Ischemic colitis: A useful clinical diagnosis, but is it ischaemic? Ann. Surg. 439–448, 1975. (○)

Wilson, R., Qualheim, R.E.: A form of acute hemorrhagic enterocolitis afflicting chronically ill individual. Gastroenterology 27, 431, 1954.

Windsberg, E.: Intestinal obstruction of the colon due to malignancy. Single stage decompression and resection. Surgery 46, 305–318, 1959. (□)

de Witte, C., Sersté, J.P., Dony, A.: Rectitis and ischemic colitis. J. Belg. Radiol. 60, 113–116, 1977. (○)

Wittenberg, J., O'Sullivan, P., Williams, L.: Ischemic colitis after abdominoperineal resection; case reports. Gastroenterology 69, 1321–1325, 1975.

Wittenberg, J., Athanasoulis, C.A., Williams, L.F., Paredes, S., O'Sullivan, P., Brown, B.: Ischemic colitis, radiology and pathophysiology. AJR 123, 2, 287–300, 1975. (○)

Wood, M.K., Read, D.R., Kraft, A.R., Baretta, T.M.: A rare cause of ischemic colitis; periarteritis nodosa. Dis. Colon & Rectum 22, 428–433, 1979.

Yoshioka, H.: A case of ischaemic enterocolitis associated with systemic lupus erythematosus (SLE). Jap. J. Clin. Radiol. 27, 291–294, 1982.

Young, J.R., Britton, R.C., De Wolf, B.G., Humphries, A.W.: Intestinal ischemic necrosis following abdominal aortic surgery. Surg. Gynec. Obstet. 115, 615, 1962. (○)

Young, J.R., Humphries, A.W., De Wolfe, V.G., le Fèvre, F.A.: Complications of abdominal aortic surgery: intestinal ischemia. Arch. Surg. 86, 51, 1963.

Zizic, T.M., Shulman, L.E., Stevens, M.B.: Colonic perforations in systemic lupus erythematosus. Medicine 54, 411–426, 1975.

Zwalenburg, C. van: Strangulation resulting from distension of hollow viscera. Ann. Surg. 46, 780, 1907.

INDEX

186